# Essentials of Radiographic Physics and Imaging

FOURTH EDITION

# Essentials of Radiographic Physics and Imaging

## James N. Johnston, PhD, RT(R)(CV), FASRT

Chancellor
Eastern New Mexico University System
President
Eastern New Mexico University Portales Campus
Radiologic Sciences Professor Emeritus
Midwestern State University

ELSEVIER

Elsevier
3251 Riverport Lane
St. Louis, Missouri 63043

ESSENTIALS OF RADIOGRAPHIC PHYSICS AND IMAGING,
FOURTH EDITION

ISBN: 978-0-323-93067-3

Previous editions copyrighted 2020, 2016, and 2012.

*Senior Content Strategist:* Luke Held
*Senior Content Development Manager:* Ranjana Sharma
*Publishing Services Manager:* Deepthi Unni
*Project Manager:* Nayagi Anandan
*Designer:* Ryan Cook

Printed in India
Last digit is the print number:  9  8  7  6  5  4  3  2  1

Working together
to grow libraries in
developing countries

www.elsevier.com • www.bookaid.org

*It is hard to believe that this labor of love is now in its fourth edition.*
*I appreciate all who continue to use this book and support my vision for it.*
*I dedicate this edition to the person without whom it would otherwise not*
*exist, the coauthor of all things in my life's journey, my wife, Stephanie.*

**JNJ**

# Section Editor and Contributor

## EDITOR

**Brian Spence, MSRS, RT(R)**
Section editor
Radiologic Technology Program Director
Division of Health Sciences
Tarrant County College
Fort Worth, Texas

## CONTRIBUTOR

**Kelly Britton, MSHS**
Instructor
Department of Radiologic Technology
Tarrant County College
Fort Worth, Texas

# Preface

## PURPOSE

The purpose of this textbook is not only to present the subjects of physics and imaging within the same cover but also to link them together so that the student understands how the subjects relate to each other and to clinical practice. This textbook follows the ASRT-recommended curriculum and covers the content specifications of the ARRT radiography examination, making it easier for faculty to ensure appropriate coverage and adequate assessment of content mastery. Equally important, it provides the knowledge and information essential to a competent radiographer. This fourth edition continues to provide up-to-date digital information relevant to today's clinical practice.

## UNIQUE FEATURES

This textbook was written by radiographers for radiographers in a simple, straightforward, level-appropriate manner. It is a comprehensive radiologic physics and imaging text that focuses on what the radiographer needs to know and understand to safely and competently perform radiographic examinations. To achieve this, the following are some of the book's unique features:

- Each chapter begins with a rationale for studying the content of that chapter, addressing the often-asked question "Why do we need to know this?" The introduction to Chapter 2 below is an example.
*The focus of this chapter is on the structure and nature of the atom. Students may wonder why such detailed study of the atom is necessary for education and training in radiographic imaging. The following bullet points address this necessity:*
- *First, the interactions in the x-ray tube that produce x-rays occur at the atomic level, and the nature of the x-ray photon produced depends on how an electron interacts with an atom.*
- *Second, the interactions between the x-ray photons and the human body also occur at the atomic level, determining both the radiation dose delivered and how the body part will be imaged.*
- *Third, the interactions between the x-ray photons exiting the patient to produce the image interact at the atomic level of the image receptor to generate the final image.*
- *Finally, other areas of study in the radiologic sciences also require a working knowledge of the atom. So it is best to develop a strong foundation at the outset.*

- "Make the Physics Connection" and "Make the Imaging Connection" are callouts that further explain and "connect" for the student the relationship of physics information to imaging, and imaging information to physics. They are placed in a chapter with reference to the appropriate physics or imaging chapter. In this way the importance of the information is emphasized. The following are examples:

 **Make the Physics Connection**

**Chapter 7**

Differential absorption is the difference between the x-ray photons that are absorbed photoelectrically and those that penetrate the body. Denser tissue such as bone has greater absorption.

 **Make the Physics Connection**

**Chapter 7**

Photoelectric interactions occur throughout the diagnostic range (i.e., 20 kVp to 120 kVp) and involve inner-shell orbital electrons of tissue atoms. For photoelectric events to occur, the incident x-ray photon energy must be equal to or greater than the orbital shell binding energy. In these events the incident x-ray photon interacts with the inner-shell electron of a tissue atom and removes it from orbit. In the process, the incident x-ray photon expends all of its energy and is totally absorbed.

 **Make the Imaging Connection**

**Chapters 9 and 11**

Kilovoltage peak influences many areas of imaging. Among other things, it determines how the beam penetrates the body part and influences subject contrast in the digital image.

 **Make the Imaging Connection**

**Chapter 11**

The quantity of radiation exposing the patient and ultimately reaching the image receptor is directly related to the product of milliamperage and exposure time (mAs). Therefore exposure to the image receptor can be increased or decreased by adjusting the amount of radiation by adjusting the mAs.

- "Theory to Practice" is a callout that explains to the student why a particular concept is important and how it will apply to their daily practice down the road. The following are examples:

**Theory to Practice**

A single-phase machine may require a higher kVp setting than a three-phase or high-frequency machine because of the difference in efficiency, but it does not expose the patient to a different dose of radiation.

**Theory to Practice**

Knowing that the average energy of brems is one third of the kVp selected and that most of the beam is made up of brems, we can predict the average energy of an x-ray beam to be one third of the kVp selected.

**Theory to Practice**

If more photoelectric events are needed to make a particular structure visible on a radiographic image (when, for example, the tissues to be examined do not have high atomic number atoms), contrast agents such as barium or iodine are added. These agents have high atomic numbers and thereby increase the number of photoelectric events in these tissues. Protective shielding is another way of using photoelectric interactions. Lead has a very high atomic number and is used as a shielding material because the odds are great that photons will be absorbed by it.

- "Critical Concept" is a special callout that further explains and/or emphasizes the key points of the chapter. The following are some examples.

**Critical Concept**

**Ability to Ionize Matter**

The highest-energy members of the electromagnetic spectrum, x-rays and gamma rays, have the ability to ionize matter. This is an extremely important differentiating characteristic in that this characteristic can cause biologic changes and harm to human tissues.

**Critical Concept**

**The Line-Focus Principle and Anode Heel Effect**

The rotating anode design uses the line-focus principle, which means that the target face is angled to create a large actual focal spot for heat dissipation and a small effective focal spot for improved image quality. But by angling the face, the "heel" of the target is partially placed in the path of the x-ray beam produced, causing absorption and reduced intensity of the beam on the anode side.

**Critical Concept**

**X-Ray Photon Absorption**

During attenuation of the x-ray beam, the photoelectric effect is responsible for total absorption of the incoming x-ray photon.

**Critical Concept**

**Digital Image Acquisition**

With digital systems, the computer creates a histogram of the data set. The data set is the exposure received to the pixel elements and the prevalence of those exposures within the image. This created histogram is compared with a stored histogram model for that anatomic part; VOI are identified and the image is displayed.

- "Math Application" is a callout that further explains and gives examples of mathematical formulas and applications important to the radiographer.

**Math Application**

**Adjusting Milliamperage and Exposure Time to Maintain mAs**

$$100 \text{ mA} \times 100 \text{ ms } (0.1 \text{ s}) = 10 \text{ mAs}$$

To maintain the mAs, use:

$$50 \text{ mA} \times 200 \text{ ms } (0.2 \text{ s}) = 10 \text{ mAs}$$

$$200 \text{ mA} \times 50 \text{ ms } (0.05 \text{ s}) = 10 \text{ mAs}$$

**Math Application**

**Using the 15% Rule**

To increase exposure to the IR, multiply the kVp by 1.15 (original kVp + 15%).

$$80 \text{ kVp} \times 1.15 = 90 \text{ kVp}$$

To decrease exposure to the IR, multiply the kVp by 0.85 (original kVp – 15%).

$$80 \text{ kVp} \times 0.85 = 68 \text{ kVp}$$

To maintain exposure to the IR, when increasing the kVp by 15% (kVp × 1.15), divide the original mAs by 2.

$$80 \text{ kVp} \times 1.15 = 92 \text{ kVp and mAs/2}$$

When decreasing the kVp by 15% (kVp × 0.85), multiply the mAs by 2.

$$80 \text{ kVp} \times 0.85 = 68 \text{ kVp and mAs} \times 2$$

- Stressed in many areas of the textbook is the radiographer's responsibility to minimize patient radiation dose and to practice radiography in a safe and ethical manner. The following are some excerpts from chapters as examples.
  **(From Chapter 10 regarding digital imaging)** *Just because digital systems automatically rescale overexposed images does not mean one should take advantage of this by routinely utilizing excessive mAs to avoid repeats. This is flawed logic and violates the radiographers' code of ethics and the ALARA principle.*

**(From Chapter 16 regarding mobile radiography)**
*A radiography suite is a "controlled" and shielded environment specially designed for radiographic imaging. In a mobile environment, however, radiographers must take responsibility for radiation protection for themselves, the patient, and other individuals within close proximity. Radiographers should wear a lead apron during the radiation exposure and stand as far from the patient and x-ray tube as possible (at least 6 feet). Shielding of the patient and other individuals who must remain in the room should be performed as in the radiology department.*

- "Critical Thinking Questions" and "Review Questions" at the end of each chapter aid the student and instructor in assessing comprehension of presented material.

# Acknowledgments

I first want to acknowledge Dr. Terri Fauber, my long-time coauthor for the first three editions. I wish her the very best in retirement and thank her for being a great collaborator and friend.

I would also like to acknowledge my friends and mentors who have influenced the course of my professional life. A simple thank you does not seem enough but is heartfelt and offered here.

A special thank you to Brian Spence for taking a leap of faith to edit content of this fourth edition with me and lending his insight and expertise to the betterment of this textbook.

To Kelly Britton, thank you for your work on the CT chapter. Your expertise has added greatly to this work.

A special thank you to Meg Benson, Content Strategist–Imaging Sciences, for getting this project approved and moving, and to Content Development Manager Ranjana Sharma for coordinating, organizing, and keeping us on schedule through this fourth edition.

Also a special thanks to Patrick Johnston for taking many of the photographs in this text.

Finally, I would like to acknowledge and thank all of the educators who continue to use this textbook to educate future generations of radiographers and offering their comments and insights to improve its content.

JNJ

# Contents

# Introduction to the Imaging Sciences

## Outline

**Discovery and Use of X-Rays**
Dr. Roentgen's Discovery
Overview of X-Ray Evolution and Use
**General Principles**

Units of Measure
**Radiographic Equipment**
**The Fundamentals of Radiation Protection**

## Objectives

- Discuss key events in the discovery and evolution of the use of x-rays.
- Apply general physics fundamentals, including recognition of units of measure and basic calculations.
- Define and use radiologic units of measure.

- Identify the general components of permanently installed radiographic equipment.
- Describe the basic role and function of the general components of a permanently installed radiographic unit.
- Apply the basic principles of radiation protection.

## Key Terms

acute radiodermatitis
cathode ray tube
derived quantities

fluoroscope
fundamental quantities
ionizing radiation

mobile equipment
permanently installed equipment
radiologic quantities

---

This chapter begins with an overview of the discovery of x-radiation and the evolution of its adoption and use in society. Presented next is an introduction to general physics and the units of measure used in radiologic science. Finally, the general components of a radiographic suite are described and illustrated, along with basic principles for safe operation of radiographic equipment.

## DISCOVERY AND USE OF X-RAYS

### DR. ROENTGEN'S DISCOVERY

Dr. Wilhelm Conrad Roentgen (Fig. 1.1) was born on March 27, 1845, in Lennep, Germany. His public education and academic career were marked by struggle, not for lack of intelligence but for want of opportunity. After an unfortunate prank perpetrated by a classmate, he was expelled from school because he would not name the perpetrator. This began his struggle to find a place in a university to study. He eventually triumphed, receiving his PhD degree from the University of Zurich in 1869. He did, however, continue to struggle initially to establish himself as a professor and academician. Again, as a credit to his scientific skill and knowledge, he achieved considerable success, most notably being named director of the then

newly formed Physics Institute at the University of Wurzburg in 1894. It was in this "state-of-the-art" (for its time) laboratory that Dr. Roentgen forever changed the world of medicine.

The story of Dr. Roentgen's discovery of x-rays has been recounted with some variability. The general and important aspects are presented here, but attempts to establish a full and detailed picture have been complicated by Dr. Roentgen himself: in his last will and testament, he requested that, on his death, all of his laboratory notes and books be destroyed unread. Many specifics of his research, however, may be found in his own publications of the discovery and in some of the biographies and stories from his friends and colleagues. What is most important to remember, beyond his discovery, is the superb investigative and scientific skill with which he researched "x-light," as he called it ($x$ being the term representing the unknown).

Late on a Friday afternoon, November 8, 1895, Dr. Roentgen was working in his laboratory. He had prepared a series of experiments involving a **cathode ray tube** of the Crookes type (it may have been a Hittorf tube, but the general design and features of both types are the same: a partial vacuum tube that produces an electron stream). The nature of cathode

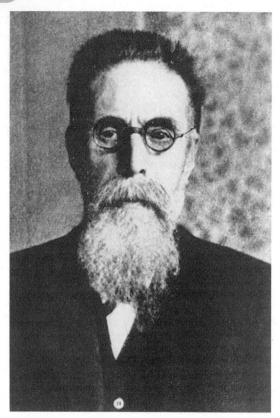

Fig. 1.1 Dr. Wilhelm Conrad Roentgen. (From Glasser O: *Wilhelm Conrad Roentgen and the early history of the roentgen rays*, 1933.)

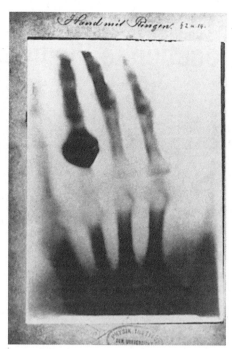

Fig. 1.2 **First Radiograph Created by Dr. Roentgen.** Image of Dr. Roentgen's wife's hand. Note the ring on her fourth digit. (From Glasser O: *Wilhelm Conrad Roentgen and the early history of the roentgen rays*, 1933.)

rays was of interest to many scientists of the day, and much experimentation was being conducted. On this particular evening, after setting up the tube and preparing for the evening's experiments, Dr. Roentgen completely covered the tube with black cardboard to continue his study of the fluorescent properties of the cathode rays. On a table a few feet away was a piece of cardboard painted with barium platinocyanide. On beginning his experiments, he noticed that the piece of cardboard fluoresced each time the tube was energized. He had already verified that the cause could not be the visible light because he had covered the tube with the black cardboard and checked to be sure no light escaped. He also knew, according to the common knowledge of the day, that the cathode rays could not penetrate the glass walls of the tube. He moved the barium platinocyanide–coated cardboard closer and started his fevered investigation of this unknown light. He was consumed by a desire to understand this phenomenon and spent the next 7 weeks investigating it. It is said that he even took his meals in his laboratory and had his bed moved there to facilitate his research. So thorough was his investigation that he described practically every property of x-rays that we know today. As a part of his investigation, he asked his wife to allow him to "photograph" her hand with this new x-light, and on December 22, 1895, he produced the first radiograph (Fig. 1.2). A profession was born.

## Critical Concept

### Discovery of X-rays

Dr. Wilhelm Roentgen discovered x-rays on November 8, 1895, while experimenting with a Crookes cathode ray tube. So thorough was his investigation that he discovered practically every property of x-rays that we know today.

He completed his investigation and wrote the first of three communications (informal papers) on the subject. He submitted the first communication to the secretary of the Wurzburg Physical Medical Society on December 29, 1895, and he asked that it be published in advance of his scheduled presentation to the society on January 23, 1896. The content of this first communication spread like wildfire through the scientific community well in advance of his oral presentation and announcement. His discovery and investigation results were received around the world with much excitement. He completed and published two more communications on the subject, concluding his initial investigation and results.

### OVERVIEW OF X-RAY EVOLUTION AND USE

As noted previously, during Dr. Roentgen's investigation of x-rays (the term we use today instead of "x-light"), he noticed in one series of experiments that the bones of his hand were visible on a barium platinocyanide screen. To capture such an image, he experimented with exposing photographic plates to x-rays and found that they did indeed expose the plate, creating a "photograph." As part of his initial communications and presentation, he included the famous "photograph" (now properly referred to as a *radiograph*) of his wife Bertha's hand. The publication of this radiograph led to an almost immediate recognition of the medical value of x-rays. Others around the world began experimenting with the radiography of different parts of the body. Physicians readily embraced this new technology and immediately put it to use to find bullets, kidney and gallbladder stones, and broken bones. The public was also fascinated by x-rays; because they produced a "photograph," most considered them a form of light.

In the early days, the cathode ray tubes and generators used for such exposures were inefficient, and the x-ray output varied considerably in quantity and quality. Exposure times were commonly in the 20- to 30-minute range; some exposures took up to 2 hours. Because of this, the early ventures into medical imaging came at a price. Many patients and operators suffered from acute radiodermatitis (radiation burns). There were even cases of electrocution of the operator in setting up the equipment for exposure because the equipment was not enclosed, grounded, and shielded as it is today (Fig. 1.3).

Initially the scientific community thought that x-rays were harmless because they did not stimulate any of the senses. Even though there were early reports of radiation injuries, physicians focused on the beneficial uses of x-rays to treat some skin conditions and ignored these warning signs. Furthermore, because radiation burns did not occur during or immediately after the exposure, many in the medical community did not make the connection and often attributed the burns to the electrical effects surrounding x-ray production, such as heat and glow from the electrical arc. Some thought that x-rays were a natural part of sunlight and the burns were just a form of sunburn.

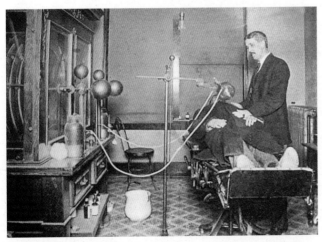

Fig. 1.3 **1900s Physician's Office.** Image of circa 1900 x-ray machine setup in a physician's office. Note the x-ray tube suspended above the patient and the open nature of the electrical wiring and tube. (Courtesy Alex Peck Medical Antiques.)

Thomas Edison brought some attention to the dangers of x-rays. He suffered a radiation burn to his face and injury to his left eye from his experimentation with x-rays and discontinued his investigations. Edison's assistant, Clarence Dally, did not cease investigation and truly suffered for it. Because of his experiments, Dally developed severe radiation burns. The only treatment of his day for such injuries was amputation, and during the course of his experiments (1897–1903) his left hand above the wrist, four fingers of his right hand, his left arm above the elbow, and finally the right arm at the shoulder were all amputated. At the end of his life, he was in such pain that he could not lie down and in 1904 died an agonizing death. Many of the early injuries were to "technicians" (as they were initially called) and doctors who worked with x-rays, and amputations and gloved hands became an identifying trait of their profession (Fig. 1.4).

By 1900, improved imaging plates, equipment, and techniques had all but eliminated acute radiodermatitis, but there was still a rather carefree attitude toward the investigation and use of x-rays. Within the medical community, recognition of the problems and early efforts to minimize them were under way, but x-rays had also captured the public's imagination in other ways. Immediately after the discovery and announcement, the public imagination went wild with speculation. Imagine a ray that could see through human flesh! Hopes abounded for this new, mysterious light, and there was speculation that it would soon be incorporated into a machine that could miraculously cure a host of mortal ills. The term *x-ray* appeared as the subject of poems, songs, and plays. It also appeared in advertisements for polishes, ointments, batteries, and powders, and the list goes on. Opportunistic advertisers and manufacturers took advantage of the glamour and mania of the word *x-ray* and incorporated it into a host of products. Advertisements claimed that "x-ray stove polish" would clean your stove better, "x-ray headache tablets" would cure your headache quickly, "x-ray prophylactics" would prevent a long list of diseases, and even "x-ray golf balls" would fly farther and straighter! Examples of such advertisements are presented in Fig. 1.5. Of course x-rays had nothing to do with any of these products' effectiveness, only their improved sales. There were, however, actual applications of x-ray machines. One such application was the shoe fitter (Fig. 1.6). This was a fluoroscope apparatus (a device that allows dynamic x-ray examination using x-rays and a fluorescent screen) placed in shoe stores to help with the proper fitting of shoes. The advertisement claimed that such machines were vital to ensure comfort through the proper alignment of the bones of the foot within the shoe. Some advertisements stated that this was of particular importance in fitting children's shoes. Consider the radiation dose that a child might have received during such a fitting or while playing with the machine as entertainment while a

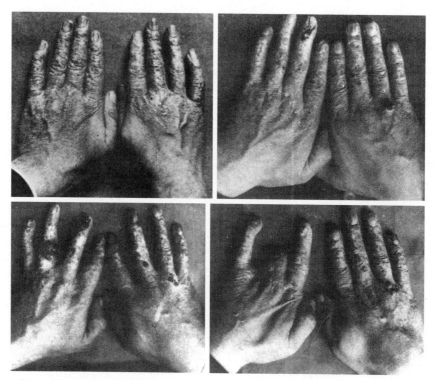

**Fig. 1.4  X-ray Dermatitis.** Picture of x-ray dermatitis and resultant amputations. Often gloves were worn to cover these injuries and amputations. (From Pancoast HK: *Amer Quart Roentgen* 1:67, 1906.)

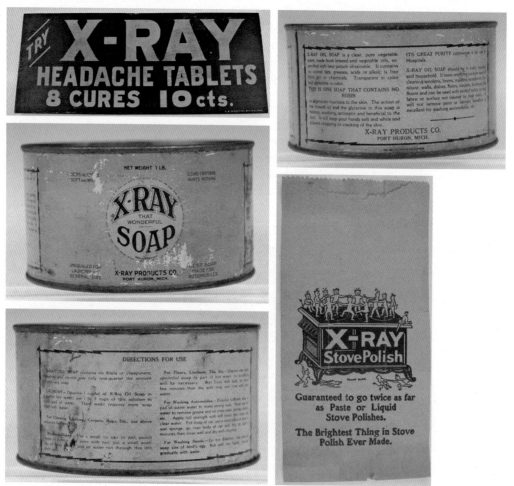

**Fig. 1.5  Products Taking Advantage of "X-ray Mania."** Advertisements using the glamour of the word *x-ray* circa 1900. Rights were not granted to include this content in electronic media. Please refer to the printed book. (Courtesy ASRT Museum & Archives.)

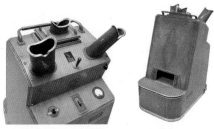

Fig. 1.6 **Shoe-Fitting Fluoroscope.** Shoe-fitting fluoroscope circa 1930 to 1940. (Courtesy Oak Ridge Associated Universities.)

mother and father shopped! The radiation dose to the salesmen, parents standing beside the device, and other customers was likely high too!

> ⚠ **Critical Concept**
>
> **Lessons Learned**
>
> The discovery of x-rays captivated the imagination of the medical community and the general public. The value of their use in medicine was quickly recognized and developed. Through trial and error, injuries, and even deaths, the medical community learned the dangers of x-rays and how to use them safely.

## GENERAL PRINCIPLES

Understanding radiologic physics is vital to the radiographer's role as a medical imaging professional and their ability to safely and responsibly use **ionizing radiation** (radiation with sufficient energy to ionize atoms) for that purpose. The primary goal of this text is to relate the x-ray production process to the imaging process. To understand radiologic physics, one must first speak the language of physics in general. Although the radiographer may not necessarily use the general physics formulas covered here, knowledge of these formulas does promote understanding of the radiologic concepts covered later in this text. The radiographer must also understand the basic and special radiologic quantities and units of measure because both are used regularly in medicine.

### UNITS OF MEASURE

In our daily lives, units of measure are a routine and important part of our communication with each other. A unit of measure must be agreed on and understood by a society to mean the same thing to all of its members. In the United States, for example, a road sign may simply present the name of the next city or town followed by a number. All licensed drivers in the United States are expected to know that the number is expressed in miles. A visitor from Europe may take this distance to be in kilometers and think the city or town is closer than it really is.

In medicine, such misinterpretations can be very dangerous to patients. When dealing with quantities in fields of medicine, it is critical to not only use a commonly understood unit of measure but to always use the correct unit. For example, there is a big difference between a dose of 1 mg and 1 g of a particular drug.

To better organize how quantities are measured, units are divided and then subdivided. The foundations of these divisions are the **fundamental quantities** of mass, length, and time. Each of these is defined using an agreed-on standard, which will be discussed shortly. By combining these fundamental quantities, the **derived quantities** of velocity, acceleration, force, momentum, work, and power are formed. These formulas form the foundation of the general language of physics. Finally, from these quantities, special categories of measure are derived for radiologic science; these are the special **radiologic quantities** of dose, dose equivalent, exposure, and radioactivity. See Fig. 1.7 for an illustration of this concept.

To give true meaning to these quantities, an agreed-on unit of measure is needed. The two systems of measure commonly used in the radiologic sciences are the Imperial system and the system international (SI) or metric system. The Imperial system uses the pound as the unit of measure for mass, the foot as the unit of measure for length, and the second as the unit of measure for time. The SI uses the kilogram to quantify mass, the meter for length, and the second to measure time.

Mass is the quantity of matter contained in an object; matter is anything that occupies space, has shape or form, and has mass. Mass does not change with gravitational force. Mass also does not change if the substance changes form. If 3 kg of water are frozen, the large ice cube created still has 3 kg of mass. If that ice is melted and boiled away, the water vapor added to the air is still 3 kg. The Imperial system uses the pound to quantify mass. The pound is actually a measure of the gravitational force exerted on a body, also known as *weight*. Such a definition varies according to the environment. For example, a person weighing 120 lb on Earth weighs 20 lb on the moon. The SI uses the kilogram to quantify mass. The kilogram is based on the mass of 1000 cm³ (cubic centimeters) of water at 4°C. This measure is a constant that does not vary with environment.

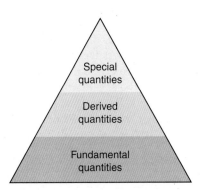

Fig. 1.7 **Quantities Pyramid.** Fundamental quantities are the foundation units. Derived quantities and special radiologic quantities are derived from these.

The SI unit of measure for length is the meter, which is now defined as the distance that light travels in 1/299,792,458 of a second. The Imperial system now bases the foot on a fraction of a meter.

The second is the unit of measure for time in both systems. This unit of measure has also gone through several definitions but is now measured by an atomic clock that is based on the vibration of cesium atoms.

By combining these fundamental quantities mathematically, one can create derived quantities. Of particular interest to radiologic physics are the derived quantities of velocity, acceleration, force, momentum, work, and power. To calculate these derived quantities, fundamental quantities and in some cases other derived quantities are used.

> ⚠ **Critical Concept**
>
> **Units of Measure**
>
> Units of measure are agreed-on standards that give meaning to specified quantities. Whether the Imperial system or SI is being used, the values and units must be understood by all parties concerned. The fundamental quantities can be combined mathematically to create derived and special quantities for more specific applications.

Velocity is equal to the distance traveled, divided by the time necessary to cover that distance. The formula is $v = d/t$, and its unit of measure (quantity) is meters per second (m/s). To determine this derived quantity (velocity), the fundamental quantities of length and time are used.

Example: What is the velocity of a baseball that travels 20 m in 2 seconds?
Answer: 20/2 = 10 m/s

 **Math Application**

Velocity is a measure of speed. In radiologic sciences, x-rays have a constant velocity equal to the speed of light, or $3 \times 10^8$ m/s. This value is used throughout the study of radiologic physics.

Acceleration is found by subtracting the initial velocity of an object from its final velocity and dividing that value by the time used. The formula is $a = (v_f - v_o)/t$ in which $v_f$ is the final velocity, $v_o$ is the original velocity, and $t$ is time. The unit of measure is meters per second squared (m/s²). Here, too, the fundamental quantities of length and time are used. Distance (length) is derived from the use of the derived quantity of velocity.

Example: What is the acceleration of a baseball if the initial velocity is 0, the final velocity is 10 m/s, and the time of travel is 2 seconds?
Answer: (10 − 0)/2 = 5 m/s²

 **Math Application**

Acceleration represents changes in velocity. In the radiologic sciences, acceleration of electrons within the x-ray tube is necessary for x-ray production.

Force is a push, a pull, or other action that changes the motion of an object. It is equal to the mass of the object multiplied by the acceleration. The formula is $F = ma$, in which $m$ is mass and $a$ is acceleration. Its unit of measure is the newton (N). In this derived quantity, the fundamental quantities of mass, length, and time are used. Distance (length) and time are derived from the use of acceleration; remember that acceleration is based on velocity. Notice how each of the derived quantities can be traced back to one or more fundamental quantities.

Example: What is the force necessary to move a 50-kg cart at a rate of 2 m/s²?
Answer: F = 50 × 2 = 100 N

Momentum is equal to the mass of the object multiplied by its velocity. The formula is $p = mv$, in which $p$ is momentum, $m$ is mass, and $v$ is velocity. Its unit of measure is kilograms-meters per second (kg-m/s). Again, mass, length, and time are used. Length (distance) and time are derived from the use of velocity.

Example: What is the momentum of an object with a mass of 15 kg traveling at a velocity of 5 m/s?
Answer: p = 15 × 5 = 75 kg-m/s

Work is an expression of the force applied to an object multiplied by the distance across which it is applied. The formula is work = Fd, and the unit of measure is the joule (J). The fundamental quantities of mass, length, and time are used. Mass and time are derived from the use of force.

Example: What is the work done if a force of 10 N is applied to a cart across a distance of 20 m?
Answer: 10 × 20 = 200 J

Power is equal to work divided by time during which work is done. The formula is P = work/t, and the unit of measure is watts (W). The fundamental quantities of mass, length, and time are used to find power. Mass and length are derived from the use of work.

Example: What is the power consumed if 100 J of work is performed in 60 seconds?
Answer: P = 100/60 = 1.67 W

Inertia is the property of an object with mass that resists a change in its state of motion. In fact, mass is a measure of the amount of inertia that a body possesses. Inertia applies to objects in motion and objects at rest. In the 17th century, Sir Isaac Newton first described the principle of inertia, which came to be known as "Newton's first law of motion." This law states that an object at rest will stay at rest unless acted on by an external force. An object in motion will remain in motion at the same velocity and in the same direction unless acted on by an external force. Inertia is solely the property of mass, and all objects with mass have inertia. Objects in motion have the additional characteristic of momentum. As noted previously, momentum is the product of mass and the velocity at which the mass is moving.

Energy is simply the ability to do work. It has two states, which are referred to as *potential energy* and *kinetic energy*. Potential energy is energy in a stored state. It has the ability to do work by virtue of state or position. A battery sitting on a shelf has potential energy in a stored state. Kinetic energy is energy being expended. In other words, it is in the act of doing work. The energy in a battery that is running an electronic device is being expended and is thus in a kinetic state.

Energy exists in a variety of forms such as electromagnetic (the form of energy with which radiologic science is most concerned), electrical, chemical, and thermal. Electromagnetic energy is a form of energy that exists as an electric and magnetic disturbance in space. Electrical energy is a form that is created by the flow of electricity. Chemical energy is a form that exists through chemical reactions. Thermal energy is a form of energy that exists because of atomic and molecular motion. In the production of a radiographic image, one is able to trace the transformation of energy from one form to another to create the image.

Practically everything can be categorized as matter, energy, or both. Albert Einstein's famous formula, $E = mc^2$, is an expression of the relationship between matter and energy. In this formula, $E$ is energy (expressed in joules); $M$ is mass (the quantity of matter contained in an object); and $C$ represents a constant, in this case the speed of light. What this equation shows us is that matter can be transformed into energy and energy can be transformed into matter.

Now we move to the special radiologic quantities. These quantities are uniquely used to quantify amounts or doses of radiation based on its effects. Increasingly the SI system is replacing the standard units as the more commonly used measures in radiologic sciences and therefore will be emphasized here. The SI units are the coulomb/kilogram (C/kg), gray (Gy), sievert (Sv), and the becquerel (Bq). The standard units are the roentgen (R), rad, rem, and curie (Ci) (note that rad stands for *radiation absorbed dose* and rem stands for *radiation equivalent man*). The coulomb/kilogram is equivalent to the roentgen. The gray is equivalent to the rad. The sievert is equivalent to the rem, and the becquerel is equivalent to the curie. Each of the units has specific applications.

## ! Critical Concept

### Radiologic Units of Measure

The radiologic units of measure are uniquely used to quantify amounts or doses of radiation based on its effects. Which unit of measure is applied depends on what is being measured. The sievert, for example, is used specifically for quantifying the dose received by radiation workers.

The coulomb/kilogram is a measure of the number of electrons liberated by ionization per kilogram of air. Ionization is the removal of electrons from atoms. More precisely, 1 C is the charge associated with $6.24 \times 10^{18}$ electrons. The roentgen is used to quantify radiation intensity. It is equal to that quantity of radiation that will produce $2.08 \times 10^9$ ion pairs in a cubic centimeter of air. An ion pair is an electron removed from an atom and the atom from which it came. The two together are an ion pair. The roentgen or coulomb/kilogram is generally used as a unit of measure for such phenomena as the output intensity of x-ray equipment or intensity in air. The relationship between the two is:

$$1\,C/kg = 3876\,R$$

or

$$1\,R = 2.58 \times 10^{-4}\,C/kg$$

To convert roentgens to coulombs/kilogram, multiply the roentgen value by $2.58 \times 10^{-4}$ (0.000258).

Example: What is the SI equivalent of 5 R?

Answer:   $5 \times 0.000258 = 0.00129$   C/kg   or   $1.29 \times 10^{-3}\,C/kg$

The gray is the unit for absorbed dose. It is an expression of the quantity of radiation energy absorbed by tissues being irradiated. The gray is equal to the absorption of 1 J of radiation energy per kilogram of tissue. The rad is used to quantify the biologic effects of radiation on humans and animals. It gives measure to the amount of energy deposited by ionizing radiation in any "target" (tissues, objects, etc.), not just air. One rad is the equivalent of 100 ergs/g. An erg is a unit of energy equal to $10^{-7}$ J. Therefore 100 ergs/g means that $10^{-5}$ J of energy are transferred per gram of mass. The relationship between the two is:

$$1\,Gy = 100\,rad$$

or

$$1\,rad = 10^{-2}\,Gy\ (0.01\,Gy)$$

To convert rad to gray, multiply the rad value by 0.01.

Example: What is the SI equivalent of 25 rad?

Answer: $25 \times 0.01 = 0.25\,Gy$

The sievert is used to quantify occupational exposure or dose equivalent. This unit specifically addresses the different biologic effects of different types of ionizing radiation to which a radiation worker may be exposed. The different types of radiation have different determined quality factors used in calculated dose equivalent. The energy range of radiation commonly encountered in radiologic sciences has a quality factor of 1. The standard unit for occupational exposure or dose equivalent is the rem, and the relationship between the two is:

$$1\,Sv = 100\,rem$$

or

$$1\,rem = 10^{-2}\,Sv\ (0.01\,Sv)$$

To convert rems to sieverts, multiply the rem value by 0.01.

Example: What is the SI equivalent of 300 rem?

Answer: 300 × 0.01 = 3 Sv

The becquerel is used to quantify radioactivity. This unit is an expression of a quantity of radioactive material, not the effect of the radiation emitted from it. The becquerel is quantifying the number of individual atoms decaying per second. Disintegration or decay is the process whereby a radioactive atom gives off particles and energy in an effort to regain a stable state. The curie is the standard unit for radioactivity. One curie is that quantity of radioactive material in which $3.7 \times 10^{10}$ atoms disintegrate every second. The relationship between the two is:

$$1\,\mathrm{Bq} = 2.70\,\mathrm{e} \times 10^{-11}\,\mathrm{Ci}$$
$$1\,\mathrm{Ci} = 3.7 \times 10^{10}\,\mathrm{Bq}$$

To convert curies to becquerels, multiply the curie value by $3.7 \times 10^{10}$ (37,000,000,000).

Example: What is the SI equivalent of 4 Ci?

Answer:    4 × 37,000,000,000 = 148,000,000,000,000    or $1.48 \times 10^{11}$ Bq

Table 1.1 summarizes the radiologic quantities. Germane to this topic is a discussion of effective dose. Effective dose is an expression of the relative risk to humans of exposure to ionizing radiation. It is a measure and concept most useful in radiation protection applications. It is measured in grays but is calculated by multiplying the absorbed dose (also in Gy) by the tissue-weighting factor. Tissue-weighting factors are used as a correction factor, because not all tissues, organs, or systems have the same level of radiosensitivity. If more than one tissue, organ, or system is exposed, the effective doses are summed. Table 1.2 is the latest International Commission on Radiological Protection (ICRP) (publication 103) recommended tissue-weighting factors.

Also germane to this topic is a discussion of kerma (the acronym for kinetic energy released per unit mass). As an expression of the energy released per unit mass, its unit of measure is joules/kg or Gy, and as you now know, this is also the unit of measure for absorbed

### Table 1.1    Special Radiologic Quantities

| USE | SI | STANDARD | CONVERSION |
|---|---|---|---|
| Output intensity/ intensity in air | Coulomb/kg | Roentgen | 1 C/kg = 3876 R |
| Absorbed dose | Gray | Rad | 1 Gy = 100 rad |
| Dose equivalent | Sievert | Rem | 1 Sv = 100 rem |
| Activity | Becquerel | Curie | 1 Bq = 2.70 e × 10⁻¹¹ Ci |

### Table 1.2    ICRP Recommended Tissue-Weighting Factors

| TISSUE | WEIGHTING FACTOR ($W_r$) |
|---|---|
| Red bone marrow, colon, lung, stomach | 0.12 |
| Breast, adrenals, extrathoracic region, gallbladder, heart, kidneys, lymph nodes, muscle, oral mucosa, pancreas, prostate, small intestine, spleen, thymus, uterus, cervix, gonads | 0.08 |
| Bladder, esophagus, liver, thyroid | 0.04 |
| Bone surface, brain, salivary glands, skin | 0.01 |

dose. Kerma is used to describe the quantity of radiation energy delivered to a given point. Kerma is a measure of energy released at a given point, whereas dose is an expression of the amount of energy absorbed at a given point. The term *air* kerma is an expression of the quantity of radiation released in air. It is in this medium (air) that we can make an easily understandable comparison. The quantity of energy released by 1 R of exposure in air is equal to the air kerma.

Radiographers routinely use these radiologic units of measure and come to know them well. Radiographers may not often use general physics units, but they serve as vehicles for understanding what is to come. All play a role in the radiography student's education.

### Theory To Practice

The radiographer must know and understand the radiologic units of measure because such things as dosimetry reports, medical physicists' reports, x-ray equipment performance specifications, and so on all use these units of measure.

## RADIOGRAPHIC EQUIPMENT

Generally, radiographic equipment may be classified as *mobile* or *permanently installed*. **Mobile equipment**, as its name implies, is a unit on wheels that can be taken to the patient's bedside, the emergency department, surgery, or wherever it may be needed. Mobile equipment is discussed in detail later in this textbook.

It is helpful to understand the basic layout of an x-ray suite before delving into the principles of x-rays and x-ray production. **Permanently installed equipment** refers to units that are fixed in place in a particular room specifically designed for the purpose and are not intended to be mobile. Lead shielding (or lead equivalent) is used in the walls, doors, and floors, and other design features are implemented to restrict the radiation produced to the confines of that room. *Permanently installed* does not mean that it can never be removed, of course, just that it cannot be wheeled to another location. Normally, when new equipment is purchased, the old unit must be uninstalled and the new unit installed. The room is generally out of use for a week or so while the process takes place, and the radiology manager must plan for this downtime in the work schedule. For the most part, such equipment is found in the radiology department, but permanently installed equipment (radiographic rooms) may also be found in large emergency departments, special surgery suites, outpatient centers, and freestanding imaging centers.

Permanently installed equipment consists of the tube, collimator, table, control console, tube stand, and wall unit. Bear in mind that all of these components are discussed specifically at the appropriate place in this textbook. A general overview is provided here, as is a discussion of equipment manipulation.

The x-ray tube, collimator, and tube stand can be discussed together as the *tube head assembly*. The x-ray tube is a special diode (two electrodes) tube that converts electrical energy into x-rays (and produces heat as a by-product). The positive electrode is called the *anode,* and the negative electrode is called the *cathode*. The tube is oriented so that generally the anode is over the head of the table and the cathode is over the foot. When facing the x-ray tube assembly, the anode is typically on the radiographer's left and the cathode is on the right (Fig. 1.8).

Because both heat and x-rays are produced, the tube is encased in a special tube housing. This housing is made of metal and has a special mounting bracket for the x-ray tube and high-voltage receptacles to deliver electricity to the x-ray tube. The housing is also filled with oil that surrounds the x-ray tube to help dissipate the heat produced. Cooling fans are also built into the housing to help dissipate heat (see Fig. 1.8).

The collimator is a box-shaped device attached to the bottom of the housing (see Fig. 1.8). The collimator serves to restrict the x-ray beam to the area of interest of the body and to help localize the beam to that area. To restrict the beam, the collimator is fitted with two pairs of lead shutters. Two buttons on the face of the collimator adjust these shutters. One button controls the shutters that adjust the width of the beam and the other button controls the shutters that adjust the length of the beam.

The collimator also contains a light source, a mirror, and a clear plastic covering over the bottom with crosshairs imprinted on it. The mirror reflects the light source through the plastic, and it casts a shadow of the crosshairs onto the patient. The shutters adjust the size of the light field, which represents the radiation field that will be produced. The light field and crosshairs show the radiographer the dimensions of the x-ray field and where it will enter the patient's body. If this tube head assembly is mishandled, the collimator mirror can, like a car's rearview mirror, be bumped out of adjustment. Periodically, a quality-control test, called a *radiation field/light field congruence test*, is conducted to check this mirror.

The tube stand or tube mount is the portion of the tube head assembly that gives mobility to the x-ray tube; this affords the radiographer the flexibility to produce an image from a variety of angles and the ability to accommodate the patient's condition. There are three basic configurations of the tube stand: the floor mount, the floor-ceiling (or floor-wall) mount, and the overhead tube assembly (sometimes called *ceiling mount*) (Fig. 1.9).

The floor mount consists of a horizontal track (rail) mounted on the floor parallel to the long axis of the table, a vertical piece that rides on the rail, and an arm

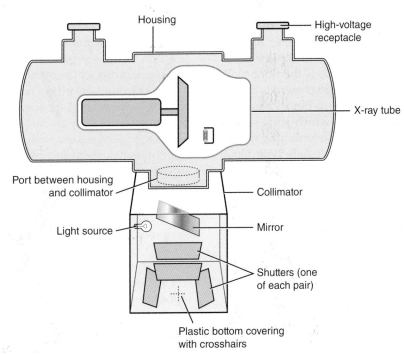

Fig. 1.8 **Tube Head Assembly.** Housing, x-ray tube, and collimator components.

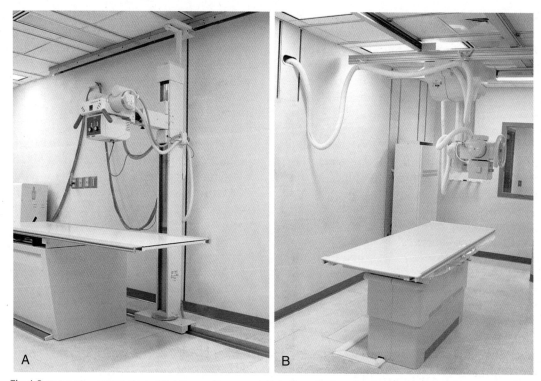

Fig. 1.9 **Tube Mount Variations.** (A) A floor-ceiling mount. Note the rails along the floor and ceiling. (B) An overhead tube assembly with ceiling-only rails and a telescoping tube crane. This is the most versatile of such designs.

to which the x-ray tube is attached. The vertical piece allows for movement along the length of the table (by riding on the horizontal track) and rotation about its axis. The arm that holds the x-ray tube moves up and down along the vertical piece and telescopes in and out across the width of the table. Finally, the tube also rotates about the axis of the arm to allow angulation of the tube. This type of assembly is fairly limited in its application and generally is best suited to low-volume workloads and basic examinations.

The floor-ceiling mount is a variation of the floor mount (Fig. 1.9A). It works basically the same, but the second point of attachment for the vertical piece adds stability. A slight modification to this is the floor-wall mount, in which the other point of attachment is a wall rail rather than a ceiling attachment. Both variations add a second point of attachment, which adds stability. The choice is merely a matter of determining which system is easier or more feasible to install. Both have the same limitations in movement as the floor mount and are best suited to the same type of environment and workload as the floor mount.

The overhead tube assembly (ceiling mount) is the most widely used in the hospital setting and the most versatile in design (Fig. 1.9B). With this design, two rails are mounted on the ceiling running along the long axis of the room. To this is attached an overhead tube crane. This device moves the length of the room (with the long axis of the table) along the rails. The crane itself allows the tube to move side to side (the width of the room and table), to telescope up and down (toward the table), rotate about its axis, and roll horizontally to

point toward a wall. It is often necessary to perform cross-table examinations and examinations requiring the tube to be angled in relation to the body part being examined. This design allows for maximum flexibility and movement of the tube to do this.

The modern table for a general radiography room permits height adjustment so that the patient can easily get on and off the table and so that the radiographer can place the table at a comfortable work height (Fig. 1.9B). It also has a four-way floating top with electromagnetic locks. The locks release with a foot pedal (not shown), and the tabletop then floats easily in any direction for ease in patient positioning. Just under the tabletop is a Bucky assembly. This device has a tray and locks to hold the image receptor in place and a grid positioned between the patient and image receptor to reduce scatter radiation in the remnant beam (x-ray beam exiting the patient) before it exposes the receptor. The grid is discussed fully in a later chapter. In direct-capture digital equipment, the Bucky assembly is different in that the receptor is built into the assembly, but its location is the same.

A variation of this table, used with fluoroscopy equipment, has a chain drive and motor to move the tabletop side to side and head to foot. It also has a mechanism to tilt the table 30 degrees toward the head and 90 degrees toward the feet. This allows the radiographer to place the patient in the Trendelenburg position (head down) or in a standing position. In these positions, it would jeopardize patient safety to release the table to float freely. It would also be very difficult to manually tilt the table. In both instances a chain-driven top allows for controlled, motor-assisted movements. The **fluoroscope** is discussed in a later chapter.

The wall unit consists of a vertical rail assembly affixed to the wall and floor and a vertical Bucky assembly. The rail allows for adjustment of the height of the vertical Bucky. The vertical Bucky is the same as the horizontal Bucky in the table and serves the same purpose. The wall unit allows the radiographer to easily perform an upright examination.

Finally, the control panel provides the radiographer with control of all the parameters necessary to produce a diagnostic image. The radiographer uses the control panel to select the kilovoltage and milliamperage that is applied to the x-ray tube to produce x-rays. There are other automated functions available to the radiographer, such as the anatomic program, the focal spot, the automatic exposure control, and the Bucky selection, and details of kilovoltage and milliamperage selection. These are discussed later in the text. For now, remember that these features of the control panel allow the radiographer to modify and fine-tune exposure parameters to obtain the best image. From a physics standpoint, note that these factors literally control the electricity applied to the x-ray tube to produce x-rays. There is nothing magical about the process. It is a simple manipulation of electricity.

## THE FUNDAMENTALS OF RADIATION PROTECTION

The following is by no means a comprehensive study of radiation protection, which is a major portion of another course you will take. Because the timing of the introduction of subject matter varies among radiography programs, what follows is intended as an introduction to guiding radiation protection principles. A central message throughout this textbook is the radiographer's responsibility to minimize radiation dose to the patient, oneself, and others in accordance with the As Low As Reasonably Achievable (ALARA) Principle. If this is the beginning of your radiography journey, this material will serve as a foundation to guide you in this effort as you begin practice. If you are well started in your studies, this material will serve to reinforce and refresh previously learned material.

 **Critical Concept**

**ALARA Principle**

It is the radiographer's responsibility to minimize radiation dose to the patient, oneself, and others in accordance with the As Low As Reasonably Achievable (ALARA) Principle.

It is often easier to learn and remember subject matter when one understands the rationale and need to do so. In this case, as previously stated, it is the radiographer's responsibility to limit radiation dose to the patient, oneself, and others, and it is a violation of

the American Registry of Radiologic Technologists/ American Society of Radiologic Technologists (ARRT/ ASRT) Code of Ethics (and, in many cases, state licensure laws) to do otherwise. This should not be taken as a negative motivator for the reader but rather a moral and professional obligation.

The ARRT certifies individuals (on passing the certifying examination) as competent to be entry-level radiographers and maintains a registry of individuals who maintain that competence through continuing education and recertification. As a part of this process, they have a Standards of Ethics document that consists of two parts: Code of Ethics and Rules of Ethics. Item number 7 of the current document (ARRT 2022) deals most directly with radiation protection. It specifically states that the radiographer is to demonstrate "expertise in minimizing radiation exposure to the patient, self, and other members of the healthcare team." With this obligation established, how does one minimize radiation dose?

 **Critical Concept**

**ARRT/ASRT Code of Ethics**

Established principles of professional conduct that articulate the radiographer's responsibility to minimize radiation exposure to the patient, self, and other members of the health care team.

Central to minimizing radiation dose to oneself and others are the cardinal principles of shielding, time, and distance. Shielding broadly refers to the use of radiopaque materials (which x-rays do NOT pass through easily) to greatly reduce radiation exposure to areas of the patient not essential to the examination being performed, to radiographers during examinations, and others. Lead-impregnated materials are a common example. Leaded/rubber sheets of varying sizes may be laid directly on the patient to shield radiosensitive areas. Lead aprons should be worn by the radiographer or other health care workers when it is necessary to be in close proximity to the patient during an exposure. Thyroid shields are also commonly used in conjunction with lead aprons during fluoroscopic examinations by those personnel who remain in the room. This collar wraps around the neck and fastens in the back to shield the entire front portion of the neck. Leaded curtains may drape from the fluoroscopy tower to provide a barrier between the fluoroscopist (the one operating the fluoroscope) and the x-ray beam during fluoroscopic examinations. The walls of the radiographic suite contain lead or lead equivalent (other materials thick enough to provide radiopaque properties equivalent to those of lead) to limit exposure to the immediate area of the radiologic examination. Primary barriers are those to which the x-ray beam is routinely directed, such as the floor beneath the x-ray table and the wall behind the upright Bucky. Primary barriers are 1/16 inch of lead or lead equivalent placed in the wall or floor where the primary beam is directed. Secondary barriers are the others, such as the wall separating the control panel from the room and the ceiling. Secondary barriers are 1/32 inch of lead or lead equivalent placed in the wall, door, or other area that may receive scatter or leakage radiation exposure. The general rule of thumb is always to maximize shielding (use as often as possible).

Time refers broadly to the duration of exposure to ionizing radiation and the time spent in a health care environment where exposure to ionizing radiation is accumulated. This may include the length of exposure and number of times the patient is exposed for a radiologic examination or the time a radiographer spends in a fluoroscopy suite (or any procedure involving fluoroscopy). Whether one is referring to the patient, the radiographer, or other health care workers, the general rule of thumb is always to minimize time (limit length of time exposed to ionizing radiation).

Distance refers to the space between oneself and the source of ionizing radiation. The reason that distance is important is simple: the intensity (quantity) of radiation diminishes over distance. This is an application of the inverse square law discussed in detail in the next chapter. Suffice it to say here that as one increases the distance from an ionizing radiation source, the intensity of that source decreases significantly. This principle is applied mostly to radiographers and others to maintain a safe distance from the source of radiation during exposure. The general rule of thumb is always to maximize distance (maintain safe distance from source during exposure).

> **! Critical Concept**
>
> **Cardinal Principles for Minimizing Radiation Dose**
>
> *Time*: Limit the amount of time exposed to ionizing radiation.
> *Distance*: Maintain a safe distance from source of ionizing radiation exposure.
> *Shielding*: Maximize the use of shielding from ionizing radiation exposure.

Another important tool in radiation protection is the limiting of the field of x-ray exposure, essentially beam restriction. The primary tool for beam restriction, the collimator, was described earlier in this chapter. This device, by limiting the area of exposure, limits the radiation dose to the patient. That is, the smaller the area of x-ray exposure, the lower the total dose to the patient. When we discuss radiation interactions in the body, we are talking about x-ray photons interacting with atoms of tissue. The greater the volume of tissue we expose, the greater the opportunity for such interactions to occur. With these interactions, the photon's energy will either be totally absorbed (which contributes to patient dose) or be scattered (which may contribute to dose

to radiographers or others if in the immediate area). See Chapter 7 for a full discussion of x-ray interactions with matter. For the purpose of this discussion, know that we must consider the total volume of tissue we expose to the x-ray beam and limit it to only the volume necessary to produce a high-quality image. It should be noted that this is not accomplished by placing lead masks (sheets of lead) beside the patient for the purpose of limiting exposure to an area of the image receptor. Such a measure, although improving image quality, does nothing to reduce the radiation dose to the patient.

> **! Critical Concept**
>
> **Beam Restriction**
>
> Limiting the size of x-ray exposure field reduces the volume of tissue irradiated and limits the radiation dose to the patient.

Next among our "tools" of radiation protection are the primary controls of the x-ray beam kilovoltage peak (kVp) and milliampere seconds (mAs). These are the factors selected by the radiographer to produce an x-ray beam of a given quality (penetrating power) controlled by kVp and quantity (number of photons) ultimately controlled by mAs. See Chapter 11 for a complete discussion of these factors. For the purposes of radiation protection, these factors control the nature of the x-ray beam to which the patient is exposed. The kVp controls the penetrating power of the x-ray beam produced. If the photons in the beam do not have sufficient energy to penetrate the anatomic part, the entire x-ray beam will contribute to patient dose. It is true that some absorption is necessary to differentiate among anatomic structures in the image; otherwise, it would be uniformly light or clear (everything absorbed) or uniformly dark (everything penetrated). But the radiographer can use this concept to their advantage. By increasing the kVp in a controlled manner, the radiographer can ensure that more photons in a given x-ray beam have the energy to penetrate the anatomic part. In so doing, more will penetrate the part and contribute to the image, and fewer photons overall will be needed to produce the image. This follows the 15% rule (see Chapter 11 for a complete discussion). The 15% rule states that, by increasing the kVp by 15%, we can reduce the mAs by one-half and still maintain optimum exposure to the image receptor. There are limitations to this that you will learn about later, but with respect to radiation protection, by using this method we cut in half the quantity of radiation to which we expose the patient. With digital imaging, this rule may be applied once and in some cases twice before significantly altering image quality. mAs ultimately control the quantity of x-ray photons produced. As you will see later, kVp has a strong influence on this, but, in general, mAs represents quantity.

8. X-ray examinations of the lower abdomen and pelvis of females in reproductive years should be limited to:
   a. the time before menstruation.
   b. the 10 days before the onset of menstruation.
   c. the 10 days after the onset of menstruation.
   d. 15 days before or after the onset of menstruation.
9. What is the power used if 2000 J of work is applied for 5 seconds?
   a. 400 W
   b. 10,000 W
   c. 2005 W
   d. 1995 W

10. What is the velocity of a car if it travels 1000 m in 4 seconds?
   a. 1004 m/s
   b. 250 m/s
   c. 1996 m/s
   d. 4000 m/s

# 2   Structure of the Atom

## Outline

## Objectives

- Discuss atomic theory.
- Describe the nature and structure of the atom.
- Identify the constituents of the atom and the characteristics of each.

- Explain classifications of the atom.
- Describe the principal types of atomic bonding.

## Key Terms

| | | |
|---|---|---|
| atom | covalent bond | molecule |
| atomic mass number | electron | neutron |
| atomic number | electron shell | nucleus |
| binding energy | element | proton |
| compound | ionic bond | |

## INTRODUCTION

The focus of this chapter is on the structure and nature of the **atom**. Students may wonder why such detailed study of the atom is necessary for education and training in radiographic imaging. The following bullet points address this necessity:

- First, the interactions in the x-ray tube that produce x-rays occur at the atomic level, and the nature of the x-ray photon produced depends on how an electron interacts with an atom.
- Second, the interactions between the x-ray photons and the human body also occur at the atomic level, determining both the radiation dose delivered and how the body part will be imaged.
- Third, the interactions between the x-ray photons exiting the patient to produce the image interact at the atomic level of the image receptor to generate the final image.
- Finally, other areas of study in the radiologic sciences also require a working knowledge of the atom. So it is best to develop a strong foundation at the outset.

The chapter begins with a brief history of the development of atomic theory that chronologically traces the progression of human understanding of the atom. This is followed by a discussion of basic atomic structure. Finally, the classification of elements based on atomic structure and how elements behave as a result of this structure is presented. Diligent study of this material is recommended because it is an important component of the radiographer's overall knowledge base.

## BASIC ATOMIC STRUCTURE

### HISTORICAL OVERVIEW

Although it is believed that some basic ideas of atomism or atomic theory predate Leucippus, his name most often is associated with the earliest atomic theory. His ideas were rather vague, and it is his student and follower, Democritus of Abdera, who provided one of the most detailed and elaborate theories and is credited with expanding on and formalizing the earliest atomic theory. Democritus lived from about 460 BCE to about 370 BCE. The word *atom* comes from the

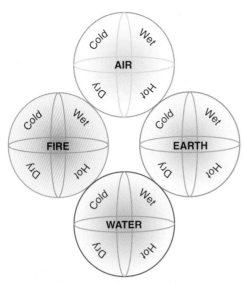

Fig. 2.1 Early Greek Theory of the Atom.

Greek word *atomos,* meaning "indivisible." Democritus hypothesized that all things were made of tiny indivisible structures called *atoms.* Fig. 2.1 illustrates the early Greek theory of atoms. Democritus believed that these atoms were indestructible and differed in their size, shape, and structure. He theorized that the nature of the object depended on its atoms. For example, sweet things are made of smooth atoms, and bitter things of sharp atoms. Solids consist of small pointy atoms, liquids of large round atoms, and so on. Such ideas and theories were debated and carried forward for another 2000 years.

The English chemist John Dalton in the early 1800s developed a sound atomic theory based not on philosophic speculation but on scientific evidence. His recognition that elements combined in definite proportions to form compounds led to questions about why this happened. This inquiry led in turn to his atomic theory. Fig. 2.2 is a photo of Dalton's original wooden models of the atom. To explain the phenomenon, he theorized that all elements were composed of tiny indivisible and indestructible particles called atoms. These

atoms were unique to each element in their size and mass. From this he theorized that compounds were formed by molecules and molecules by fixed ratios of each type of constituent atom, resulting in a predictable mass. Finally, his theory stated that a chemical reaction was a rearrangement of atoms. His theory is now more than 200 years old but remains fundamentally valid. We know now that we can destroy the atom in a nuclear reaction, but his basic ideas were correct. Later Dmitri Mendeleev advanced Dalton's work by organizing the known elements into the periodic table, which demonstrates that elements, arranged in order of increasing atomic mass, have similar chemical properties.

The next significant advancement in atomic theory came with Joseph John "J.J." Thomson's discovery of the **electron**. This discovery resulted from the scientific community's fascination with the cathode ray tube, the very fascination that led Dr. Roentgen to his discovery of x-rays. Thomson was studying the well-known glowing stream that is visible when an electric current is passed through the cathode ray tube. This glowing stream was familiar to scientists, but no one knew what it was. Thomson discovered that the glowing stream was attracted to a positively charged electrode. Through his investigation of this phenomenon, he theorized that these glowing particles were actually negatively charged pieces of atoms (later named *electrons*). Based on his understanding, he described the atom as a positively charged sphere with negatively charged electrons embedded in it, much like the raisins in a plum pudding—hence its name: the "plum pudding model" (see Fig. 2.3).

Thomson's theory was further advanced by one of his students, Ernest Rutherford. Marie and Pierre Curie had recently discovered radioactivity, and Henri Becquerel discovered radioactive rays. Rutherford was conducting scattering experiments by bombarding a

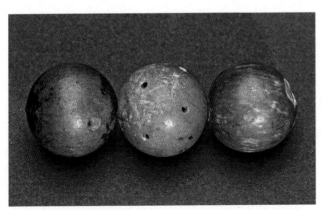

**Fig. 2.2 Dalton's Atom Model.** Dalton's wooden models of the atom. (Courtesy Science Museum London).

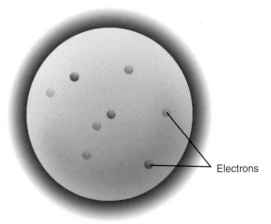

Sphere of positive charge

**Fig. 2.3 Thomson Model.** Sometimes called the "plum pudding model."

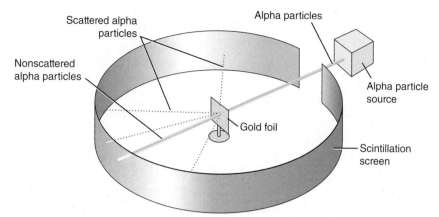

Fig. 2.4 **Rutherford's Experiment.** Ernest Rutherford's scattering experiment setup.

very thin sheet of gold with alpha particles. Alpha particles are made up of two protons and two neutrons (basically the nucleus of a helium atom) and have a positive charge. He placed a zinc sulfide screen in a ring around the gold sheet and observed the experiment with a movable microscope (Fig. 2.4). He observed that most particles passed straight through the sheet, but some were deflected at varying angles from slight to 180 degrees back along the path they had traveled. To Rutherford, this suggested that there were tiny spaces, or holes, at the atomic level. This space allowed most of the particles to pass through, but some particles hit parts of the atoms. Such an idea contradicted his teacher's model and, based on his experiments, he proposed a new, rather different model of the atom. His model resembled a tiny version of our solar system. He described a positively charged and very dense nucleus with tiny electrons orbiting it in defined paths. This model explained how some of the alpha particles could pass right through the gold sheet (between the nuclei of the atoms and missing the orbiting electrons), whereas others were deflected (repelled by the strong, positively charged nucleus). His version was a radically new idea, but it did not explain a couple of physical principles of nature. The 20th-century Danish physicist Niels Bohr refined Rutherford's work, bringing us to the theory and model of the atom with which we are most familiar.

## MODERN THEORY

The atom is considered the basic building block of matter. Bohr's theory describes the atom as having three fundamental components: **electrons**, **neutrons**, and **protons** (Fig. 2.5). These particles are generally referred to as the *fundamental particles*. The quantity of each is unique to the matter or element it composes. That is, a hydrogen atom is different from lead, which is different from tungsten, and so on. In radiology, we select elements for use because of their atomic structure and how they interact with x-rays. Today the quantum theory, which is based on mathematics and wave properties,

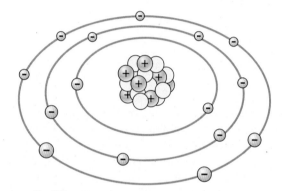

Fig. 2.5 **Bohr Atom.** The Bohr model of the atom.

**Structure of atom**

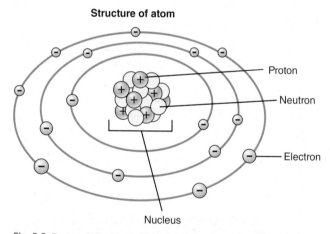

Fig. 2.6 **Parts of the Atom.** The atom is made up of protons and neutrons in the nucleus orbited by electrons in defined energy levels.

more accurately describes the atom, but for radiologic science purposes, the following discussion suffices.

The atom has a **nucleus** made up of protons and neutrons (collectively called *nucleons*); orbiting that nucleus are electrons in defined energy levels and distances from that nucleus (Fig. 2.6). The proton is one component of the nucleus. It has one unit of positive electrical charge and a mass of $1.673 \times 10^{-27}$ kg. The neutron is the other component of the nucleus; it has no electrical charge and a mass of $1.675 \times 10^{-27}$ kg. The primary difference between protons and neutrons is that protons have a positive electrical charge. An easy way to remember the difference is to think of the *pro* in proton, which suggests "positive," whereas the word *neutron* sounds like "neutral." The neutron is in fact neutral; it has no electrical charge. Protons and neutrons compose the majority of the mass of an atom. The electron is the third principal part of the atom. It has one unit of negative electrical charge and a mass of $9.109 \times 10^{-31}$ kg. Compared with the mass of a nucleus, an electron has very little mass, yet each electron is moving extremely fast in its orbit, and thus it has significant kinetic energy.

 **Critical Concept**

### Atomic Structure

The atom is composed of three fundamental particles: protons, neutrons, and electrons. The nucleus is central to the atom and is made up of protons and neutrons (collectively called *nucleons*). The electrons orbit the nucleus in defined energy bands or shells.

Electrical charge is a characteristic of matter, whether it is a subatomic particle, an atom, or a large object. Remember that each proton has one unit of positive charge and each electron has one unit of negative charge (neutrons are neutral; they have no charge). If an atom has an equal number of protons and electrons, it has no net charge (the positives and negatives are equal and cancel each other out, making it electrically neutral). If this balance is disrupted, the atom's charge becomes positive if there are more protons or negative if there are more electrons. Because the protons are generally very strongly bound in the nucleus, the cause of the electrical change (acquisition of a net charge) usually involves the gain or loss of electrons. If the atom gains an extra electron, the negative charges will outnumber the positives and the atom will have a net negative charge, which is called a *negative ion*, or *anion*. If the atom loses an electron, the positive charges will outnumber the negative charges and the atom will have a net positive charge, which is called a *positive ion*, or *cation*.

 **Critical Concept**

### Atomic Charge

Within each atom, each proton has one unit of positive charge, each electron has one unit of negative charge, and neutrons have no charge.

The nucleus is held together by a strong nuclear force, creating a **binding energy**. This energy creates a very strong attraction in the nucleus that overcomes even the natural tendency for like charges to repel (a law of electrostatics: like charges repel each other, opposites attract). This is what holds the protons and neutrons together to form the nucleus of the atom.

The mass of the nucleus is always less than the sum of the masses of nucleons that make up the nucleus. This difference in mass is called the mass defect and represents the energy necessary to hold the nucleus together. That is, if one added the masses of all of the protons and neutrons of a particular atom together (atomic mass) and then compared it with the mass of the nucleus itself, the sum of the individual masses would be greater. That is because some mass is converted to energy (recall Einstein's famous equation $E = mc^2$) to hold the nucleus together. Binding energy is also a measure of the amount of energy necessary to split an atom (break it apart). If a particle strikes the nucleus with energy equal to the nucleus's binding energy, the atom could break apart. This force is referred to as *nuclear binding energy* and is expressed in megaelectron-volts (MeV).

Electrons orbit the nucleus at very high velocities. The force of attraction between the negatively charged electrons and positively charged protons keeps the electrons in orbit. Just as neutrons and protons are held together in the nucleus by nuclear binding energy, the electrons are held in their orbits by electron-binding energy. This electron-binding energy depends on several factors, including how close the electron is to the nucleus and how many protons are in the atom. The closer the electron is to the nucleus, the stronger its binding energy (expressed in electron-volts [eV]).

Both nuclear binding energy and electron binding energy are key determinates of x-ray production. There are two types of atomic interactions in the x-ray tube that produce x-rays: characteristic and bremsstrahlung. Both are discussed in detail in Chapter 6. Because it relates to the present discussion, note that characteristic interactions involve the removal of orbital electrons from atoms. The penetrating strength (energy) of the x-ray photon produced depends on the difference in electron-binding energies of the electron shells involved. Bremsstrahlung interactions involve attraction to the nucleus of the atom, and the penetrating strength (energy) of the x-ray photon produced depends on nuclear binding energy. (The beginning pages of Chapter 6 explain x-ray production in relation to atomic structure, and it may be helpful to read this material at this point and also review it later in your studies.)

The following description of electron orbit completes the discussion of the structure of the atom. Electrons do not all occupy the same orbit at the same distance from the nucleus. An atom has defined energy levels, each at a different distance from the nucleus. These energy levels are called **electron shells** and describe a sphere around the nucleus (Fig. 2.7). Electrons orbit three-dimensionally around the nucleus. They are not simply orbiting the nucleus in a single plane (although in many discussions of radiologic science, we illustrate them this way for simplicity).

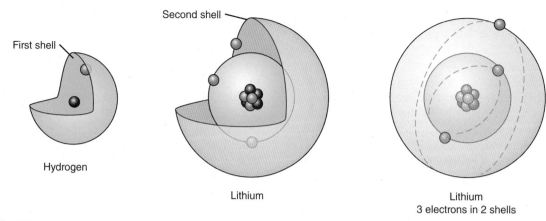

Fig. 2.7 **Electron Shells.** Atoms have defined energy levels, called *electron shells*, which describe spheres around the nucleus.

Each electron shell of an atom is lettered beginning with *K* nearest to the nucleus and moving outward with *L, M, N, O, P,* and so on. Generally, these shells fill from the K shell outward, with the outermost shells not necessarily filling completely, depending on the stability and nature of the atom. Each shell has a limit to the number of electrons that it can hold. The first shell can hold only two electrons. If an atom has three electrons, two electrons will occupy the K shell and one the L shell. An easy way to determine the maximum number of electrons that will fit in an electron shell is the formula $2n^2$, in which *n* is the shell's number (K becomes 1, L becomes 2, M becomes 3, and so on). For example, for the K shell $n = 1$, so the number of electrons that will fit is 2 because 1 squared is 1 and $1 \times 2 = 2$ ($2 \times 1^2 = 2$). For the L shell, $n = 2$, 2 squared is 4, and $2 \times 4 = 8$, so the number of electrons that will fit is 8 ($2 \times 2^2 = 8$). For the M shell, $n = 3$, 3 squared is 9, and $2 \times 9 = 18$, so the number of electrons that will fit is 18 ($2 \times 3^2 = 18$).

> ### ⚠ Critical Concept
>
> **Binding Energy**
>
> The K shell has the greatest electron-binding energy. Binding energy decreases with each subsequent shell. The maximum number of electrons that may occupy each shell can be found by using the formula $2n^2$, in which *n* represents the shell number, beginning with the K shell as 1.

The outermost shells of atoms may or may not have a full complement of electrons. Although shells can hold a certain number of electrons, they are not necessarily full. Except for the first (K) shell, a maximum of eight electrons can exist in the outermost shell of any atom (octet rule). Some inner shells may hold more than eight electrons. For example, the M shell can contain 18 electrons; if there are more electrons present, they will be in an N shell. If M is the outermost shell, however, it can hold a maximum of only eight electrons. It is important to note that the outermost shell may hold fewer, but no more than eight electrons.

Keep the following in mind regarding atomic structure as you continue your studies. Think of atoms as archery targets with the nucleus as the bull's-eye and the electron shells as the rings. Whether we are discussing atomic interactions in the x-ray tube to produce x-rays or interactions between human tissue atoms and x-ray photons, atoms represent "targets" for interactions. There is a greater opportunity for interactions with very large, complex atoms because their nucleus is larger and there are more electron shells and electrons in orbit around the nucleus (more complex atoms are physically larger) (Fig. 2.8). There is less opportunity for interactions with very small and less complex atoms because the nucleus is smaller and there are fewer shells and electrons in orbit around the nucleus (less complex atoms are physically smaller in size). Continuing with the archery target analogy, it would be easier for an archer to hit a target that is 3 feet in diameter than one that is 3 inches in diameter. Of course, binding energies and photon energies are critical parts of this interaction equation, but one also has to consider the fact that the greater the complexity of the atom, the greater the opportunity for interactions to occur.

## CLASSIFICATION AND BONDING

Before discussing classification and bonding, a few definitions must be understood: **atomic number, atomic mass number, elements,** and **compounds.** The atomic number of an atom refers to the number of protons it contains in its nucleus. (Remember that in a stable atom the number of electrons is equal to the number of protons, so the atomic number *indicates* the number of electrons.) The atomic mass number is the number of protons *and* neutrons an atom has in its nucleus. Elements are the simplest forms of substances that compose matter. Each element is made up of one unique type of atom with an

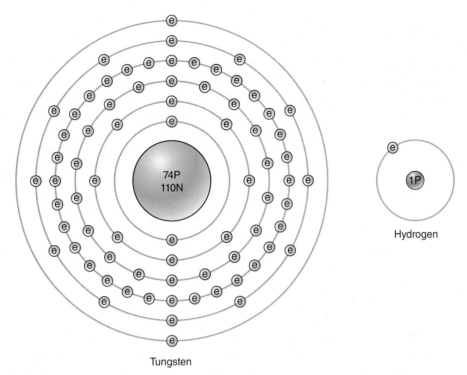

Tungsten

Fig. 2.8 **Atom Complexity.** Comparison of the complexity and size of a hydrogen atom versus a tungsten atom.

unchanging number of protons. The number of atoms that form a molecule of an element varies. Ninety-two different elements exist in the natural world, and almost two dozen others have been created artificially. Familiar elements include oxygen, carbon, and chlorine. Two or more atoms bonded together form a **molecule**. Most naturally occurring elements exist independently in nature—that is, in a pure form not combined with other elements. For example, iron, zinc, nickel, oxygen, carbon, hydrogen, and so on all exist as pure elements. But when you look at the world around you, most of what you see is in the form of chemical compounds, which are combinations of elements bonded together. For example, the most common substance on the earth's surface is water, which is a compound of two atoms of hydrogen and one atom of oxygen.

In chemical shorthand, the chemical symbol is an abbreviation of the element, such as *H* for hydrogen. The superscript number that appears with it is the atomic mass number, and the subscript number below it is the atomic number. So the top number (superscript) is the number of protons and neutrons in the atom, and the bottom number (subscript) is the number of protons in the atom. It appears in the format illustrated in Fig. 2.9.

## CLASSIFICATION

We now move to what are sometimes called the *isos*. This refers to isotopes, isotones, isobars, and isomers and is a way of classifying elemental relationships based on the number of protons, neutrons, and electrons in their constituent atoms. An *isotope* refers to elements whose

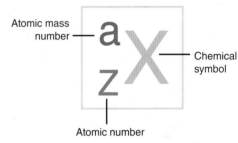

Fig. 2.9 **Chemical Shorthand.** Format for chemical shorthand.

atoms have the same number of protons but a different number of neutrons. An *isotone* refers to elements whose atoms have the same number of neutrons but a different number of protons. An *isobar* refers to elements whose atoms have a different number of protons but the same total number of protons and neutrons (atomic mass number). An *isomer* refers to elements whose atoms have the same number of protons and neutrons but with different amounts of energy within their nuclei. Isomers have the same atomic number and same atomic mass number but vary in the amount of energy within the nuclei because of differences in how the protons and neutrons are arranged.

### ⚠ Critical Concept

**The Isos**

The *isos* are a way of classifying elements based on the number of protons, neutrons, and electrons in each of their constituent atoms. The second-to-last letter in the name of each may be used as a prompt for what stays the same.

So what stays the same with isos? The names of these variants—*isotope, isotone, isobar,* and *isomer*—can serve as an easy way to remember their characteristics. The second-to-last letter in the name of each suggests which characteristic stays the same. In isoto*p*e, the *p* reminds you that the number of protons stays the same. In isoto*n*e, the *n* reminds you that the number of neutrons stays the same. In isob*a*r, the *a* reminds you that the atomic mass number is the same (total number of neutrons and protons). In isom*e*r, the *e* reminds you that everything (that is, all the fundamental particles of the atoms) remains the same (but with different amounts of energy).

Apply the definitions to the following examples:

$_{1}^{1}$H, and $_{1}^{2}$H; $_{53}^{131}$I and $_{54}^{132}$Xe; $_{3}^{7}$Li and $_{4}^{7}$Be; and $^{99m}$Tc

The first two, $_{1}^{1}$H, and $_{1}^{2}$H, are isotopes of hydrogen (note that they have the same atomic number and a different atomic mass number). The next two, $_{53}^{131}$I and $_{54}^{132}$Xe, are isotones. (Note that the isotone has the same number of neutrons and a different number of protons. The number of neutrons is found by subtracting the atomic number from the atomic mass number.) The next two, $_{3}^{7}$Li and $_{4}^{7}$Be, are isobars (same atomic mass number, different atomic number). Finally, $^{99m}$Tc is an isomer. As indicated by the superscript *m*, which stands for "metastable," it will decay to a stable form of technetium.

Another means of classifying elements is according to the periodic table, as in Fig. 2.10. The periodic table is organized by periods and groups. There are seven periods arranged as rows of the table and eight groups arranged as columns of the table. Elements in each period and group have certain characteristics.

Atoms in each period have the same number of electron shells, and the number of shells increases as one moves from the top row (period 1) to the bottom row (period 7). This means that the atoms of the element become increasingly larger and more complex.

Atoms in each group have the same number of electrons in the outermost shell. The number of electrons in the outermost shell increases as one moves from left (group 1) to right (group 8) on the table.

The periodic table is not perfectly uniform. In the middle of the chart are a number of elements that do not easily fit into the eight groups. In these elements, called the *transitional metals*, inner electron shells are being filled. These elements have some characteristics different from other elements.

There are additional elements that do not readily fit into the eight groups. They are the two series of inner transitional metals, which are not shown at all on a simplified version of the periodic table. The elements with the atomic numbers 57 to 71 and 89 to 103 are the inner transitional metals. They generally have special qualities; many are radioactive.

## BONDING

To this point, atoms have been discussed as individual entities, but as the building blocks of matter, it is the chemical bonds between atoms that allow complex matter (such as living tissue) to exist. As already mentioned, a molecule is formed when two or more atoms join together chemically. Some elements naturally exist as molecules (e.g., H$_{2}$). A **compound** is a molecule that contains at least two different elements. Thus all compounds are molecules, but not all molecules are compounds. There are two primary ways atoms bond to form molecules and subsequently more complex structures. One type of bond is called the **ionic bond** and the other is called a **covalent bond**.

Ionic bonding is based on the attraction of opposing charges. Recall that generally atoms are electrically neutral—that is, each has the same number of protons (positive electrical charges) and electrons (negative electrical charges). When in the presence of other atoms, however, some atoms have a tendency to lose electrons, whereas others have a tendency to gain electrons. An atom that loses an electron (a cation) has a net positive electrical charge. An atom that gains an electron (an anion) has a net negative electrical charge. In an ionic bond, one of the atoms gives up an electron and the other takes the extra electron; the difference in their electrical charge attracts and bonds the two together (see Fig. 2.11).

Covalent bonding is based on two atoms sharing electrons that then orbit both nuclei. Recall that as the electron shells of atoms fill, they do so from the one nearest the nucleus outward, and the outermost shells are not always full. In a covalent bond, an outermost electron from one atom begins to orbit the nucleus of another adjacent atom in addition to its original nucleus. Think of this electron as creating a figure eight as it orbits first one nucleus, then the other (see Fig. 2.12).

 **Critical Concept**

**Bonding**

There are two ways in which atoms bond to form molecules. Ionic bonds occur when one atom gives up an electron and becomes positively charged and another atom takes on that electron, acquiring a negative charge. It is the difference in charge that bonds the two together. In a covalent bond, two atoms share electrons that then orbit both nuclei, completing the outermost shell of each.

The bonding of various atoms to form molecules permits the highly complex matter about us to exist.

| 1 hydrogen H 1.0079 | | | | | | | | | | | | | | | | | 2 helium He 4.0026 |
|---|---|---|---|---|---|---|---|---|---|---|---|---|---|---|---|---|---|
| 3 lithium Li 6.941 | 4 beryllium Be 9.0122 | | | | | | | | | | | 5 boron B 10.811 | 6 carbon C 12.011 | 7 nitrogen N 14.007 | 8 oxygen O 15.999 | 9 fluorine F 18.998 | 10 neon Ne 20.180 |
| 11 sodium Na 22.990 | 12 magnesium Mg 24.305 | | | | | | | | | | | 13 aluminium Al 26.982 | 14 silicon Si 28.085 | 15 phosphorus P 30.974 | 16 sulfur S 32.065 | 17 chlorine Cl 35.453 | 18 argon Ar 39.948 |
| 19 potassium K 39.098 | 20 calcium Ca 40.078 | 21 scandium Sc 44.956 | 22 titanium Ti 47.867 | 23 vanadium V 50.942 | 24 chromium Cr 51.996 | 25 manganese Mn 54.938 | 26 iron Fe 55.845 | 27 cobalt Co 58.933 | 28 nickel Ni 58.693 | 29 copper Cu 63.546 | 30 zinc Zn 65.39 | 31 gallium Ga 69.723 | 32 germanium Ge 72.61 | 33 arsenic As 74.922 | 34 selenium Se 78.96 | 35 bromine Br 79.904 | 36 krypton Kr 83.80 |
| 37 rubidium Rb 85.468 | 38 strontium Sr 87.62 | 39 yttrium Y 88.906 | 40 zirconium Zr 91.224 | 41 niobium Nb 92.906 | 42 molybdenum Mo 95.94 | 43 technetium Tc (98) | 44 ruthenium Ru 101.07 | 45 rhodium Rh 102.91 | 46 palladium Pd 106.42 | 47 silver Ag 107.87 | 48 cadmium Cd 112.41 | 49 indium In 114.82 | 50 tin Sn 118.71 | 51 antimony Sb 121.76 | 52 tellurium Te 127.60 | 53 iodine I 126.90 | 54 xenon Xe 131.29 |
| 55 caesium Cs 132.905 | 56 barium Ba 137.327 | 57-70 * | 71 lutetium Lu 174.97 | 72 hafnium Hf 178.49 | 73 tantalum Ta 180.95 | 74 tungsten W 183.84 | 75 rhenium Re 186.21 | 76 osmium Os 190.23 | 77 iridium Ir 192.22 | 78 platinum Pt 195.084 | 79 gold Au 196.97 | 80 mercury Hg 200.59 | 81 Thallium Tl 204.38 | 82 lead Pb 207.2 | 83 bismuth Bi 208.98 | 84 polonium Po (209) | 85 astatine At (210) | 86 radon Rn (222) |
| 87 francium Fr (223) | 88 radium Ra (226) | 89-102 ** | 103 lawrencium Lr (262) | 104 rutherfordium Rf (261) | 105 dubnium Db (262) | 106 seaborgium Sg (266) | 107 bohrium Bh (264) | 108 hassium Hs (269) | 109 meitnerium Mt (276) | 110 ununnillium Uun (271) | 111 unununium Uuu (272) | 112 ununbium Uub (277) | | 114 ununquadium Uuq (289) | | | |

Key: element name, atomic number, Symbol, atomic weight (mean relative mass)

*lanthanoids: 57 lanthanum La 138.91 | 58 cerium Ce 140.116 | 59 praseodymium Pr 140.90 | 60 neodymium Nd 144.24 | 61 promethium Pm (145) | 62 samarium Sm 150.36 | 63 europium Eu 151.96 | 64 gadolinium Gd 157.26 | 65 terbium Tb 158.93 | 66 dysprosium Dy 162.50 | 67 holmium Ho 164.93 | 68 erbium Er 167.26 | 69 thulium Tm 168.93 | 70 ytterbium Yb 173.04

**actinoids: 89 actinium Ac (227) | 90 thorium Th 232.04 | 91 protactinium Pa 231.04 | 92 uranium U 238.03 | 93 neptunium Np (237) | 94 plutonium Pu (244) | 95 americium Am (243) | 96 curium Cm (247) | 97 berkelium Bk (247) | 98 californium Cf (251) | 99 einsteinium Es (252) | 100 fermium Fm (257) | 101 mendelevium Md (258) | 102 nobelium No (259)

Fig. 2.10 **Periodic Table.** Note that on the periodic table, each element is abbreviated with a chemical symbol. The superscript number with the symbol is the atomic number and the bottom number is the elemental mass. The elemental mass is the characteristic mass of an element determined by the relative abundance of the constituent atoms and their respective masses.

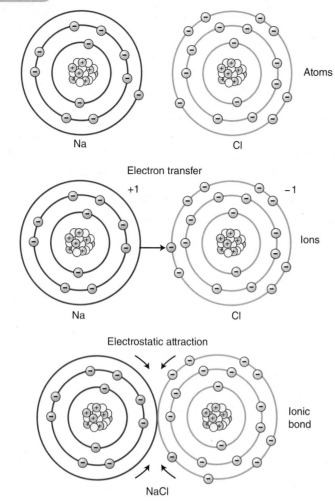

**Fig. 2.11 Ionic Bonding.** Note that one atom gives up an electron, becoming positively charged, and the other takes on an electron, becoming negatively charged; the opposing charges attract the two atoms together.

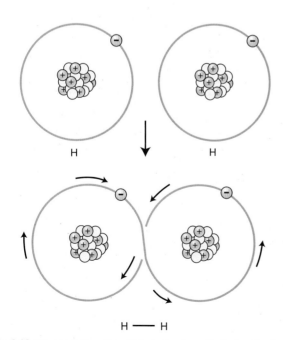

**Fig. 2.12 Covalent Bonding.** Note in the lower illustration the figure-eight orbital path of the shared electron.

## On the Spot

- The basic ideas of atomism or atomic theory most often are ascribed to Leucippus. However, his student and follower, Democritus of Abdera, is credited with formalizing and elaborating on the earliest atomic theory.
- In the early 1800s, John Dalton proposed an atomic theory based on scientific investigation that remains fundamentally sound today. The work of Thomson, Rutherford, and Bohr furthered Dalton's atomic theory, giving us the solid understanding we have today.
- The atom is the basic building block of matter and consists of three fundamental particles: protons and neutrons, which compose the nucleus, and electrons, which orbit around the nucleus. Protons have one unit of positive charge, electrons have one unit of negative charge, and neutrons have no charge.
- The atom is held together by a strong nuclear force (nuclear binding energy) and by electrostatic attraction between the nucleus and orbiting electrons (electron-binding energy).
- The *isos*—isotopes, isobars, isotones, and isomers—are a way of classifying elements based on the number of protons, neutrons, and electrons in their constituent atoms.
- There are two ways in which atoms chemically bond to form molecules. Ionic bonds occur when two atoms of opposite charge are held together by their mutual attraction. In a covalent bond, two atoms share electrons that then orbit both nuclei, completing the outermost shell of each.

## CRITICAL THINKING QUESTIONS

1. How does atomic structure complexity affect x-ray interactions in the human body and patient dose?
2. Describe the atom in terms of its physical organization, electrical charge (if present and under what circumstance), binding energy, and bonding nature.

## REVIEW QUESTIONS

1. Which of the following is considered a nucleon?
   a. proton
   b. electron
   c. alpha particle
   d. beta particle
2. What is the maximum number of electrons permitted in the M shell?
   a. 8
   b. 18
   c. 32
   d. 50
3. How many protons does $^{131}_{53}$I have?
   a. 131
   b. 53
   c. 78
   d. 184

4. How many nucleons are in $\binom{39}{19}K$)?
   a. 39
   b. 19
   c. 20
   d. 58
5. $^{132}_{54}Xe$ and $^{131}_{53}I$ are:
   a. isomers.
   b. isotopes.
   c. isobars.
   d. isotones.
6. $^{130}_{53}I$ and $^{131}_{53}I$ are:
   a. isotopes.
   b. isobars.
   c. isotones.
   d. isomers.
7. What is the maximum number of electrons that will occupy the outermost shell of an atom?
   a. 2
   b. 8
   c. 18
   d. 32

8. The maximum number of electrons that can occupy the P shell is:
   a. 8
   b. 32
   c. 72
   d. 98
9. Atoms that bind together because of their opposite charges form:
   a. covalent bonds.
   b. convalescent bonds.
   c. ionic bonds.
   d. nonionic bonds.
10. The horizontal periods of the periodic table contain elements with:
    a. the same number of electron shells.
    b. the same number of electrons.
    c. the same chemical properties.
    d. the same number of protons.

# 3 Electromagnetic and Particulate Radiation

## Outline

## Objectives

- Describe the nature of the electromagnetic spectrum.
- Discuss the energy, wavelength, and frequency of each member of the electromagnetic spectrum and how these characteristics affect its behavior in interacting with matter.
- Explain the relationship between energy and frequency of electromagnetic radiation.
- Explain wave-particle duality as it applies to the electromagnetic spectrum.
- Calculate the wavelength or frequency of electromagnetic radiation.

- Differentiate between x-rays and gamma rays and the rest of the electromagnetic spectrum.
- Identify concepts regarding the electromagnetic spectrum important for the radiographer.
- Describe the nature of particulate radiation.
- Differentiate between electromagnetic and particulate radiation.
- Discuss sources of ionizing radiation constituting human exposure.

## Key Terms

| | | |
|---|---|---|
| alpha particles | infrared light | radioactivity |
| beta particles | inverse square law | radiowaves |
| electromagnetic radiation | ionization | ultraviolet light |
| electromagnetic spectrum | microwaves | visible light |
| frequency | particulate radiation | wavelength |
| gamma rays | photon | x-rays |
| hertz (Hz) | Planck's constant | |

## INTRODUCTION

This chapter introduces the nature of electromagnetic and particulate radiation. Students may wonder why it is necessary for the radiographer to understand the entire spectrum of radiation. This question can be answered both broadly and specifically. In general, it is the radiographer's role to be familiar with the different types of radiation to which patients may be exposed and to be able to answer questions and educate patients. The radiographer should consider themselves as resources for the public and should be able to dispel any myths or misconceptions about medical imaging in general. Both ends of the electromagnetic spectrum are used in medical imaging. **Radiowaves** are used in conjunction with a magnetic field in magnetic resonance imaging (MRI) to create images of the body. **X-rays** and **gamma rays** are used for imaging in radiology and nuclear medicine, respectively. One difference between the "ends" of the spectrum is that only high-energy radiation (x-rays and gamma rays) has the ability to ionize matter. This property is explained in this chapter. More specifically, the radiographer should be able to explain to a patient the nature of ionizing radiation and any risks and benefits, and they should be an advocate for the patient in such discussions with other professionals. They should also understand the nature of radiation well enough to safely use it for medical imaging purposes. With this rationale in mind, the electromagnetic spectrum is discussed first, followed by a discussion of particulate radiation.

## ELECTROMAGNETIC RADIATION

### NATURE AND CHARACTERISTICS

In the latter half of the 19th century, the physicist James Maxwell developed his electromagnetic theory, significantly advancing the world of physics. In this theory, he explained that all **electromagnetic radiation** is very similar in that it has no mass, carries energy in waves as electric and magnetic disturbances in space, and travels at the speed of light (Fig. 3.1). His work is considered by many to be one of the greatest advances of physics. *Electromagnetic radiation* may be defined as "an electric and magnetic disturbance traveling through space at the speed of light." The **electromagnetic spectrum** is a way of ordering or grouping the different electromagnetic radiations. All of the members of the electromagnetic spectrum have the same velocity (the speed of light or $3 \times 10^8$ m/s) and vary only in their energy, **wavelength**, and **frequency**. The members of the electromagnetic spectrum from lowest energy to highest are radiowaves, **microwaves**, infrared light, **visible light**, ultraviolet light, x-rays, and gamma rays. The wavelengths of the electromagnetic spectrum range from $10^6$ to $10^{-16}$ m, and the frequencies range from $10^2$ to $10^{24}$ **Hz**. Wavelength and frequency are discussed later. The ranges of energy, frequency, and wavelength of the electromagnetic spectrum are continuous—that is, one constituent blends into the next (Fig. 3.2).

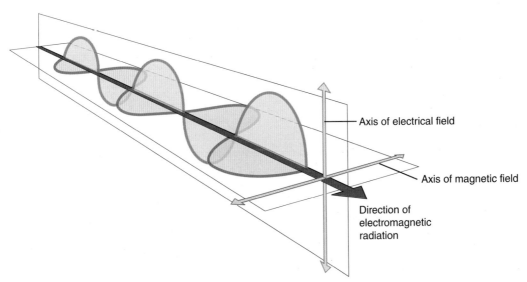

**Fig. 3.1 Electromagnetic Radiation.** Electromagnetic radiation is energy traveling at the speed of light in waves as an electric and magnetic disturbance in space.

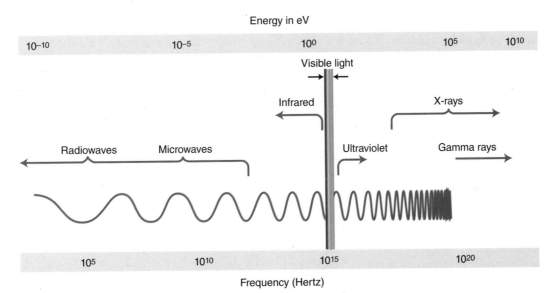

**Fig. 3.2 Electromagnetic Spectrum.** The electromagnetic spectrum energy, frequency, and wavelength ranges are continuous, with energies from $10^{-12}$ to $10^{10}$ eV.

## Critical Concept

### The Nature of Electromagnetic Radiation

All electromagnetic radiations have the same nature in that they are electric and magnetic disturbances traveling through space. They all have the same velocity—the speed of light— and vary only in their energy, wavelength, and frequency.

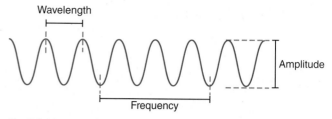

**Fig. 3.3 Electromagnetic Wave Measures.** An electromagnetic wave may be described by its wavelength (distance from one peak to the next), amplitude (maximum height of a wave), or frequency (the number of waves that pass a given point per second).

Electromagnetic radiation is a form of energy that originates from the atom. That is, electromagnetic radiations are emitted when changes in atoms occur, such as when electrons undergo orbital transitions or atomic nuclei emit excess energy to regain stability. Unlike mechanical energy, which requires an object or matter to act through, electromagnetic energy can exist apart from matter and can travel through a vacuum. For example, sound is a form of mechanical energy. The sound from a speaker vibrates molecules of air adjacent to the speaker, which then pass the vibration to other nearby molecules until they reach the listener's ear. In the absence of the intervening air molecules, no sound would reach the ear. With electromagnetic radiation, it is the energy itself that is vibrating as a combination of electric and magnetic fields; it is pure energy. In fact, energy and frequency of electromagnetic radiation are related mathematically. The energy of electromagnetic radiation can be calculated by the following formula:

$$E = hf$$

In this formula, $E$ is energy, $h$ is **Planck's constant** (equal to $4.135 \times 10^{-15}$ eV seconds; $6.626 \times 10^{-34}$ J seconds), and $f$ is the frequency of the **photon**. The energy is measured in electron volts (eV). The physicist Max Planck first described the direct proportionality between energy and frequency; that is, as the frequency increases, so does the energy. Planck theorized that electromagnetic radiation can only exist as "packets" of energy, later called *photons*. The constant, $h$, which is named for Planck, is a mathematical value used to calculate photon energies based on frequency. The energy of the electromagnetic spectrum ranges from $10^{-12}$ to $10^{10}$ eV.

## Critical Concept

### Difference Between Electromagnetic and Mechanical Energy

Electromagnetic energy differs from mechanical energy in that it does not require a medium in which to travel. Rather, the energy itself vibrates.

Electromagnetic radiation exhibits *properties* of a wave or a particle depending on its energy and, in some cases, its environment. This phenomenon is called *wave-particle duality,* which is essentially the idea that there are two equally correct ways to describe electromagnetic radiation. Conceptually, we can talk about electromagnetic radiation based on its wave characteristics of velocity, amplitude, wavelength,

and frequency. As previously stated, the velocity for all electromagnetic radiation is the same: $3 \times 10^8$ m/s. The *amplitude* refers to the maximum height of a wave. *Wavelength* is a measure of the distance from the peak of one wave to the peak of the next wave. *Frequency* refers to the number of waves that pass a given point per second (Fig. 3.3).

Because all electromagnetic radiation travels at the same velocity, the relationship between wavelength and frequency is inverse. That is, the longer the wavelength, the lower the frequency, and vice versa. Wavelength is generally expressed in meters. Because we are dealing with very large to very small wavelengths in the electromagnetic spectrum, the actual measure is typically in exponential form (e.g., $10^{-11}$ m). Frequency is generally expressed in Hz. One hertz is defined as one cycle per second. Long-wave AM radiowaves have frequencies from 500 to 1600 kHz, or 0.5 to 1.6 MHz. One kilohertz is 1000 cycles per second; 1 MHz is 1,000,000 cycles per second. Shorter FM radiowaves have frequencies in the hundreds of megahertz. As with electromagnetic radiation wavelengths, frequencies are also very large or very small and are generally expressed in exponential form. Electromagnetic radiation with very short wavelengths, such as x-rays, has frequencies measured in million-trillions of hertz (e.g., $10^{19}$ Hz).

The basic formula for calculating wavelength or frequency is velocity = frequency × wavelength ($v = f\lambda$). This formula is simplified when applied to electromagnetic radiation because the velocity of the spectrum is the same for all. So we replace $v$ with $c$ (the constant symbol for the speed of light: $3 \times 10^8$ m/s), and our formula becomes $c = f\lambda$. When solving for frequency, this formula becomes $f = c/\lambda$; this is simply a mathematical rearrangement to isolate the unknown value. When solving for wavelength, the formula becomes $\lambda = c/f$—again, just to isolate the unknown value.

## Math Application

The speed of light is a known value and is used in other formulas encountered in studies of radiologic science. It is commonly represented by the letter $c$, and its value is equal to $3 \times 10^8$ m/s.

## Math Application

To find the frequency of electromagnetic radiation, divide the speed of light by the wavelength measure:

$$f = c/\lambda$$

For example, what is the frequency of electromagnetic radiation if the wavelength is $1 \times 10^{-11}$ m? The problem is set up like this:

$$f = c/\lambda = 3 \times 10^8 \text{ m/s}/1 \times 10^{-11} \text{ m} = 3 \times 10^{19} \text{ Hz}$$

## Math Application

To find the wavelength of electromagnetic radiation, divide the speed of light by the frequency measure:

$$\lambda = c/f$$

What is the wavelength of electromagnetic radiation if the frequency is $1.5 \times 10^{12}$ Hz? The problem is set up like this:

$$\lambda = c/f = 3 \times 10^8 \text{m/s}/1.5 \times 10^{12} \text{ Hz} = 2 \times 10^{-4} \text{ m}$$

Electromagnetic radiation can also be characterized by how it interacts with matter. When discussed in this way, electromagnetic radiation may exhibit more characteristics of particles, depending on its energy. An individual particle or photon of electromagnetic radiation has an energy given by the Planck formula presented earlier. Higher-energy photons (e.g., x-rays, gamma rays) act more like particles, whereas lower-energy radiation (e.g., radiowaves, microwaves) acts more like waves.

The intensity of electromagnetic radiation diminishes over distance. This should be a familiar observation with sources of light or perhaps a campfire. This is an application of the **inverse square law**: the intensity of electromagnetic radiation diminishes by a factor of the square of the distance from the source. This concept is illustrated with a light source in Fig. 3.4 and is important to medical imaging as the reader will see in later chapters. The formula is:

$$\frac{I_1}{I_2} = \frac{(D_2)^2}{(D_1)^2}$$

If the formula is applied to a light source, "I" represents luminosity (measured in lumens or candela) and "D" represents distance. If applied to x-rays, the "I" represents coulombs per kilogram (C/kg), which is a measure of radiation intensity (number of electrons liberated by ionization per kilogram of air) with "D" again representing distance. The calculation is the same and involves solving for the unknown value. As you continue in your studies, you will have many x-ray

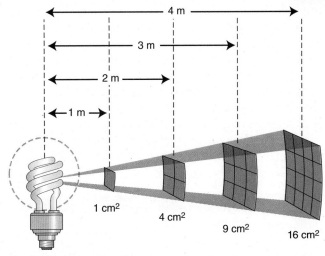

Fig. 3.4 **Inverse Square Law.** Illustration of the inverse square law using a grid pattern from a source.

problems with which to practice, so in keeping with Fig. 3.4, let's continue with a light source example. If a light source has an output of 1000 lumens at 2 m, what will the intensity be at 4 m? Inserting the values into the inverse square law formula we get:

$$1000/I_2 = 4^2/2^2$$
$$1000/I_2 = 16/4$$
$$1000/I_2 = 4$$
$$I_2 = 1000/4 = 250 \text{ lumens}$$

## Critical Concept

**Wave-Particle Duality**

Electromagnetic radiation exhibits properties of both a particle and a wave, depending on its energy and environment. Higher-energy electromagnetic radiation tends to exhibit more particle characteristics, and lower-energy electromagnetic radiation tends to exhibit more wave characteristics.

## Make the Imaging Connection

**Chapter 11**

The inverse square law is also used to calculate the change in the intensity (quantity) of radiation reaching the image receptor with changes in distance.

## X-RAYS AND GAMMA RAYS

X-rays and gamma rays have characteristics of both waves and particles, but because of their high energy, they exhibit more particulate characteristics than those at the other end of the electromagnetic spectrum. They do exhibit the wave characteristic of transmission. But they can also burn the skin, and their intensity varies according to the inverse square law, both of which are particulate characteristics. One additional particulate characteristic unique to the highest two members of the electromagnetic spectrum (x-rays and gamma rays) is the ability to ionize matter. When a photon possesses sufficient energy, it can remove electrons from the orbit of atoms during interactions. This removal of an electron from an atom is called **ionization**. The atom and the electron that was removed from it are called an *ion pair*. Ionization is the characteristic of x-rays and gamma rays that make them dangerous in general and harmful to the patient if misused. When tissue atoms are ionized, they can damage molecules and DNA and cause chemical changes in cells.

**Critical Concept**

**Ability to Ionize Matter**

The highest-energy members of the electromagnetic spectrum, x-rays and gamma rays, have the ability to ionize matter. This is an extremely important differentiating characteristic in that it can cause biologic changes and harm to human tissues.

What differentiates x-rays from gamma rays is that each originates from a different energy source. Gamma rays originate in the nuclei of atoms and represent the excess energy the atom is giving off to reach a stable state. X-rays originate through interactions between electrons and atoms. X-rays are produced when fast-moving electrons within the x-ray tube strike the atoms of the metal in its target. This subject is discussed in greater detail in later chapters.

## THE REST OF THE SPECTRUM

Readers should now understand the nature of x-rays and gamma rays. This section discusses the rest of the spectrum. As mentioned earlier, radiographers do encounter the other members of the electromagnetic spectrum and should be able to explain the difference to patients.

The low end of the energy spectrum begins with **radiowaves**. One common use of radiowaves (aside from transmitting our favorite music to our radios) is in MRI. The basic principle of operation of MRI hinges on the fact that the nuclei of hydrogen atoms are magnetic: when placed in a strong magnetic field, the nuclei will absorb and reemit radiowaves of a particular frequency. Through sophisticated processing of these emitted radiowaves, images can be constructed. Because human tissue contains large amounts of hydrogen (in molecules of water, fat, etc.), a substantial signal is observed. It is important to note that radiowaves do *not* ionize atoms.

**Microwaves** are used routinely to transmit cell phone signals and heat food. Microwave towers can be seen across the landscape, and microwaves generally provide a reliable signal. In microwave ovens, a microwave generator is used to create microwaves (electromagnetic waves at a frequency of about 2500 MHz) that are directed at the food. Microwaves hit the atoms of the food, giving them excess energy. This

energy causes "vibration" of the atoms and molecules. The atoms release this excess energy as heat, which increases the temperature of the food to the point of cooking or warming it. Microwave ovens work because microwaves are readily absorbed by water, sugars, and fats, but not by glass or plastic. Metals reflect microwaves and prevent them from being absorbed by the food and could damage the generator (which is why metals cannot be used in microwave ovens). Although microwaves can cause heating of tissues, they do not ionize atoms.

**Infrared light** is a low-energy electromagnetic radiation just above microwaves. It is sometimes used to "beam" information between electronic devices. For example, the signal sent from the television remote to change channels or settings on the television is infrared light. It may also be used to send information between portable electronic devices, such as between cell phones, between cell phones and computers, or between personal digital assistants and computers. Again, infrared light does not ionize atoms.

**Visible light** is likely the most familiar member of the electromagnetic spectrum. It represents the colors visible to the human eye. White light consists of all of the colors of the visible spectrum together. Therefore, an object perceived as white is reflecting all of the wavelengths of light at once. When we see a particular color, the object is absorbing all of the wavelengths of light except the one we see. The color black represents absorption of all of the color wavelengths. The visible spectrum is a very tiny portion of the electromagnetic spectrum and, again, visible light does not ionize atoms.

**Ultraviolet light** has energies approaching those of x-rays and gamma rays. Ultraviolet light–emitting bulbs are used in tanning beds because it is that part of sunlight that causes darkening of the skin (or burning if exposure is excessive). Ultraviolet light can be harmful, and routine exposure has been demonstrated to cause skin cancer. Ultraviolet light stimulates melanin production in skin cells, causing the darkening of or damage to the melanocytes, resulting in cancer, but it does not ionize the atoms.

All of these are members of the electromagnetic spectrum, but each behaves differently depending on its energy, and none has the ability to ionize matter. See Table 3.1 for a summary of the electromagnetic spectrum.

**Theory to Practice**

The radiographer should be able to explain the electromagnetic spectrum to patients or others for the purpose of education and reassurance during examinations.

## PARTICULATE RADIATION

**Particulate radiation—alpha particles** and **beta particles—** is important to know and understand because, like

**Table 3.1** Summary of Electromagnetic Spectrum

| ELECTROMAGNETIC RADIATION | COMMON USE | IONIZE MATTER? |
|---|---|---|
| Radiowaves | Broadcasting of music, MRI | No |
| Microwaves | Cell phone signals, microwave ovens | No |
| Infrared light | Communication between electronic devices | No |
| Visible light | The part of the spectrum the human eye perceives as colors | No |
| Ultraviolet light | Tanning beds | No |
| X-rays | Medical imaging, radiation therapy | Yes |
| Gamma rays | Nuclear medicine imaging, radiation therapy | Yes |

*MRI,* Magnetic resonance imaging.

x-rays and gamma rays, alpha and beta particles have the energy to ionize matter. Particulate radiation is more often dealt with in nuclear medicine or radiation therapy. But imaging professionals are obliged to understand its nature to fulfill their role as a source of information and an advocate for patients and the public.

> **! Critical Concept**
>
> **The Nature of Particulate Radiation**
>
> Particulate radiation—alpha and beta particles—are physical particles originating from radioactive atoms with the ability to ionize matter, much like x-rays and gamma rays.

To understand particulate radiation, one must first understand radioactivity. *Radioactivity* is a general term for the process by which an atom with excess energy in its nucleus emits particles and energy to regain stability. This process of a radioactive element giving off excess energy and particles to regain stability is known as *radioactive decay.* Elements that are composed of atoms with unstable nuclei are said to be *radioactive.* Some radioactive elements, such as radium and uranium, exist in nature, whereas others, such as technetium, are artificially produced for various purposes. (Technetium is produced for nuclear medicine studies.) A radioactive substance does not suddenly decay all at once. Decay is a process that may last minutes or billions of years. One term used to describe the rate at which a radioactive substance decays is *half-life.* A half-life is the length of time it takes for half the remaining atoms in a quantity of a particular radioactive element to decay. The half-life of radium 226, for example, is 1620 years. Half the unstable atoms are left after that time, and half of that amount (or one-fourth) is left after another 1620 years, and so on. Half-lives are used to measure radioactivity because that is how radioactive substances happen to decay. Chapter 1 noted that

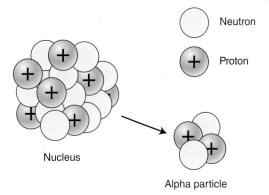

Fig. 3.5 **Alpha Particle.** An alpha particle is composed of two protons and two neutrons, the same makeup of the nucleus of a helium atom.

the unit of measure for radioactive decay is the becquerel (or curie). The electromagnetic photons emitted in this process (gamma rays) have already been discussed. That leaves the two common particles: alpha and beta.

An alpha particle is actually two protons bound to two neutrons (the same makeup of the nucleus of a helium atom; Fig. 3.5). Alpha particles have a net positive charge, two protons giving a charge of plus two. For example, uranium 238 is naturally radioactive. Each uranium atom has 92 protons and 146 neutrons. When it decays and emits an alpha particle, uranium then has 90 protons and 144 neutrons and becomes an atom of the element thorium. Alpha particles do not travel very far because they are relatively large and cannot penetrate most objects (tissue penetration is about 0.1 mm). Even in passing through air, they quickly pick up electrons that are attracted to their net positive charge and become helium atoms. A helium atom has two protons, two neutrons, and two electrons. When an alpha particle picks up the two electrons, it becomes a neutral helium atom.

A beta particle is an electron that is emitted from an unstable nucleus; it does not originate in an electron shell (Fig. 3.6). A beta particle is much lighter and

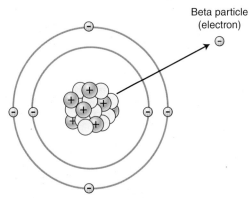

Fig. 3.6 **Beta Particle.** A beta particle is an electron emitted from an unstable nucleus; it does not originate from one of the electron shells.

| Table 3.2 | Range of Ionizing Radiation Constituting Human Exposure | |
|---|---|---|
| **RADIATION** | **CLASSIFICATION** | **SOURCE** |
| Cosmic | Natural/background | Sun and celestial events in space-emitting particulate or electromagnetic radiation |
| Terrestrial | Natural/background | Minerals in the soil such as uranium and thorium, or gases such as radon from decay of radioactive minerals |
| Internal | Natural/background | Isotopes such as potassium-40 and carbon-14 found naturally in the body |
| X-rays | Manmade | Electromechanically produced with an x-ray tube or similar device |
| Radiopharmaceuticals for nuclear medicine | Manmade | Most common are I-131, Tc-99m, Co-60, Ir-192, Cs 137 |
| Gamma | Natural/background | Electromagnetic from decay of radioisotopes, also created by cosmic events. |
| Alpha | Natural/background | Particulate, from process of radioactive decay |
| Beta | Natural/background | Particulate, from process of radioactive decay |

smaller than an alpha particle and thus can penetrate light materials (tissue penetration is up to 2 cm). Betas have a much larger range and may ionize many atoms along their path. They may have a positive or negative charge. The negatively charged beta particle differs from an electron only in that it originated in the nucleus of the atom, not an orbital shell. The positively charged beta particle is called a *positron*. When beta particles are stopped by collisions with other atoms, they join with atoms, just as electrons do.

To complete our study of electromagnetic and particulate radiation and complete the radiographer's understanding of ionizing radiation exposure to humans, a general overview of sources is in order. When the layperson considers radiation exposure, they may think of a nuclear event or, more commonly, radiation from medical uses. But in fact, we are exposed to ionizing radiation every day. These sources may be discussed as natural, or background, and manmade. Through further division of these, we can categorize them as cosmic, terrestrial, internal, and medical. Those constituting natural or background come from cosmic, terrestrial (radioactive decaying of minerals in the earth), internal (ingestion of foods and minerals with trace radioactivity), and medical sources (x-rays or nuclear medicine studies). Table 3.2 provides a general summary of some of the most common of these sources. The total dose from these sources varies according to geographic location. It is sometimes helpful when explaining radiation dose to a patient to indicate that we are exposed to small doses of ionizing radiation every day and some exposure or dose is okay. It is our responsibility as radiographers to effectively use medical sources so that the benefit of the examination outweighs any potential adverse effects of exposure.

### On the Spot

- Radiographers serve as advocates for patients and resources of information regarding the nature, benefits, and risks of the use of radiation. They should understand electromagnetic and particulate radiation and safely use the ionizing forms for medical imaging.

- Electromagnetic radiation is an electric and magnetic disturbance traveling through space at the speed of light. The members of the electromagnetic spectrum vary only in their energy, wavelength, and frequency.
- Electromagnetic energy differs from mechanical energy in that it does not require a medium in which to travel.
- Electromagnetic radiation exhibits properties of both a particle and a wave depending on its energy and environment. Higher-energy electromagnetic radiation tends to exhibit more particle characteristics than lower-energy electromagnetic radiation.
- The wavelength or frequency of electromagnetic radiation may be calculated using the following formula: $c = f\lambda$.
- The crucial difference between x-rays and gamma rays and the rest of the electromagnetic spectrum is that these two members have the ability to ionize matter.
- Radiographers should be aware of the nature and characteristics of all members of the electromagnetic spectrum and be able to explain such differences to the public.
- Particulate radiation includes alpha and beta particles, which originate from radioactive nuclei and have the ability to ionize matter.
- Particulate radiation is emitted from radioactive nuclei through decay, the process by which radioactive nuclei emit excess particles and energy in an effort to regain stability.
- As inhabitants of this planet, we are exposed to small doses of ionizing radiation every day.

### CRITICAL THINKING QUESTIONS

1. A patient states that they work around microwave ovens every day and is concerned about the additional radiation from the examination you are about to perform. How would you explain the electromagnetic spectrum (difference in microwaves versus x-rays) to them and inform them of the risks versus benefits of the examination?
2. Using your understanding of electromagnetic energy and its properties, explain why health care providers continue to struggle with the safe use of x-rays.

# REVIEW QUESTIONS

1. As the frequency of electromagnetic radiation decreases, wavelength will:
   a. increase.
   b. decrease.
   c. remain the same.
   d. frequency and wavelength are unrelated.
2. Which of the following members of the electromagnetic spectrum has the ability to ionize matter?
   a. Radiowaves
   b. X-rays
   c. Microwaves
   d. Ultraviolet light
3. Which of the following is not within the wavelength range of electromagnetic radiation?
   a. $10^{-24}$
   b. $10^{-12}$
   c. $10^{7}$
   d. $10^{-16}$
4. Which member of the electromagnetic spectrum has the longest wavelength?
   a. Microwaves
   b. Visible light
   c. Radiowaves
   d. X-rays
5. A diagnostic x-ray photon has a frequency of $2.42 \times 10^{19}$ Hz. What is its wavelength?
   a. $12.4 \times 10^{-11}$ m
   b. $12.4 \times 10^{27}$ m
   c. $1.24 \times 10^{-11}$ m
   d. $1.24 \times 10^{27}$ m

6. A photon has a wavelength of $3 \times 10^{-12}$ m. What is its frequency?
   a. $3 \times 10^{-4}$ Hz
   b. $3 \times 10^{20}$ Hz
   c. $1 \times 10^{-4}$ Hz
   d. $1 \times 10^{20}$ Hz
7. Which of the following do not originate from an unstable nucleus?
   a. Alpha particles
   b. Beta particles
   c. X-rays
   d. Gamma rays
8. How much activity will remain in a dose of 20 mCI $^{99m}$TC after 24 hours? (The physical half-life of $^{99m}$Tc is 6 hours.)
   a. 5 mCi
   b. 10 mCi
   c. 0.05 mCi
   d. 1.25 mCi
9. The intensity of a source at 15 inches is 10 R. What will the intensity be at 45 inches?
   a. 1.11 R
   b. 0.74 R
   c. 90 R
   d. 304 R
10. The intensity of a source is 25 R at 40 inches. What will the intensity be at 20 inches?
    a. 6.25 R
    b. 62.5 R
    c. 100 R
    d. 1000 R

## Outline

## Objectives

- Discuss the nature of electricity in terms of electrostatics and electrodynamics.
- Explain electric potential, current, and resistance.
- Demonstrate an understanding of Ohm's law and apply it to series and parallel circuits.
- Describe conductors and insulators and give examples of each.
- Identify electronic devices important to the understanding of the x-ray circuit.
- Demonstrate a basic understanding of magnetism.

- Explain electromagnetism.
- Explain electromagnetic induction (both mutual induction and self-induction).
- Describe basic generators, motors, and transformers.
- Identify the components of the x-ray circuit as being in the primary, secondary, or filament circuits.
- Explain the role and function of each major part of the x-ray circuit.
- Explain the basic principles of operation of the x-ray circuit from incoming power to x-ray production.

## Key Terms

| | | |
|---|---|---|
| alternating current (AC) | electromagnetic induction | magnetism |
| automatic exposure control (AEC) | electromagnetism | motors |
| conductor | electrostatics | primary circuit |
| current | filament circuit | resistance |
| direct current (DC) | generators | secondary circuit |
| electric potential | grounding | transformers |
| electrodynamics | insulator | |

## INTRODUCTION

This chapter provides a concise overview of the nature of electricity, electrical devices, and the basics of x-ray circuitry and principles of operation. It is true that many types of x-ray equipment are automated (Fig. 4.1). However, a radiographer is not someone who merely "pushes buttons." Rather, they have an understanding of the principles of x-ray production and have mastered the art of producing quality images with minimal radiation exposure to the patient. To reach this level of mastery, the radiographer must understand the basic elements of the x-ray machine and the steps in the process. Consider a pilot who flies a jet. A pilot untrained for that aircraft may be able to get it off the ground and

flying, but without some understanding of the jet's instrumentation, they are not likely to stay in the air very long. The safety of the passengers aboard that aircraft rests with the training and knowledge of that pilot. Similarly, the radiographer is responsible for the safety of the patient; the radiation dose that patient receives depends on the radiographer's understanding and safe operation of the x-ray machine. The concepts presented here are important to the radiographer because they ground the radiographer's practice in a fundamental understanding of what is happening each time they operates the x-ray machine. By understanding what happens within the x-ray machine with each selection made at the operating console, the radiographer is able

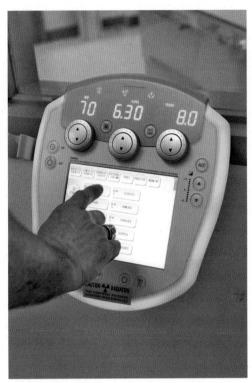

**Fig. 4.1 X-Ray Machine Control Panel.** Touch-screen control panel of a typical radiographic unit.

to use the machine with maximum efficiency and minimal radiation exposure to the patient. The knowledgeable radiographer is also able to make adjustments in exposure technique with variations in machines and daily operation.

## NATURE OF ELECTRICITY

The nature of electricity may be understood through a discussion of **electrostatics** and **electrodynamics**. Electrostatics is the study of stationary electric charges, and electrodynamics is the study of electric charges in motion. The latter is most often considered "electricity." A few fundamental concepts must first be discussed.

Electric charge is a property of matter. The smallest units of charge exist with the electron and the proton. Each electron has one unit of negative charge, and each proton has one unit of positive charge. Electrical charges are measured in the systeme internationale (SI) unit "coulomb." One coulomb is equal to the electrical charge of $6.25 \times 10$ electrons. A measure of electrons is used because electricity most often results from their movement. Except in decaying radioactive elements, protons are generally fixed in their position inside the nucleus of the atom. Electrons, on the other hand, are relatively free to move about, depending on the material. Some materials, such as copper and gold, have a very large number of free electrons, making them good **conductors** of electricity. Glass and plastic, on the other hand, have very few free electrons, making them good

insulators. This is discussed in greater detail later in this chapter.

Although an understanding of the laws of electrostatics is not the primary focus of this chapter, it is helpful in understanding the nature of electricity. There are five general principles of electrostatics. They are as follows:

- Like charges repel and unlike charges attract.
- The electrostatic force between two charges is directly proportional to the product of their quantities and inversely proportional to the square of the distance between them (also known as *Coulomb's law*).
- Electric charges reside only on the external surface of conductors.
- The concentration of charges on a curved surface of a conductor is greatest where the curvature is greatest.
- Only negative charges (electrons) are free to move in solid conductors.

In electrostatics, electrification of objects occurs when they gain either a net positive or a net negative charge. An object may be electrified in three ways: by friction, by contact, or by induction. The classic physics experiment involving rubbing a rubber rod with fur is an example of electrification by friction. Once charged, the rod can be discharged by placing it in contact with a conductor. This is an example of electrification by contact. Electrification by induction is the process by which an uncharged metallic object experiences a shift of electrons when brought into the electric field of a charged object. Induction occurs as a result of the interaction of the electric fields around two objects that are not in contact with each other. This is very useful in the design of the x-ray tube, as is discussed in Chapter 5.

*Electrodynamics* describes electrical charges in motion. This movement is associated with "electricity," and it is the intended meaning for all further discussions of electricity in this text. For electric current to move, an electric potential must exist. Electric potential is the ability to do work because of a separation of charges. If one has an abundance of electrons at one end of a wire and an abundance of positive charges at the other end (separation of charges), electrons will flow from abundance to deficiency.

 **Theory to Practice**

By design, the x-ray tube creates a separation of charges, and the exposure factors the radiographer selects on the control panel determine the number of electrons that will flow and the magnitude of their attraction to the positive side.

 **Critical Concept**

**Nature of Electricity**

The smallest units of charge rest with the proton and the electron. However, only electrons are free to move in solid conductors. Therefore "electricity" is most often associated with the flow of electrons.

# ELECTRIC POTENTIAL, CURRENT, AND RESISTANCE

**Electric potential, current,** and **resistance** are expressions of different phenomena surrounding electricity. Electric potential is the ability to do work because of a separation of charges. Current is an expression of the flow of electrons in a conductor. Finally, resistance is that property of an element in a circuit that resists or impedes the flow of electricity. There is nothing magical about the production of x-rays; it is simply the manipulation of electricity. Of course, significant engineering and technological knowledge is required to design and manufacture the equipment, but, when viewed at its most basic level, x-ray production is achieved through the manipulation of electricity. In fact, the units of measure for electric potential (the volt) and current (the ampere) are the factors selected on the operating console of the x-ray machine to produce x-rays. They are expressed in thousands and thousandths, respectively, but they are electrical terms and are not exclusive to radiology.

## Critical Concept

### Expressions of Electrical Phenomena

Electric potential, current, and resistance are expressions of different phenomena surrounding electricity. Electric potential is the ability to do work because of a separation of charges. Current is an expression of the flow of electrons in a conductor. Resistance is that property of an element in a circuit that resists or impedes the flow of electricity.

Electric potential is measured in volts, named for the Italian physicist Volta, who invented the battery. A *volt* may be defined as "the potential difference that will maintain a current of 1 ampere in a circuit with a resistance of 1 ohm" (amperes and ohms are discussed next). It is the expression of the difference in electric potential between two points. The volt is also equal to the amount of work in joules that can be done per unit of charge. (Refer to Chapter 1 for a review of the definition and calculation of work.) A volt is the ratio of joules to coulombs (volt = joules/coulombs). For example, a battery that uses 6 joules of energy to move 1 coulomb of charge is a 6-volt battery.

Again, one of the exposure factors selected on the control panel of the x-ray machine is kilovoltage peak (kVp). The role of kVp within the machine and in image production is discussed later in this text. For now, note that the radiographer is literally selecting the thousands of volts that will be applied to the x-ray tube to produce x-rays. kVp is the peak kilovoltage, and its selection represents the highest intensity of an x-ray photon possible for that setting. An understanding of this unit of measure and the concepts presented here are vital to the competent and safe operation of the x-ray machine.

## Make the Imaging Connection

### Chapters 11 and 13

Kilovoltage peak influences many areas of imaging. Among other things, it determines how the beam penetrates the body part and influences contrast in the digital image.

Current is measured in amperes, named for André-Marie Ampere, a French physicist who made significant contributions to the study of electrodynamics. The *ampere* may be defined as "1 coulomb flowing by a given point in 1 second." Reflecting its relationship to the definition of *volt* (discussed previously), it may also be defined as "the amount of current flowing with an electric potential of 1 volt in a circuit with a resistance of 1 ohm." For electric current to flow, there must be a potential difference between two electrodes and a suitable medium through which it can travel. With regard to potential difference, electrons flow from abundance to deficiency and will continue to do so as long as that difference exists. Electricity behaves differently depending on the medium through which it travels. Suitable media are conductors, and those resisting electric current flow are insulators. Both types of media are important to the production of x-rays. Two in particular, vacuums and metallic conductors, are of particular usefulness in x-ray production. In a vacuum tube, electrons tend to jump the gap between oppositely charged electrodes. This is part of the environment that exists inside an x-ray tube. With metallic conductors, electrons from the conductor's atoms will move out of the valence shell to a higher energy level just beyond, called the *conduction band*, where they are free to drift along the external surface of the conductor (refer to Chapter 2 for a discussion of atomic structure). Copper is particularly useful as a conductor and is commonly used as such in electronic devices. Other metals with this characteristic are used extensively in x-ray machine and x-ray tube design.

The two types of current, **direct current (DC)** and **alternating current (AC),** are also important to x-ray production and should be understood before moving on. DC is a type of current that flows in only one direction. A battery is a good example: It has a positive and a negative electrode, and, when placed in an electrical circuit, electrons flow from the negative terminal to the positive terminal (current flows in the opposite direction, a topic clarified later). AC is current that changes direction in cycles as the electric potential of the source changes (the negative and positive "terminals" alternate). In the United States, the electricity that flows into homes alternates at 60 cycles per second. This is expressed as a frequency of 60 Hz (see Chapter 3 for a definition and discussion of hertz). Both AC and DC are used in basic x-ray production.

**Critical Concept**

### Types of Current

There are two types of electric current. DC is a type that flows in only one direction (from positive to negative, opposite of the direction of electron flow). AC is a type that changes direction in cycles as the electric potential of the source changes (the negative and positive or polarity changes). In the United States, electricity alternates at 60 cycles per second.

Resistance is measured in ohms, named for the physicist Georg Simon Ohm, who discovered the inverse relationship between current and resistance. The *ohm* may be defined as "the electrical resistance equal to the resistance between two points along a conductor that produces a current of 1 ampere when a potential difference of 1 volt is applied." Ohm's law states that the potential difference (voltage) across the total circuit or any part of that circuit is equal to the current (amperes) multiplied by the resistance. It is expressed by the formula $V = IR$, in which $V$ is voltage, $I$ is current, and $R$ is resistance. Further discussion and examples of uses of Ohm's law are provided with examples of circuits later in this chapter.

 **Critical Concept**

### Relationship of Voltage, Current, and Resistance

The relationship among voltage, current, and resistance may be expressed through Ohm's law, which states that the potential difference (voltage) across the total circuit or any part of that circuit is equal to the current (amperes) multiplied by the resistance (ohms) ($V = IR$).

Resistance is that property of a circuit element that impedes the flow of electricity. The amount of resistance of a particular conductor depends on four things: material, length, cross-sectional area, and temperature.

Material: Some materials allow a free flow of current because they have an abundance of free electrons, whereas other materials have tremendous resistance because they have virtually no free electrons.

Length: Resistance is directly proportional to the length of the conductor; that is, a long conductor has more resistance than a short one.

Cross-sectional area: A conductor with a large cross-sectional area has a lower resistance than one with a small cross-sectional area because there is a greater external surface area on which electrons can travel.

Temperature: With metallic conductors, the resistance becomes greater as the temperature of the conductor rises.

Although resistance may sound like a hindrance to the x-ray production process, it is quite useful and is an important part of the process of x-ray production.

## CONDUCTORS, INSULATORS, AND ELECTRONIC DEVICES

Conduction and insulation are properties of elements and materials used in daily life. As previously stated, conductors are those materials with an abundance of free electrons that allow a relatively free flow of electricity. Although any such material conducts electricity, metals are typically used to serve this purpose. Copper typifies a conductive material. Its valence electrons are relatively free and will readily move to the conduction band, allowing a free flow of electricity. Gold is also a good conductor but is considerably more expensive because it is a precious metal and not widely used for this purpose. Water is also a good conductor of electricity because of the mineral impurities it often contains.

In contrast, most nonmetallic elements are made up of atoms with tightly bound electrons and do not conduct electricity well, even when attracted by a potential difference. Such materials are **insulators**. Insulators have virtually no free electrons and, as such, are very poor conductors of electricity. But it is this very property that makes them particularly useful in containing the flow of electricity. Covering a copper wire with rubber or plastic "insulates" the wire and restricts the flow of electricity to the copper wire; such is the case with an electric cord (extension cord). Glass, ceramic, and wood are also good insulators. This combination of conductors and insulators is prevalent in daily life.

In between these extremes are semiconductors. These materials will conduct electricity but not as well as conductors, and they will insulate but not as well as insulators. Silicon, germanium, and diamond are examples of semiconductors. Semiconductor properties are very useful and widely used in electronics.

 **Critical Concept**

### Conductors and Insulators

Conductors are materials with an abundance of free electrons that allow a relatively free flow of electricity, whereas insulators have virtually no free electrons and are therefore very poor conductors of electricity.

An electric circuit is a closed pathway composed of wires and circuit elements through which electricity may flow. This pathway for electricity must be closed (complete) for electricity to flow. This is what is meant by a *closed circuit*. In contrast, an *open circuit* is one in which the pathway is broken, such as when a switch is turned off. Turning off a switch opens the pathway and turning on a switch closes the pathway. The elements of a circuit may be arranged in series (called a series circuit), in parallel (called a parallel circuit), or a combination (called series-parallel). A series circuit is one in which the circuit elements are wired along a single conductor. A parallel circuit is one in which the circuit elements "bridge" or branch across a conductor. The

| Box 4.1 | Rules for Calculating Voltage, Current, and Resistance Based on Circuit Type |
|---|---|

**RULES FOR SERIES CIRCUITS**

Total voltage is equal to total current × total resistance.

$$V_T = I_T R_T$$

Resistance is equal to the sum of the individual resistances.

$$R_T = R_1 + R_2 + R_3$$

Current is equal throughout the circuit. $I_T = I_1 = I_2 = I_3$

Voltage is equal to the sum of the individual voltages.

$$V_T = V_1 + V_2 + V_3$$

**RULES FOR PARALLEL CIRCUITS**

Total voltage is equal to the total current × the total resistance.

$$V_T = I_T R_T$$

Total current is equal to the sum of the individual currents.

$$I_T = I_1 + I_2 + I_3$$

Voltage is equal throughout the circuit. $V_T = V_1 = V_2 = V_3$

Total resistance is inversely proportional to the sum of the reciprocals of each individual resistance. $1/R_T = 1/R_1 + 1/R_2 + 1/R_3$

calculation of voltage, current, and resistance differ between the two, and the rules for each are summarized in Box 4.1. An x-ray circuit is a complex version that has different voltages and currents flowing through different sections.

The following provides an overview and examples of calculations for voltage, current, and resistance. In a series circuit, the total voltage is determined by multiplying the total current by the total resistance or by summing the individual voltage values. The total resistance is found by summing the values of the individual resistances. The current in a series circuit is equal throughout the circuit. In a parallel circuit, the total voltage is again determined by multiplying the total current by the total resistance or by measuring voltage anywhere in the circuit because voltage is equal throughout the circuit. The total current is found by summing the values of the individual current values. The total resistance is a little different in parallel circuits. It is inversely proportional to the sum of the reciprocals of each individual resistance value. Use Box 4.1 and the following example circuits to practice these concepts.

Use the following circuit to answer the next six questions.

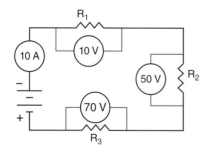

1. What is the resistance of R1?
2. What is the resistance of R2?
3. What is the resistance of R3?
4. What is the total voltage?
5. What is the total resistance?
6. What is the total current?

Use the following circuit to answer the next six questions.

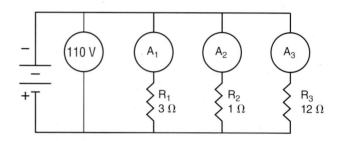

7. What is the current through $A_1$?
8. What is the current through $A_2$?
9. What is the current through $A_3$?
10. What is the total current?
11. What is the total resistance?
12. What is the total voltage?

One final note regarding these problems is that when you are working with a series-parallel circuit, apply and solve the parallel element first and then use those values to solve the series problems.

The term *electronic devices* may mean a number of things depending on the context. Music players, cell phones, video gaming systems, televisions, and so on are all referred to as *electronic devices*. This same definition can be applied to many devices used in health care. An understanding of seven electronic devices—battery, capacitor, diode, protective devices (fuses and circuit breakers), resistor or rheostat, switch, and transformer—facilitates understanding of the x-ray circuit.

A battery is a device that produces electrons through a chemical reaction, stores an electric charge for the long term, and provides an electric potential. A capacitor is like a battery in that it stores an electric charge, but it works very differently in that it cannot produce new electrons and stores the charge only temporarily. A diode (e.g., solid-state rectifier) is a "one-way valve" device that allows electrons to flow in one direction only. Protective devices, such as fuses and circuit breakers, act as emergency devices that "break" or open the circuit if there is a sudden surge of electricity to the circuit or device. This act of opening the circuit protects the other circuit elements and the device as a whole. A fuse is simply a section of special wire usually encased in glass that quickly melts if the current flow rises excessively, thus opening the circuit. A circuit breaker acts in the same manner as a fuse. If the current flow rises excessively, the circuit breaker's internal switch is tripped (opened), stopping the flow of electricity. A resistor is a device designed to inhibit the flow of electrons, thereby precisely regulating the flow of electricity through that part of the circuit where it is placed. A rheostat is simply an adjustable or variable form of resistor. A switch is a device that opens a circuit (breaks the pathway). Finally, a transformer is a device that can increase or decrease voltage by a predetermined amount.

Table 4.1 provides a summary of these devices and the symbols of each. Several of these symbols were used in the example circuits previously.

A term you may see in relation to circuits and electricity is **grounding**. Grounding, a process of connecting the electrical device to the Earth via a conductor, is a protective measure. The Earth is essentially an infinite reservoir of electrons. Any charged object can be neutralized if it is grounded. Positively charged objects take on electrons from the Earth and negatively charged objects give up electrons to the Earth until neutral. Inside electrical equipment, the grounding wire connects to metal parts that are not a part of the circuit, such as the housing. If a "live" wire happens to touch the housing, the current is conducted away by the grounding wire. This "short circuit" into the ground wire trips the circuit breaker, shutting off the electricity to the circuit. With these concepts and components in mind, electromagnetism and electromagnetic induction can now be discussed.

### Table 4.1  Common Circuit Devices

| DEVICE | USE | SYMBOL |
|---|---|---|
| Battery | Produces electrons through a chemical reaction, stores an electric charge long term, and provides an electric potential. | |
| Capacitor | Temporarily stores an electric charge. | |
| Diode | A "one-way valve" device; allows electrons to flow in only one direction. | |
| Protective devices (fuses, circuit breakers) | Emergency devices that break or open the circuit if there is a sudden surge of electricity to the circuit or device. | Fuse / Circuit breaker |
| Resistor (and rheostat) | Inhibits the flow of electrons, thereby precisely regulating the flow of electricity through that part of the circuit where it is placed. A rheostat is simply an adjustable or variable form of resistor. | Resistor / Rheostat |
| Switch | A device that opens a circuit (breaks the pathway). | |
| Transformer | A device that can increase or decrease voltage by a predetermined amount. | |

> **⚠ Critical Concept**
>
> **Grounding**
>
> Grounding is a process of neutralizing a charged object by placing it in contact with the Earth. Positively charged objects take electrons from the Earth until neutral and negatively charged objects give up electrons to the Earth until neutral.

## ELECTROMAGNETISM AND ELECTROMAGNETIC INDUCTION

### MAGNETISM

Electricity and **magnetism** are two different parts of the same phenomenon known as **electromagnetism**. *Magnetism* may be defined as "the ability of a material to attract iron, cobalt, or nickel." The magnetic properties of cobalt and nickel assume their pure form. The U.S. nickel coin does not exhibit strong magnetic properties because it contains only 25% nickel; the rest is copper.

Iron is relatively abundant and is used extensively in the creation of magnets and magnetic fields.

The nature of magnetic materials is such that the orbital electrons of their atoms spin in predominately one direction. Such atoms create tiny magnets called *magnetic dipoles*. When these dipoles, or "atomic magnets," form groups of similarly aligned atoms, they create magnetic domains. These domains exist in magnetic materials but are not "coordinated" with each other. When such magnetic materials are placed in a strong magnetic field, the domains align with the external field, which organizes them and "magnetizes" the material, creating a magnet.

A magnetic field consists of lines of force in space called *flux* and has three basic characteristics. First, the lines of flux travel from the south pole to the north pole *inside* the magnet and from the north pole to the south pole *outside* the magnet, creating

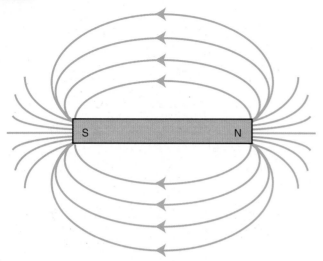

**Fig. 4.2 Magnetic Flux.** A magnetic field consists of lines of force in space called flux.

elliptical loops (Fig. 4.2). Second, lines of flux in the same direction repel each other, and lines of flux in the opposite direction attract each other. Third, magnetic fields are distorted by magnetic materials and are unaffected by nonmagnetic materials. There are three laws of magnetism that may promote an understanding of electromagnetism. The first law is that every magnet has a north and south pole. The second law states that like poles repel each other and opposite poles attract each other. The third law states that the force of attraction or repulsion varies directly with the strength of the poles and inversely with the square of the distance between them. The strength of the magnetic field is measured in the SI unit tesla (T), named for the American physicist Nikola Tesla. Magnetic resonance imaging units used for medical imaging are referred to by their magnetic field strength and operate with fields from 0.5 to 5 T (5 T is currently experimental).

Just as materials can be classified as conductors or insulators, they may also be classified by their magnetic properties. There are four categories: Nonmagnetic materials (e.g., glass, wood, plastic) are not attracted to magnetic fields at all, diamagnetic materials (e.g., water, mercury, gold) are weakly repelled by magnetic fields, paramagnetic materials (e.g., platinum, gadolinium, aluminum) are weakly attracted to magnetic fields, and ferromagnetic materials (e.g., iron, cobalt, nickel) are strongly attracted to magnetic materials.

## ELECTROMAGNETISM

With an understanding of electricity and magnetism, they can be discussed together as electromagnetism. As previously stated, electricity and magnetism are two parts of the same basic force. That is, any flow of electrons, whether in space or in a conductor, is surrounded by a magnetic field.

Likewise, a moving magnetic field can create an electric current.

 **Critical Concept**

**Electromagnetism**

Electricity and magnetism are two parts of the same basic force. That is, any flow of electrons, whether in space or in a conductor, is surrounded by a magnetic field. Likewise, a moving magnetic field can create an electric current.

The principle of electromagnetism was first identified by the Danish physicist Hans Oersted when he discovered that the needle of a compass is deflected when placed near a conductor carrying electric current. It was later discovered that the magnetic field surrounding the conductor could be intensified by fashioning it into a coil (called a *solenoid*) and intensified further by adding an iron core to the coil (called an *electromagnet*). Shortly after Oersted's discovery, British scientist Michael Faraday found that moving a conductor (such as copper wire) through a magnetic field induces an electric current in that conductor. This phenomenon is called **electromagnetic induction**. Fashioning the conductor into a coil and passing it through the magnetic field increases the induced voltage, and this voltage increases with an increasing number of coils. Increasing the strength of the magnetic field or the speed with which the conductor is passed through the magnetic field also increases the induced voltage.

 **Critical Concept**

**Electromagnetic Induction**

Current may be induced to flow in a conductor by moving that conductor through a magnetic field or by placing the conductor in a moving magnetic field.

Two forms of electromagnetic induction are used in the operation of the x-ray machine: mutual induction and self-induction. Mutual induction is the induction of electricity in a secondary coil by a moving magnetic field (Fig. 4.3).

The coil on the left in Fig. 4.3 is connected to an AC source. As previously discussed, a magnetic field is associated with the flow of electricity, and AC switches direction of flow in cycles. Each time AC switches direction, the associated magnetic field also changes. That is, the north and south poles of the magnetic field are directionally oriented to the current flow, and when the current changes direction, the previous magnetic field dies away and a new one is created that is opposite in orientation and properly oriented to the new current flow direction. The

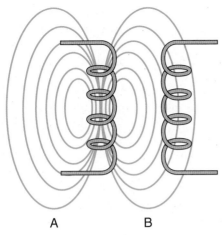

**Fig. 4.3 Mutual Induction.** Coil A is the primary coil connected to an AC power source. Coil B is the secondary coil, and as the fluctuating magnetic field from A moves back and forth through the turns of B, a secondary current is induced.

important part of this phenomenon is that a "moving" magnetic field is created. The previous field collapses and a new one expands, then current changes direction again and the process starts over. When this moving magnetic field is placed near a secondary coil (the coil on the right in Fig. 4.3), electricity is induced to flow in that coil. This is also the case for AC because it, too, switches with the changing magnetic fields.

Self-induction is a bit more complex, requiring an understanding of Lenz's law, which states that an induced current flows in a direction that opposes the action that induced it. In this case, that action is the changing magnetic field. Returning to the example of the primary coil illustrated in Fig. 4.3, the magnetic field is created in this coil and expands

outward from the center of the coil. As it does so, it "cuts" through the turns of the coil. This act of "cutting" creates a current within the same conductor that opposes the original (Lenz's law). Using DC, this phenomenon is short-lived, because the magnetic field reaches maximum strength and the cutting action stops. But with AC, this process repeats with each change of direction. The result is a fluctuating magnetic field cutting back and forth through a single coil, inducing a constant secondary current that opposes the original. This process is called *self-induction* and is used in the x-ray circuit in the autotransformer design (discussed shortly).

## GENERATORS, MOTORS, AND TRANSFORMERS

Electromagnetism and electromagnetic induction have many applications in electrical equipment. Of particular interest in understanding the x-ray circuit are electric **generators**, electric **motors**, and **transformers**. Each is described briefly here and is then placed in context in the discussion of the x-ray circuit.

Electric generators are devices that convert some form of mechanical energy into electrical energy. Examples include the force of water through a dam; steam, which is created by burning some type of fuel, turning a turbine; or the wind turning a windmill turbine. In its simplest form, rotating a loop of wire in a magnetic field induces a current in that loop through electromagnetic induction. Remember: When the loop cuts the magnetic flux lines, a current is induced (Fig. 4.4).

The more complex design uses coils of wire forming an armature that is rotated in a magnetic field by some mechanical means.

Electric motors are devices that convert electrical energy to mechanical energy through electromagnetic

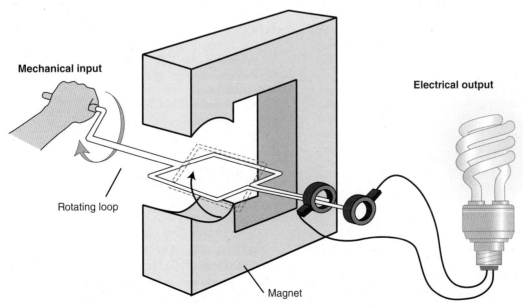

**Fig. 4.4 Generator.** As the loop is rotated in the magnetic field, a current is induced in the loop.

induction. In a simple motor, an armature is placed in an external magnetic field and the armature is supplied with AC. As discussed previously, every flow of current has an associated magnetic field. This magnetic field associated with the armature is oriented such that the north pole is next to the north pole of the external field and the south pole is next to the external south pole. Because like poles repel, the armature flips to orient itself to the external field. At the same instant that the two magnetic fields align, the AC current changes direction. A new magnetic field is created in the armature, which, again, is not aligned to the external field, and the armature rotates again. This process is continuous, converting electrical energy to mechanical energy. A more sophisticated variation of this design, called the *induction motor*, is discussed with the x-ray tube in Chapter 5. Transformers are devices used to increase or decrease voltage (or current) through electromagnetic induction. They are named for their effect on voltage. A step-up transformer is one that increases voltage and a step-down transformer is one that decreases voltage. The change in voltage and current is an inverse relationship. As voltage is increased, current decreases, and vice versa. This relationship is expressed using the transformer laws for voltage and current as follows where V = voltage; I = current; N = number of turns in the coil; s = secondary coil; p = primary coil.

Transformer law for voltage is:

$$V_s / V_p = N_s / N_p$$

This is a direct relationship.

Example: If a transformer has 10 turns in the primary, 50 turns in the secondary, and 110 volts is applied, what is the output voltage?

Answer: $V_s / 110 = 50/10$; $V_s = 5 \times 110$; $V_s = 550$

Transformer law for current is:

$$I_s / I_p = N_p / N_s$$

This is an inverse relationship.

Example: If a transformer has 10 turns in the primary, 50 turns in the secondary, and 5 amps is applied, what is the output current?

Answer: $I_s / 5 = 10/50$; $I_s = 5 \times 0.2$; $I_s = 1$

The relation of voltage to current in a transformer is:

$$I_s / I_p = V_p / V_s$$

This is an inverse relationship.

Example: If a transformer has an input voltage of 110, an input current of 5 amps, and an output voltage of 550, what is the output current?

Answer: $I_s / 5 = 110/550$; $I_s = 110/550 \times 5$; $I_s = 1$

Note that these expressions assume ideal circumstances in a transformer and do not take into account eddy current loss (heat loss in the core) or hysteresis loss (loss because the voltage is applied in a nonlinear fashion to the core), but they suffice for the sake of understanding their role in the x-ray circuit. In some instances, a transformer may be used to increase or decrease voltage, and in others, it may be used to increase or decrease current. Both uses occur in the x-ray circuit. The example presented with the explanation of electromagnetic mutual induction (see Fig. 4.3) is the simplest transformer design, consisting of two coils placed next to each other with one connected to an AC source. When AC is flowing through the primary coil, it has an associated "fluctuating" magnetic field. This collapsing and expanding magnetic field induces electricity in the secondary coil. The difference in the voltage induced in the secondary coil depends on the ratio of the number of turns of wire in the two coils. For example, if there are twice as many turns in the secondary coil as in the primary, the voltage in the secondary coil is twice that of the primary coil. If there are half as many turns in the secondary coil, the voltage is half that in the primary coil. Much more sophisticated designs are used in x-ray equipment, such as closed-core and shell-type transformers that incorporate a ferromagnetic core to maximize efficiency (Fig. 4.5).

---

 **Critical Concept**

**Inverse Relationship of Current and Voltage**

The change in voltage or current through a transformer is an inverse relationship: If voltage is increased, current decreases, and vice versa.

---

One final type of transformer important to the x-ray machine is the autotransformer. This transformer operates on the principle of self-induction, as described earlier. This transformer has only one coil of wire around a central magnetic core (not to be confused with the shell type, which has *two* coils of wire). This coil is used as both the primary and secondary coil. The outside wires are attached at different points along the coil, and the induced voltage varies, depending on where the connections are made (Fig. 4.6).

## GENERAL X-RAY CIRCUIT

Fig. 4.7 is a general drawing of an x-ray circuit. This is a greatly simplified version, but it is sufficient to understand the principles of operating the x-ray machine. The x-ray circuit may be divided into three sections: the **primary circuit**, the **secondary circuit**, and the **filament circuit**. Each section has specific components and roles to play. The primary circuit consists of the main power switch (connected

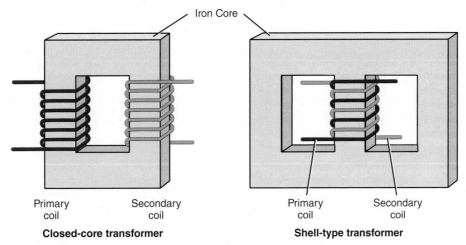

**Fig. 4.5 Transformer Types.** The basic design of a closed-core and shell-type transformer. The iron cores of each increases magnetic field strength and transformer efficiency.

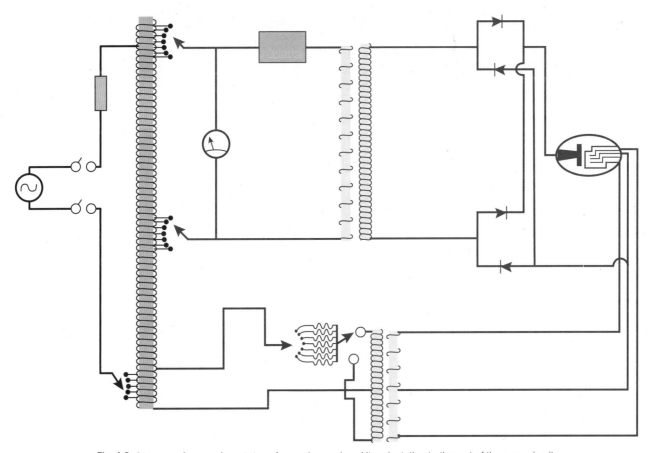

**Fig. 4.6 Autotransformer.** An autotransformer (orange) and its orientation to the rest of the x-ray circuit.

to the incoming power supply), circuit breakers, the autotransformer, the timer circuit, and the primary side of the step-up transformer. The secondary circuit consists of the secondary side of the step-up transformer, the milliampere meter, a rectifier bank, and the x-ray tube (except for the filaments). The filament circuit consists of a rheostat, a step-down transformer, and the filaments.

## PRIMARY CIRCUIT

Fig. 4.8 is a labeled version of the basic x-ray circuit. Beginning in the primary circuit, the main power switch is simply an on-off switch for the unit and is connected to the power supply of the facility. Because the incoming power is not a consistent 220 V, a line compensator is also used. This device is usually wired to the autotransformer and automatically

**X-ray circuit**

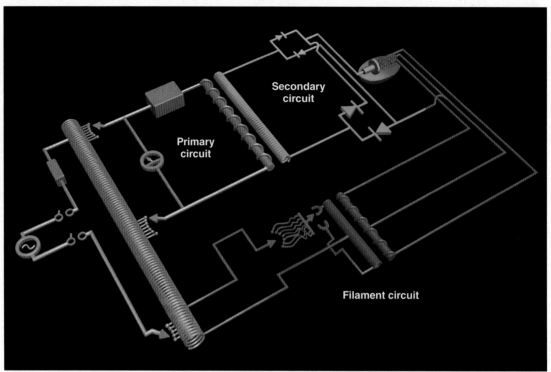

Fig. 4.7 **Basic X-Ray Circuit.** The primary circuit is indicated in orange, the secondary circuit is in blue, and the filament circuit is in *purple*.

**X-ray circuit**

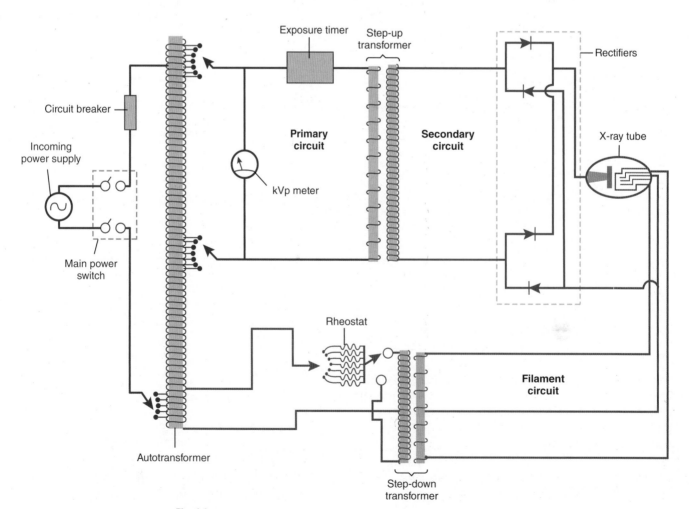

Fig. 4.8 **Parts of the X-Ray Circuit.** Labeled version of a basic x-ray circuit.

adjusts the power supplied to the x-ray machine to precisely 220 V. The circuit breakers are included in the primary circuit to protect against short circuits and electric shock. The autotransformer (see Fig. 4.8) is an adjustable transformer controlled by the kilovoltage peak selector on the operating console. When the radiographer selects a kVp setting, they are controlling this transformer. As stated earlier, this transformer operates on the principle of self-induction. When the radiographer selects a kVp setting, they determine the number of turns on the secondary side to be included in the circuit element and, with it, the output voltage. Because of its function, the autotransformer is sometimes called the *kVp selector.* Its primary purpose is to provide a voltage that will be increased by the step-up transformer to produce the kilovoltage selected at the operating console.

---

 **Critical Concept**

**The Autotransformer**

The radiographer controls the autotransformer through the kVp selector on the operating console, and through this, directly determines the voltage applied to the x-ray tube to produce x-rays.

---

The step-up transformer (Fig. 4.8) is used to increase the voltage from the autotransformer to the kilovoltage necessary for x-ray production. This transformer is the dividing line between the primary and secondary circuits. The primary coil is in the primary circuit and the secondary coil is in the secondary circuit (hence the names). Unlike the autotransformer, this transformer is not adjustable and increases the voltage from the autotransformer by a fixed amount. The timer circuit (exposure timer) is located in this section because it is easier to control (turn on and off) low voltage than a very high one. There are several variations of the exposure timer. The first variation is a synchronous timer, which is based on a synchronous motor. The motor is designed to turn a shaft at precisely 60 revolutions per second. This shaft turns a disk, which is connected to on-off switches, through reduction gears. The exposure time selected determines the reduction gear used and therefore the time it takes the disk to move from the on switch to the off switch. The second variation, the electronic timer, is a very sophisticated and accurate timer that is the most widely used today. This timer is based on the time it takes to charge a capacitor through a variable resistor. Once the capacitor receives its preprogrammed charge, it terminates the exposure. The time it takes to charge this capacitor to its preprogrammed level is controlled by the variable resistor. To achieve a 1-second exposure, the resistance is increased so

that it takes longer to charge the capacitor (including inherent electrical delays, the total time is 1 second). To achieve a 1-millisecond exposure, there is virtually no resistance; the capacitor charges very quickly and the timer terminates the exposure. This is one application for a resistor in the x-ray circuit. The mAs timer is a variation of the electronic timer, but it monitors the current passing through the x-ray tube and terminates the exposure when the desired mAs is reached. Because of the way it functions, this timer is located in the secondary circuit instead of the primary circuit.

Serving the same role as a timer is the **automatic exposure control (AEC)** device. This device operates somewhat differently from the others in that it uses a patient's body part as the variable in determining when to terminate exposure. The AEC uses a device called an *ionization chamber.* This is a radiolucent device placed between the patient and the image receptor. When x-rays interact with this chamber, its atoms are ionized (electrons removed), creating an electric charge. This charge becomes a signal that terminates the exposure. The AEC can be adjusted (calibrated) so that more or less of a charge is needed before the signal to terminate exposure is sent. AEC calibration is performed by installation personnel by exposing phantoms until the desired density (image quality factor) is achieved. This amount of exposure varies with the image receptor, and the AEC must be recalibrated if that receptor changes (e.g., from one cassette-based digital system to another). Once the AEC is calibrated, the patient becomes the variable. As x-rays exit the patient on the way to the image receptor, they pass through the ionization chamber, causing ionization. Once the preprogrammed magnitude of electric charge is reached, the exposure is terminated. The length of the exposure is then determined by the thickness and density of the area of the patient placed over the ionization chamber. For example, an infant abdomen and an adult abdomen could be placed over the ionization chamber and, although both are abdomens, the exposure time is very different because of the differences in tissue thickness of the two patients. That is, it takes longer for enough x-rays to exit the larger abdomen to create the signal in the chamber.

*At the console.* To this point, the radiographer has selected the exposure factors (kVp and mAs) among other parameters and pressed the exposure button. In the primary circuit, this results in a voltage being determined by the autotransformer and applied to the primary side of the step-up transformer. A voltage is also selected from the autotransformer and applied to the filament circuit. With the voltage and current selected and traveling, the stage is set for the rest of the circuit.

## Make the Imaging Connection

### Chapter 11

AEC controls only the quantity of radiation reaching the image receptor and therefore has no effect on other image characteristics such as contrast. The radiographer must still select kVp and in many cases mA.

## Critical Concept

### Automatic Exposure Control

The AEC is a device that serves to terminate exposure (like a timer). It consists of an ionization chamber that is placed between the patient and image receptor. As the radiation exits the patient and passes through the chamber, ionization occurs. When sufficient ionization occurs in the chamber, a signal is sent to terminate exposure. The thickness and density of the body part of interest becomes the "timer" variable.

## SECONDARY CIRCUIT

The secondary circuit begins with the rest of the step-up transformer. The role of the step-up transformer was presented previously. The milliampere meter is simply a device placed in the secondary circuit that monitors x-ray tube current. The rectifiers are needed to convert AC to DC and require a more detailed discussion. In a general x-ray circuit, AC is necessary for transformers to operate correctly (provide the "moving" magnetic field). However, to allow the x-ray tube to be exposed to AC would be disastrous. Within the x-ray tube, current must always flow from anode to cathode and electrons from cathode to anode (this process is covered in detail in Chapter 5). To achieve this, rectifiers are used.

The rectifier commonly used in today's x-ray circuit is a solid-state rectifier. This device is made of two semiconducting crystals. One is a p-type crystal and the other is an n-type crystal. The p-type crystal has an abundance of "electron traps," whereas the n-type has an abundance of freely moving electrons. These two crystals are joined to form a solid-state diode.

When a positive charge is placed on the p-type crystal and a negative charge is placed on the n-type crystal, the solid-state diode will conduct electricity. To do this, both the traps from the p-type crystal and the electrons from the n-type crystal move toward and across the p-n junction, allowing current to flow. When the AC cycle reverses, and the p-type crystal receives the negative charge and the n-type crystal receives the positive charge, the solid-state diode will not conduct. This is because the traps and electrons "stay at home" (do not move to the junction) and no current is conducted (Fig. 4.9).

To be used most effectively, rectifiers are arranged in pairs so that the AC cycle has an open "path" from each direction. The symbol for the solid-state rectifier is the same as that for the diode in general: Using this symbol, current flow is *with* the direction of the arrow and electron flow is *against* the arrow of the symbol. It is possible to use only two rectifiers, but this suppresses (wastes) the negative half of the cycle only and simply serves to protect the x-ray tube during that phase. One-half of the AC cycle flows through the x-ray tube, and the other half, which would otherwise flow through the x-ray tube the wrong way, is suppressed (blocked). This type of waveform is called *half-wave rectification*.

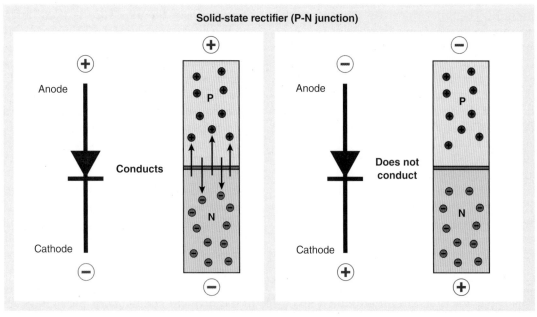

**Fig. 4.9 Solid-State Rectifier.** Solid-state rectifier showing its conduction and nonconduction phases. Note the change in polarity in each half of the illustration.

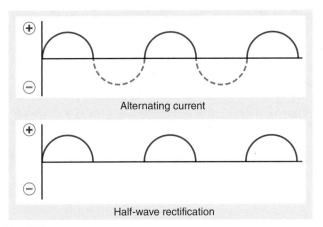

**Fig. 4.10 Rectification of Alternating Current.** Alternating current and half-wave rectification waveforms.

Figure 4.10 shows AC (*top*) and what the waveform would look like with only two rectifiers (half-wave rectification, *bottom*).

When four rectifiers are used, full-wave rectification is achieved. Notice the arrangement of the four rectifiers in Fig. 4.11. They are highlighted to show which two are in use with each half of the cycle. With four rectifiers arranged in this way, both halves of the AC cycle are used. The resulting waveform is illustrated in Fig. 4.12. Note that we, in effect, "invert" the negative half of the cycle, thereby making use of the entire cycle. Note also that the energy fluctuates from zero (on the line) to the maximum voltage (peak of wave). This is called *ripple*, and, in the case of single-phase full wave, it is 100% ripple. Although single-phase, full-wave power is much more desirable and certainly less wasteful, this 100% ripple is a problem because the x-rays vary in energy from the kVp selected on the operating console (maximum energy available) to zero. One solution is to use three AC waveforms at the same time. With a bit of engineering, three waveforms can be phased or synchronized. Each is generated independently and then phased so that each one is 120 degrees out of step with the next (i.e., out of step by one-third). The result is a waveform like that shown in Fig. 4.13. It would be a terrible waste not to rectify this waveform. When we do rectify each one as if they were a single-phase waveform, the x-ray tube "sees" a waveform like the one in Fig. 4.14. This is referred to appropriately as *three-phase power*. Although this obviously has less ripple than the single-phase waveform, it still has ripple. Depending on the number of rectifiers and engineering, it will have anywhere from 13% ripple (three-phase 6 pulse) to 3.5% ripple (three-phase 12 pulse). This translates into x-rays being produced with anywhere from 87% to 100% of the kVp selected on the operating console for three-phase 6 pulse to 96.5% to 100% for three-phase 12 pulse.

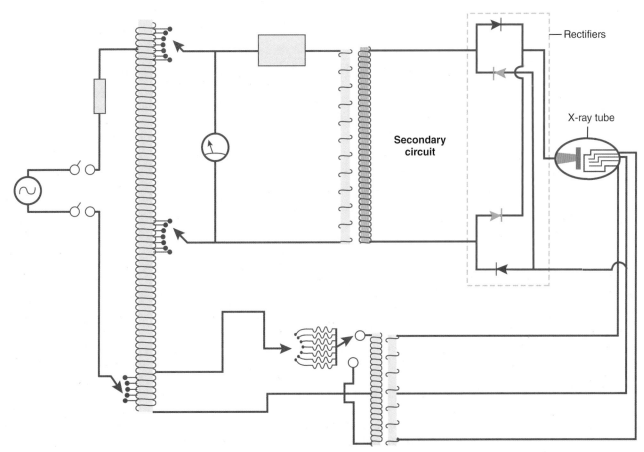

**Fig. 4.11 Rectifier Bank.** A four-rectifier bank. Note the color coding of the pair that operates together in each half of the cycle.

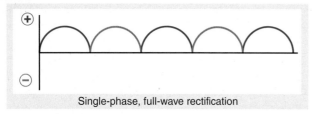

Fig. 4.12 **Single-Phase Alternating Current.** Single-phase, full-wave waveform.

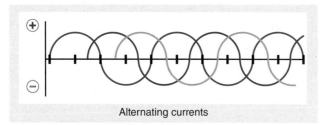

Fig. 4.13 **Three Single-Phase Waveforms.** Three single-phase waveforms unrectified.

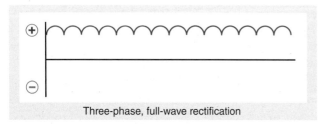

Fig. 4.14 **Three-Phase Waveform.** Three single-phase waveforms rectified.

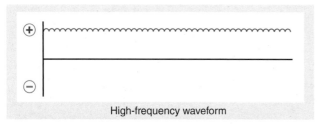

Fig. 4.15 **High frequency, full-wave rectification.**

The next evolution in the quest to improve the waveform is the use of high-frequency generators in place of the standard 60-Hz generators. The standard 60-Hz incoming power is first fully rectified and then sent through a capacitor bank, where it is smoothed. From there it passes through an inverter circuit that "chops" this DC waveform and converts it to high-frequency AC. This low-voltage, high-frequency AC is then passed through a step-up transformer, converting it to high-voltage AC. It is again passed through rectifiers, where it is again fully rectified, and finally through high-voltage capacitors, where it is smoothed to provide the x-ray tube with a near-constant potential

voltage waveform. These generators reduce the ripple "seen" by the x-ray tube to less than 1%. Fig. 4.15 demonstrates the resulting waveform. In general, these generators are smaller, lighter, less costly, and offer better exposure reproducibility.

Keep in mind that through all of this, rectifiers—the one-way valves—are necessary to route the electricity through the x-ray tube correctly.

> ### ⇄ Theory to Practice
> A single-phase machine may require a higher kVp setting than a three-phase or high-frequency machine because of the difference in efficiency but does not expose the patient to a different dose of radiation.

The x-ray tube, with the exception of the filaments, is also a part of this section. Because the x-ray tube head assembly is the subject of Chapter 5, it is addressed in detail there.

*At the console.* Within the secondary circuit, pressing the exposure button has sent voltage through the step-up transformer, increasing it to the kilovoltage selected and indicated on the control console. This kilovoltage is passed through a series of rectifiers so that it travels through the x-ray tube correctly to produce x-rays. A large positive charge now resides with the anode, and a large negative charge with the cathode within the x-ray tube. All that is lacking is the source of electrons on which this kinetic energy will ride, which brings us to the filament circuit.

## FILAMENT CIRCUIT

The filament circuit begins with the rheostat (Fig. 4.16). This variable resistor is controlled by the mA selector on the operating console. The milliampere parameter is called *tube current* because it reflects the rate of flow of electrons passing through the x-ray tube during an exposure. When the radiographer adjusts milliamperage on the operating console, they are adjusting this rheostat and thus the amount of resistance in the filament circuit, and ultimately the amount of current applied to the filament (called *filament current*) in the x-ray tube. The higher the milliamperage station number, the lower the resistance. A 1000-mA station will have very little resistance to the flow of electricity, whereas a 100-mA station will have considerable resistance. The goal of the filament circuit is to literally boil electrons out of the filament wire. Normally, a rather large filament current of 5 to 7 amperes is required to produce a tube current in the range of milliamperes. The thermionically emitted electrons are needed for x-ray production and represent one more step in the manipulation of electricity. However, in the filament circuit, we are boiling these electrons off of a very small wire and must precisely control the current that is applied. If the current is too high, this tiny wire will be damaged or destroyed.

**X-ray circuit**

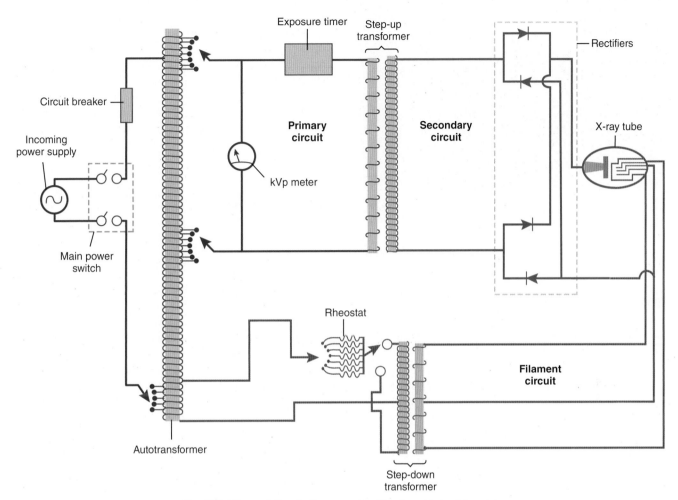

Fig. 4.16 **Filament Circuit.** Components of the filament circuit (purple).

 **Make the Imaging Connection**

**Chapter 11**

The quantity of radiation exposing the patient and ultimately reaching the image receptor is directly related to the product of milliamperage and exposure time (mAs). Therefore, exposure to the image receptor can be increased or decreased by adjusting the amount of radiation by adjusting the mAs.

 **Critical Concept**

**Milliamperage Selector**

The radiographer controls the rheostat through the milliamperage selector of the operating console, which directly determines the current that is ultimately applied to the selected filament and the number of electrons boiled off and available for x-ray production.

The exposure timer, discussed previously, works in concert with the rheostat. The rheostat controls filament temperature and the rate at which electrons are boiled off of the filament. The timer determines the duration

of this process. Together, they determine the quantity of electrons boiled off of the filament and available for x-ray production (this subject is addressed in detail in Chapter 5).

A step-down transformer is used in the filament circuit to increase the current by reducing the voltage that is applied to the filament. The purpose of the filament circuit is to control the degree and duration that the filament is heated, which in turn controls the number of electrons boiled off that will ultimately become the tube current. Although the step-down transformer reduces the voltage that is applied to the filament, because we are concerned with the current through the filament, we generally talk about the output current of this transformer rather than voltage. Remember that as voltage decreases, current increases.

The final piece of the filament circuit is the filaments (Fig. 4.17). A general-purpose radiographic tube typically has two filaments. These are tiny coils of wire housed in the cathode of the x-ray tube. The design and purpose of the filaments is covered later. They are represented on the operating console by the "large focal spot" and "small focal spot." When selecting one

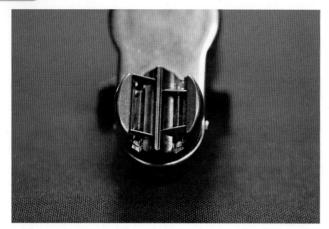

**Fig. 4.17 Filaments.** Filaments (small wire coils) within the cathode focusing cup.

of these, the radiographer is literally selecting the filament to be heated and used for that exposure.

*At the console.* Within the filament circuit, when the exposure button is pressed, a voltage and current is sent through the filament circuit. The quantity is precisely controlled by a rheostat to reflect the mA selected and indicated on the control console. A step-down transformer is used to reduce this voltage and increase current (recall that this is an inverse relationship: as voltage decreases, current increases). This current heats the filament chosen by the radiographer and begins boiling off electrons. The time selected by the radiographer controls the duration that the voltage and current in the x-ray tube is applied (as described with timers).

## PRINCIPLES OF CIRCUIT OPERATION

Now that all of the pieces and parts have been covered, it is helpful to walk through the x-ray circuit's operation from incoming power supply to x-ray tube. The discussion of the events in the x-ray tube is brief here, but they are covered in detail in Chapters 5 and 6.

The appropriate place to begin is the operating console. Like the controls of an automobile, options and arrangement vary, but all have basic options in common. The operating console offers options for selecting kVp, mA, exposure time, and focal spot size. If the unit is equipped with AEC or anatomic programming, those options are also displayed. The same is true for Bucky selection if both a table and a wall Bucky are available. The process begins when the radiographer selects an exposure technique, which specifies kVp, mA, exposure time, and focal spot. From here it is easiest to follow the sequence of events in two parts. This discussion first follows voltage through the primary and secondary circuits, then follows current through the filament circuit.

The kVp selected adjusts the autotransformer and determines the number of turns on the secondary side necessary to produce a voltage, through self-induction, which will be sent to the step-up transformer. The step-up transformer increases this voltage by a fixed amount and, through mutual induction, produces the kilovoltage selected on the operating console. This transformer represents the transition from the primary circuit to the secondary circuit.

Once kilovoltage is created, it must be rectified for the x-ray tube. Where the x-ray tube is concerned, the electrons must always flow from cathode to anode. Solid-state rectifiers are used to route electricity through the x-ray tube correctly. The number of rectifiers used depends on the circuit type. These "one-way valves" route current from positive to negative and electrons from negative to positive. After passing through the rectifiers, the electricity creates a large positive charge on the anode of the x-ray tube and a large negative charge on the cathode focusing cup (part of the tube that surrounds the filaments).

It is now necessary to return to the autotransformer to cover the other half of the process. The filament circuit draws electricity from the autotransformer, which then travels to the rheostat. The rheostat is a variable resistor controlled by the mA selector on the operating console and is tied to the focal spots. The focal-spot selector represents the two filaments in the x-ray tube: one large and one small. When the mA station was selected, the appropriate filament was also selected (small for small mA stations and large for large mA stations). The selected mA station sets the resistance in the filament circuit. From the rheostat, electricity then travels to the step-down transformer. Recall that we are more concerned with the current output in this case than with the voltage, and as voltage decreases, current increases. The adjusted current from the step-down transformer then travels directly to the filament located within the focusing cup of the x-ray tube. This current heats the filament to the point at which electrons are literally boiled off.

Now the two halves of the process can be joined. A group, or cloud, of electrons is created by the filament circuit (heating of the filament). The kilovoltage applied to the x-ray tube creates a large positive charge on the anode and a large negative charge on the cathode (focusing cup). The large positive charge attracts the electrons boiled off the filament, giving them tremendous kinetic energy in the process. Opposites attract, and in the short 1- to 3-centimeter gap between cathode and anode the electrons from the filament reach speeds of about one-half the speed of light. The large negative charge on the cathode serves to keep the electrons crowded together; otherwise they would repel each other and scatter throughout the tube. The electrons travel across to the anode and interact there to produce x-rays until the timer circuit terminates the process.

## ON THE SPOT

- The smallest units of charge rest with the proton (one unit of positive charge) and the electron (one unit of negative charge).
- Only electrons are free to move in solid conductors; "electricity" is most often associated with the flow of electrons. Electrical charge is measured in coulombs. One coulomb is equal to $6.25 \times 10^{18}$ electrons.
- Electric potential, current, and resistance are expressions of different phenomena surrounding electricity. Electric potential (measured in volts) is the ability to do work because of a separation of charges; current (measured in amperes) is an expression of the flow of electrons in a conductor; resistance (measured in ohms) is that property of an element in a circuit that resists or impedes the flow of electricity.
- Electricity behaves differently depending on the medium. In a vacuum, electrons jump the gap between electrodes; in a metallic conductor, electrons move to the conduction band and flow.
- There are two types of electric current. DC is a type that flows in only one direction (from positive to negative, opposite of the direction of electron flow), and AC is a type that changes direction in cycles as the electric potential of the source changes (the negative and positive or polarity changes). In the United States, the electricity alternates at 60 cycles per second.
- The relationship between voltage, current, and resistance may be expressed through Ohm's law, which states that the potential difference (voltage) across the total circuit or any part of that circuit is equal to the current (amperes) multiplied by the resistance.
- Resistance of a conductor depends on the material, length of the conductor, cross-sectional area, and temperature.
- Conductors are materials with an abundance of free electrons that allow a relatively free flow of electricity, whereas insulators have virtually no free electrons and therefore are very poor conductors of electricity.
- Grounding is a process of neutralizing a charged object by placing it in contact with the Earth.
- Electricity and magnetism are two parts of the same basic force. That is, any flow of electrons, whether in space or in a conductor, is surrounded by a magnetic field. Likewise, a moving magnetic field can create an electric current.
- Current may be induced to flow in a conductor by moving that conductor through a magnetic field or by placing the conductor in a moving magnetic field. There are two forms: mutual induction and self-induction.
- Electric generators are devices that convert mechanical energy into electrical energy.
- Electric motors are devices that convert electrical energy into mechanical energy.
- Transformers are devices that increase or decrease voltage (or current) through electromagnetic induction. A step-up transformer increases voltage and a step-down transformer decreases voltage.
- The x-ray circuit is divided into three main sections: the primary circuit, the secondary circuit, and the filament circuit.
- The radiographer controls the autotransformer through the kVp selector of the operating console, which creates a voltage through self-induction that, when passed through the step-up transformer, becomes the kilovoltage applied to the x-ray tube to produce x-rays.
- The exposure timer is generally located in the primary section, and the electronic timer is the most sophisticated, most accurate, and most commonly used today.
- The AEC terminates exposure (like a timer). It consists of an ionization chamber that is placed between the patient and image receptor. As the radiation exits the patient and passes through the chamber, ionization occurs. When sufficient ionization occurs in the chamber, a signal is sent to terminate exposure.
- Solid-state rectifier banks are arranged to route current through the x-ray tube the same way each time, in effect "converting" AC to DC. This process is called *rectification.*
- By combining three single-phase waveforms, three-phase power is created and the percentage of ripple in the waveform is reduced. Through the use of high-frequency generators, this ripple is reduced further still.
- When the radiographer adjusts milliamperage on the operating console, he or she is adjusting this rheostat and thus the amount of resistance in the filament circuit, and ultimately the amount of current applied to the filament in the x-ray tube. The higher the mA station number, the lower the resistance.
- Following the sequence of events through the primary and secondary circuits, voltage flows from the autotransformer to the step-up transformer, through the rectifiers to the x-ray tube. Following the sequence of events through the filament circuit, current flows from the autotransformer through the rheostat, to the step-down transformer, and to the selected filament within the cathode of the x-ray tube. Both halves of this sequence happen simultaneously to set up the environment in the x-ray tube that produces x-rays.

## CRITICAL THINKING QUESTIONS

1. What are the sequences of events through the primary, secondary, and filament sections of the x-ray circuit when a set of exposure factors are selected?
2. How is electricity manipulated and used in an x-ray machine to ultimately produce x-rays?

## REVIEW QUESTIONS

1. An x-ray tube is an example of current flow in a/an:
   a. gas.
   b. vacuum.
   c. metallic conductor.
   d. ionic solution.
2. Which of the following increases or decreases voltage by a fixed amount?
   a. capacitor
   b. rheostat
   c. diode
   d. transformer

3. Which of the following is Coulomb's law?
   a. Like charges repel, unlike charges attract.
   b. Electrostatic force between charges is directly proportional to product of quantities and inversely proportional to square of distance between them.
   c. Electric charges reside only on the external surface of conductors.
   d. Only positive charges can move in solid conductors.

4. A rheostat will:
   a. provide electric potential.
   b. vary resistance.
   c. increase or decrease voltage.
   d. provide infinite resistance.

5. In a metallic conductor:
   a. electrons move on external surface.
   b. electrons move internally.
   c. protons move on external surface.
   d. protons move internally.

6. Nearly all discussion of electricity deals with the movement of:
   a. positive charges.
   b. negative charges.
   c. neutrons.
   d. all of the above.

7. Which of the following conditions or environments will provide the least resistance?
   a. glass material
   b. long conductor
   c. large cross-sectional area
   d. high temperature of conductor

8. The potential difference that will maintain a current of 1 ampere in a circuit with a resistance of 1 ohm is the definition of:
   a. ampere.
   b. volt.
   c. ohm.
   d. coulomb.

9. The removal of electrons from an object by rubbing it with another is electrification by:
   a. contact.
   b. friction.
   c. induction.
   d. grounding.

10. Which of the following allows electrons to flow in only one direction?
    a. transformer
    b. rheostat
    c. battery
    d. diode

11. Which of the following is a unit of measure of current?
    a. ampere
    b. volt
    c. coulomb
    d. ohm

12. Magnetic flux is:
    a. magnetic material.
    b. groups of smaller magnets.
    c. curved lines of force in space.
    d. the magnetizing of other materials.

13. What is the magnetic classification of materials weakly attracted to magnets?
    a. nonmagnetic
    b. ferromagnetic
    c. paramagnetic
    d. no such classification

14. The unit of measure for electric potential is:
    a. A
    b. V
    c. Ω
    d. W

# The X-Ray Tube

5

## Outline

## Objectives

- Describe the construction and purpose of the x-ray tube housing.
- Identify the principal parts of the x-ray tube and their purposes.
- Describe the operation of the principal parts of the x-ray tube.
- Discuss anode designs and construction.
- Explain the line-focus principle.

- Explain the anode heel effect.
- Discuss cathode designs and construction.
- Trace the path of electricity through the x-ray circuit and x-ray tube, connecting the selections on the operating console to the functions within the unit.
- Employ methods of safe x-ray tube operation and extending x-ray tube life.

## Key Terms

| | | |
|---|---|---|
| actual focal spot | focusing cup | rotor |
| anode | heat units (HUs) | space charge |
| anode heel effect | induction motor | space-charge effect |
| cathode | leakage radiation | stator |
| effective focal spot | line-focus principle | target window |
| filament | protective housing | thermionic emission |

## INTRODUCTION

Chapter 1 provided a general discussion of the x-ray tube head assembly and the function of the major parts of the design. Chapter 4 discussed the components of the x-ray circuit and the events that lead to the production of x-rays in the x-ray tube. This chapter examines the x-ray tube itself (Fig. 5.1), its general construction, and how it works. The sole purpose for manipulating electricity in an x-ray circuit is to create the environment in the x-ray tube necessary for x-ray production. The need for the radiographer to understand the x-ray tube is twofold. First, as was described in Chapter 4, the radiographer must have a basic understanding of how the tube works to competently and safely formulate exposure techniques and minimize patient radiation dose. Second, such an understanding is critical to extending the life of the tube and to avoid damaging it.

A thorough discussion of each part of the x-ray tube is presented here, including how each selection made at the control panel affects the corresponding part of

the x-ray tube. Several procedures and considerations to protect the tube are also presented. Finally, quality-control considerations to extend the life of the tube are discussed. The safe operation and proper maintenance of the x-ray unit rest with the radiographer; appropriate operation and maintenance of the x-ray unit stem from the knowledge of how it works.

## GENERAL TUBE CONSTRUCTION

### HOUSING

The general construction of the tube head assembly is discussed first. Recall that the x-ray tube is situated in a **protective housing** that provides solid, stable mechanical support. This housing is a lead-lined metal structure that also serves as an electrical insulator and thermal cushion for the tube itself (Fig. 5.2). X-ray production is a rather inefficient process, and much of the electrical energy that goes into it is converted to heat. The design of the housing incorporates an oil bath and cooling fans

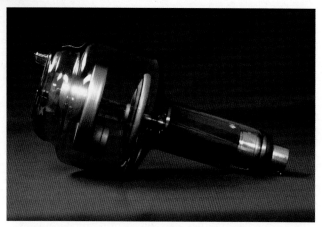

Fig. 5.1 **Photograph of X-Ray Tube.** A basic rotating anode x-ray tube.

to help dissipate heat away from the tube, protecting it from thermal damage. The tube is immersed in the oil bath, which draws heat away from the tube. The cooling fans circulate air around the assembly, which also helps dissipate heat. Because of the large current and voltage needed to produce x-rays, electrical insulation is necessary. Two large electrical cables enter the housing and are securely attached to the x-ray tube through special high-voltage receptacles. Finally, although x-rays are perceived as being produced and traveling in one direction out through the collimator to the patient and image receptor, this is not the case. X-rays are produced isotropically (in all directions), and another role of the housing is to absorb most of the photons traveling in directions other than toward the patient. The housing design reduces this radiation, called **leakage radiation**, to less than 100 mR/h (0.0258 millicoulomb/kg/h) at a distance of 1 m, as required by regulation.

Two notes of caution about the housing are necessary. First, with extended "on" times, the housing can become rather hot. This is most likely to occur with fluoroscopic

units, and most permanently installed units have the tube located under the tabletop, which limits the possibility of contact. But mobile fluoroscopic units can be easily touched; caution should be used when they are involved in very long cases in which heating is considerable. Second, the high-voltage cables are *not* "handles." Some radiographers develop the bad habit of using them as such, but doing so poses a risk to the radiographer and potential for damage to the equipment.

## ⚠ Critical Concept

### The Protective Housing

The housing protects the x-ray tube by serving as an electrical insulator and thermal cushion. The radiographer should take care not to touch it after long "on times" and not to use the high-voltage cables as "handles" for maneuvering the tube.

## X-RAY TUBE

Although there are several specialty designs of the x-ray tube, they do have basic components in common. This text focuses on the design used for general medical radiography. The general-purpose x-ray tube is an electronic vacuum tube that consists of an **anode**, a **cathode**, and an **induction motor** all encased in a glass or metal enclosure (envelope). Fig. 5.3 provides a labeled illustration of this design. Recall that the anode is the positive end of the tube and the cathode is the negative end of the tube. The anode incorporates an anode target and an induction motor, half of which is inside and half of which is outside the protective enclosure; the anode is discussed in detail shortly. The cathode consists of the **focusing cup** and **filaments** with its supporting wires.

The main purpose of the enclosure is to maintain a vacuum within the tube. Because the production of x-rays involves the interaction between filament

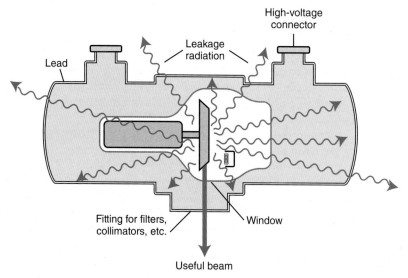

Fig. 5.2 **X-Ray Tube Inside Protective Housing.** Protective housing with the x-ray tube situated inside. The design of the housing serves as an electrical insulator and thermal cushion for the x-ray tube in addition to being a protective device against physical damage.

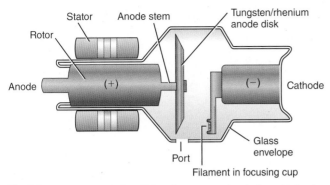

**Fig. 5.3 Parts of the X-Ray Tube.** A cross-sectional view of a basic rotating anode x-ray tube.

electrons and the anode target, if any air were present, the electrons from the air would contribute to the electron stream, causing arcing and damage to the tube. The glass envelope variety is generally made of borosilicate glass because it is very heat resistant. However, as these tubes age, vaporized tungsten from the filament deposits on the inside of the glass (called "sun tanning" because of the bronze discoloration of the glass), which causes problems with arcing and damage. The metal envelope variety provides a constant electric potential between the electron stream from the cathode and the enclosure, thereby avoiding the arcing problem and extending tube life. Both enclosure types have a specially designed **target window** for the desired exit point of the x-rays produced. The target window is fashioned to minimally interfere with (absorb) the x-rays. It is usually about 5 cm square and is a place on the enclosure that has been made thinner than the rest. This thinned section reduces the amount of absorption by the enclosure.

 **Critical Concept**

**The Enclosure or Envelope**

> The primary purpose of the glass or metal enclosure of the x-ray tube is to maintain a vacuum so that electrons from the air do not contribute to the electron stream, which would disrupt the x-ray production process and damage the tube.

## ANODE

The anode is the positive end of the tube. It provides the target for electron interaction to produce x-rays and is an electrical and thermal conductor. Remember that electricity is flowing through the x-ray tube, and the electrons flowing from cathode to anode are a part of that flow of electricity. Some of the electrons interact with the target to produce x-rays (see Chapter 6), and the rest continue as current flow through the x-ray circuit. Remember, too, that a tremendous amount of heat is also generated during the process. The anode is designed to dissipate this heat.

There are two designs for the anode. One is the stationary anode (Fig. 5.4A). This is basically a tungsten button embedded in a copper rod. It is called *stationary*

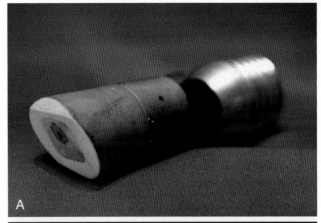

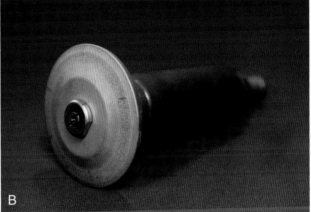

**Fig. 5.4 Anode Types. (A)** A stationary anode removed from the glass envelope. Note the silver-colored tungsten button and the discolored area where electrons interacted with it. **(B)** A rotating anode removed from the glass envelope. The focal track along the edge of the disc and some damage from extensive use are visible.

because the target does not move. Stationary anodes were used in old tube designs and may still be found in dental x-ray units or those requiring very small exposure techniques. The primary disadvantage of this design is that, because the electrons always hit the same small target area, heat builds up rapidly and can damage the tube. This problem limits the exposure technique factors that can be used. This limitation spurred the development of rotating-anode designs.

The rotating-anode design is used in general-purpose tubes today (Fig. 5.4B). It consists of a rotating disc made of molybdenum as a core material coated with tungsten and mounted on a copper shaft with a molybdenum core. Copper is used as part of the shaft because it has excellent thermal and electrical conductive properties. Molybdenum is used as the disc base and core because it has a low thermal conductivity, which slows migration of heat into the rotor bearings (minimizing heat damage), and it is a light but strong alloy, making it easier to rotate the anode. The target material (coating) is made of tungsten because it has a very high melting point (3400°C [6152°F]), and its thermal conductivity is almost equal to that of copper. Furthermore, it has a high atomic number (74), improving the efficiency of x-ray production. Rhenium may also be added to the tungsten to increase thermal capacity and tensile strength. The anode is rotated using an induction motor. The two major parts of this motor are the **stator** and the **rotor** (see Fig. 5.3). The stator is made up of electromagnets arranged in pairs around the rotor. The stator is outside the tube enclosure. The rotor is made of an iron core (iron bars embedded in the copper shaft) surrounded by coils and located in the center of the stator but within the enclosure. The rotor does not touch the stator, nor is it supplied with electric current. It is operated through mutual induction. The stators are energized in opposing pairs and induce an electric current in the rotor with an associated magnetic field. This induced field opposes that of the stator pair, and the rotor turns to correct that orientation. Just as the two fields align, the next pair of stators is energized and again a new electric current and magnetic field is induced, causing the rotor to turn again. This process continues with the energizing of each pair of stators in sequence. The response of the rotor is to continuously turn as the induced magnetic fields try to orient with the ever-changing external fields. Fig. 5.5 illustrates this concept. Using an induction motor allows for the rotation of the anode in a vacuum without engineering a motor into the vacuum. Such motors are capable of rotating the anode at speeds of 3400 revolutions per minute (rpm) for general purpose tubes and 10,000 rpm for specialty tubes.

The purpose of rotating the anode is to spread the tremendous heat produced during x-ray production over a larger surface area. Instead of electrons always striking the same small surface area (as with stationary anodes), the electrons strike only a small part of the total anode surface area at any one time, and that area changes. The focal "spot" becomes a focal "track," with the rotating anode and the heat build-up spread over the focal track circumference rather than on one spot. This greatly increases the heat-load capacity and the exposure techniques that can be used.

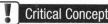

### Critical Concept

### The Rotating Anode

The rotating anode is turned using an induction motor that operates through electromagnetic mutual induction. The rotation of the anode spreads the heat produced during x-ray production over a larger surface area, greatly increasing the thermal and exposure technique capacity of the tube.

Notice in Fig. 5.6 that the face of the target is angled. This makes use of the **line-focus principle**. The line-focus principle states that by angling the face of the anode target, a large **actual focal spot** size (area actually bombarded with filament electrons) can be maintained and a small **effective focal spot** size (the x-ray beam area as seen from the perspective of the patient) can be created. The

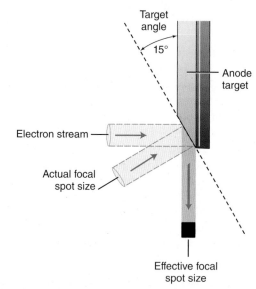

**Fig. 5.6 Line-Focus Principle.** By angling the face of the target, a large actual focal spot is maintained to spread heat load and create a small effective focal spot to improve image detail.

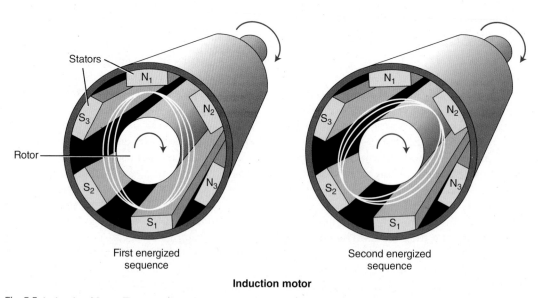

**Fig. 5.5 Induction Motor.** The operation of opposing pairs of stators in sequence ultimately causes rotation of the rotor.

actual focal spot is the area being bombarded by the filament electrons. The size of the electron stream depends on the size of the filament. The smaller this stream, the greater the heat generated in a small area; therefore, it is desirable to have a larger actual focal spot area. The effective focal spot is the origin of the x-ray beam and is the area as seen from the patient's perspective. The smaller this area of origin, the sharper the image will be. It is desirable to keep this as small as practical to improve image quality. When the angle of the target face is less than 45 degrees, the effective focal spot will be smaller than the actual focal spot. The target angles are 7 to 18 degrees for a general-purpose tube, with 12 degrees being the most common. The smaller the anode angle, the smaller the effective focal spot will be, while maintaining a large actual focal spot area. Again, this means that a large actual focal spot for heat dissipation is maintained, but a small effective focal spot to improve image quality is created. The smaller the effective focal spot, the sharper the image will be (Fig. 5.7). Anode target angle is determined based on the intended use of the tube and is not something the radiographer "selects" at the operating console. For example, the angles are optimized for mammography units, angiographic units, general radiography units, etc.

Although the line-focus principle achieves this goal of balance between heat area and projected focal spot, it is not without tradeoffs. When the target angle becomes too small, the x-ray beam area may not be large enough to fully expose a 14 × 17-inch image receptor at a 40-inch source-to-image receptor distance. Such angle limitations are taken into consideration when the x-ray tube is designed and manufactured. Additionally, the angle causes the intensity of the x-ray beam to be less on the anode side because the "heel" of the target is in the path of the beam. This means that the x-rays on the anode side must first penetrate a portion of the target before exiting the tube. Some do not have the energy to do so and are absorbed in the target heel, reducing the intensity on the anode side. This phenomenon is called the **anode heel effect** (Fig. 5.8).

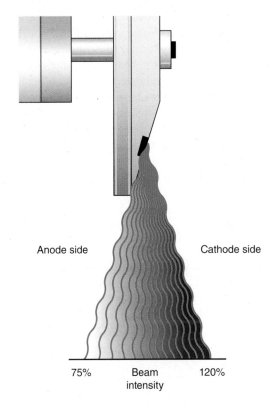

**Fig. 5.8 Anode Heel Effect.** The anode heel effect is simply caused by photons produced on the anode side, which must penetrate the heel of the target before exiting the tube. This causes some photons to be weakened and some to be absorbed. The net effect is a reduced intensity of the beam on the anode side.

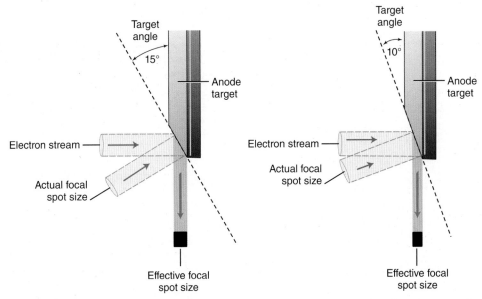

**Fig. 5.7 Target Angle and Line-Focus Principle.** Two different target angles illustrate the effect of target angle on effective focal spot size. The smaller the target angle, the smaller the effective focal spot.

Notice in Fig. 5.8 the percentage difference in x-ray beam intensity from cathode side to anode side. This lowering of intensity on the anode side of the beam can cause the image to be "lighter" on that end. This is because there are fewer high-energy x-ray photons on the anode side, and not enough penetrate the patient to expose the image receptor. This was particularly true of film/screen technology, and for some examinations, placing the thinner or less dense portion of the patient's anatomy under the anode end would partially compensate for this and improve image quality. This is less of an issue with digital technology, because these systems can record and display many shades of gray, a characteristic called *dynamic range*. Digital systems have a wide dynamic range, meaning that they can accurately detect, record, and display very high and very low x-ray photon intensities. In the case of the anode heel effect, the lower intensities on the anode side will still be detected and accurately displayed on the final image. However, it is still useful for the radiographer to be mindful of and understand the anode heel effect.

 **Critical Concept**

**The Line-Focus Principle and Anode Heel Effect**

The rotating anode design uses the line-focus principle, which means that the target face is angled to create a large actual focal spot for heat dissipation and a small effective focal spot for improved image quality. But by angling the face, the "heel" of the target is partially placed in the path of the x-ray beam produced, causing absorption and reduced intensity of the beam on the anode side.

## CATHODE

The cathode is the negative end of the tube; it provides the source of electrons needed for x-ray production. The cathode is made up of the filaments and the focusing cup (Fig. 5.9) and is connected to two different parts of the x-ray circuit. Recall that the filaments are connected to the filament circuit and the focusing cup is connected to the secondary circuit.

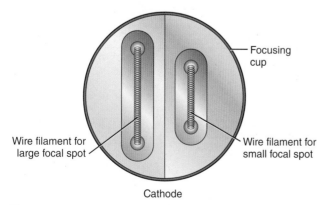

Cathode

**Fig. 5.9 Cathode.** Front view of the cathode focusing cup with two filaments situated within.

Most general-purpose tubes have two filaments and are referred to as *dual-focus tubes*. These filaments are represented by the large and small focal-spot options on the operating console. Each filament is a coil of wire usually 7 to 15 mm long and 1 to 2 mm wide. They are usually made of tungsten with 1% to 2% thorium added. Here, too, tungsten is used because it has a very high melting point and does not vaporize easily. Thorium is a radioactive metallic element that is added to increase **thermionic emission** (boiling off of electrons) and extend filament life. The filaments are situated parallel to each other in the focusing cup and share a common ground wire.

 **Make the Imaging Connection**

**Chapter 11**

The filament (focal spot size) only affects recorded detail. The smaller the focal spot, the greater the recorded detail in the image.

The focusing cup is made of nickel and surrounds each filament on its back and sides, leaving the front open and facing the anode target. The focusing cup receives a strong negative charge from the secondary circuit that forces the electrons together into a cloud as they are boiled off of the filament. The size, shape, and charge of the focusing cup and how the filaments are designed and placed within it affect how well it "focuses" the electrons on the target. All of these things are taken into consideration in the design for optimum performance. The focusing cup serves its function through electrostatic repulsion. That is, its negative charge is greater than the negative charges of the electrons and thus forces them together. Otherwise, the individual electron-negative charges would cause them to repel each other and scatter as they are boiled off of the filament.

 **Critical Concept**

**The Cathode**

The cathode, the negative end of the x-ray tube, consists of filaments and the focusing cup and provides the source of electrons necessary for x-ray production.

## PRINCIPLES OF OPERATION

This section begins with a discussion of the operating console, retraces the steps to the x-ray tube, and then adds the details of x-ray tube operation. At the operating console, the radiographer selects the desired exposure factors (i.e., kVp, mAs, and focal-spot size [on some units, focal spot size may be an automated function]). Whether selection is made through anatomic programming or any other form of automation is unimportant for the moment. When the exposure switch is first pressed, some of the electricity is diverted to the induction motor of the x-ray tube to bring the rotor up to speed. (Some radiographers call this "hitting the rotor.") Inside the x-ray tube, the induction motor turns the anode at approximately 3400 rpm (or faster depending on the tube type and purpose) to spread the generated heat over a larger total surface area. At the same time that the rotor is spinning up, the selected filament is energized until the desired degree of thermionic emission is achieved. Prepping the rotor is the first phase of a two-phase switch. The second phase actually initiates the x-ray production process. The process from rotor preparation to exposure lasts only a few seconds, with the actual exposure generally measured in milliseconds.

When the exposure switch is pressed, the voltage from the autotransformer (controlled by the kVp selector) passes to the step-up transformer (or in the case of high-frequency generators, to capacitor banks, then the inverter circuit, to the step-up transformer). This voltage (and current) then passes through a rectifier bank before passing to the anode and cathode of the x-ray tube so that the anode is always positive and the cathode is always negative. This voltage creates a huge potential difference between the electrodes. Previously, with the preparation phase, some power from the autotransformer was diverted to the filament circuit, where it passes through a rheostat (controlled by the mA selector) to a step-down transformer, then to the selected filament (determined on the control panel) within the cathode focusing cup. This current heats the filament to a point of incandescence (white hot), and electrons are literally boiled off of the filament by thermionic emission. The focusing cup forms them into a cloud. This cloud is called a **space charge**. This space charge is self-limiting. Once the space charge reaches a size commensurate with the current used, it becomes difficult for additional electrons to be emitted. This self-limiting factor is called the **space-charge effect**. The three things needed to produce x-rays are now present: (1) a large potential difference to give kinetic energy to the filament electrons (provided by the kVp setting), (2) a vehicle on which kinetic energy can ride (a quantity of electrons provided by mAs), and (3) a place for interaction (the target of the anode).

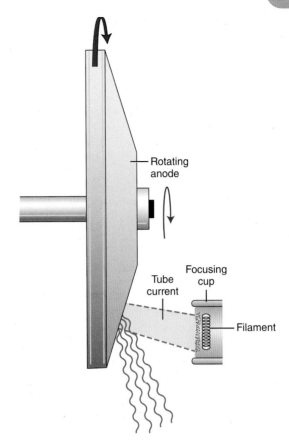

**Fig. 5.10 X-Ray Production.** In the process of x-ray production electrons are boiled off of the filament and are attracted to the anode, where they interact with target atoms, producing heat and x-rays.

The electron cloud is attracted to the anode target because of the huge potential difference. In fact, these filament electrons will reach speeds of about half the speed of light in the short 1 to 3 cm between the focusing cup and anode target. Because the electron cloud flows from cathode to anode, it is a continuation of the flow of electricity through the x-ray circuit. There is one very important "detour" in this flow of electrons. As they penetrate the target surface, these filament electrons interact with the atoms of tungsten, generating heat and x-rays (Fig. 5.10). The two types of interactions that produce x-rays at the atomic level are discussed in detail in Chapter 6. The current chapter continues to follow the effects of this process on the x-ray tube itself.

## QUALITY CONTROL AND EXTENDING TUBE LIFE

Several factors can shorten the life of an x-ray tube or damage it. Most have to do with the thermal characteristics of x-ray production and are within the radiographer's control. In particular, the frequent use of very high or maximum exposure factors, use of lower but very long exposure factors (maintaining the tube at high temperatures), and overload of the filament (prolonged excessive heating caused by prepping the rotor unnecessarily or arcing from filament) are the major causes of tube failure.

### ! Critical Concept

**Environment for X-Ray Production**

Three things are needed in the x-ray tube for x-ray production: a large potential difference to give kinetic energy to filament electrons (provided by the kVp setting), a vehicle on which kinetic energy can ride (source of electrons provided by mAs), and a place for interaction (the anode target).

## Critical Concept

### Major Causes of X-Ray Tube Failure

The major causes of tube failure are the frequent use of very high or maximum exposure factors, the use of lower but very long exposure factors (maintaining the tube at high temperatures), and overload of the filament (prolonged excessive heating or arcing from filament).

As noted at the beginning of this chapter, built-in methods help dissipate heat (i.e., oil bath and cooling fans). Additionally, rotating anodes spread heat over a larger surface area, helping with the heat-load problem. The use of heat-tolerant materials in the construction of the tube also helps deal with heat load. Radiational cooling of the anode is also used. That is, the anode "radiates" heat within the tube away from itself. Therefore, three processes of heat transfer are at play: conduction of heat by heat-tolerant materials, radiation of heat energy from the anode to the oil bath, and convection of heat into the room by the cooling fans. Finally, modern x-ray machines have protective circuits built in that prevent the use of unsafe exposure techniques and heat overloads of the x-ray tube. However, even with all of these safety measures, the radiographer must understand anode thermal capacity and keep in mind that the production of x-rays is a very inefficient process, with almost 99% of the energy used being converted to heat.

To better understand how much heat may be produced during an exposure, students should first be aware of the concept of **heat units (HUs)**. HUs are a measure of the amount of heat stored in a particular device. For the x-ray tube, HUs are calculated using the following formula:

$$kVp \times mA \times s \times c$$

*kVp* is the kilovoltage selected, *mA* is the milliamperage station selected, and *s* is the exposure time in seconds. The *c* represents a correction factor and depends on the generator type. Its value is as follows:

Single-phase = 1.0
Three-phase, 6 pulse = 1.35
Three-phase, 12 pulse = 1.41
High-frequency = 1.45

If multiple exposures are made using a given technique, the answer from this formula is multiplied by the number of exposures. One can quickly see that heat is a major factor in the damage done to an x-ray tube over thousands of exposures.

For example, how many heat units are produced if 80 kVp, 200 mA, 0.2 seconds is used with a high-frequency generator?
Answer:
$80 \times 200 \times 0.2 \times 1.45 = 4640$

What if 10 exposures were made using the previous factors?
Answer:
$4640 \times 10 = 46,400$

To extend tube life, simple procedures and guidelines should be followed. First, the warm-up steps specific to the unit should be followed completely and routinely. This is akin to warming up a car on a very cold day. Doing so warms the engine slowly and prepares it for normal operation. Similarly, the x-ray tube should be warmed before normal operation. Note that newer units may have automatic warm-up protocols. Second, do not prep the rotor excessively. This preexposure phase maintains the filament in an energized state and thus shortens its useful life. In fact, it is usually preferable to press both the rotor and exposure buttons almost simultaneously, so that the filament is heated for the minimum time necessary. The machine will not apply the high voltage until the rotor reaches full operating speed. Third, do not routinely use extremes of exposure factors. Consistently using single, very high-exposure values results in pitting the anode (small areas of melting), which can then cause irregular outputs. By the same token, consistently using low but very long exposures also results in uneven heating and wear. Excessive heating may also cause heat transfer to the bearings of the rotor. This heating can damage the bearings, resulting in uneven rotation speed and damage to the tube.

### On the Spot

- The protective housing of the x-ray tube serves as an electrical insulator, a thermal cushion, and an x-ray shield (lead lining) to reduce leakage radiation to less than 100 mR/h.
- The glass or metal enclosure of the x-ray tube serves to maintain a vacuum so that electrons from air do not contribute to the electron stream. It also has a target window made thinner than the rest to minimally absorb x-rays as they exit the tube.
- There are two basic anode designs. The stationary anode is basically a target embedded in a copper rod and has a very limited heat-load capacity. The rotating anode design is used today and incorporates a rotating target to dissipate heat, greatly increasing its heat-load capacity.
- Copper is used in the construction of the rotating anode because of its thermal and electrical conductivity. Molybdenum is used because of its low thermal conductivity and tensile strength. Tungsten is used because of its high atomic number and thermal capacity (high melting point).
- The rotating anode is turned using an induction motor that operates through electromagnetic mutual induction. The rotor of the induction motor is within the glass or metal enclosure, and the stators are outside the enclosure around the neck of the tube.
- The rotating anode design uses the line-focus principle, which means that the target face is angled to create a large actual focal spot for heating and a small effective

focal spot for improved image quality. But by angling the face, the "heel" of the target is partially placed in the path of the x-ray beam produced, causing absorption and reduced intensity of the beam on the anode side.

- The cathode of the x-ray tube is typically made up of two filament coils made of a tungsten-thorium alloy and a surrounding focusing cup made of nickel. The cathode is designed to provide a source of electrons needed for x-ray production.
- Once the radiographer selects the exposure factors on the operating console, electricity is manipulated using various x-ray circuit components to create the proper environment for x-ray production.
- Three things are needed in the x-ray tube for x-ray production: a large potential difference to give kinetic energy to filament electrons (provided by kilovoltage peak setting), a vehicle on which kinetic energy can ride (source of electrons provided by milliamperage/second setting), and a place for interaction (the anode target).
- Several factors can shorten the life of an x-ray tube. Most have to do with the thermal characteristics of x-ray production, particularly the frequent use of very high exposure factors, the use of lower but very long exposure factors, and the overload of the filament.
- HUs are a measure of the amount of heat stored in a particular device. For the x-ray tube, HUs are calculated using the following equation: $kVp \times mA \times s \times c$.
- Always follow warm-up and recommended exposure guidelines specific to the x-ray machine being used.

## CRITICAL THINKING QUESTIONS

1. How does each part of the x-ray tube contribute to maximizing x-ray production and extending the life of the tube?
2. Focusing on x-ray tube operation, explain the effect of each factor selected at the control console on the x-ray tube.

## REVIEW QUESTIONS

1. Which of the following reduces leakage radiation to required standards?
   a. X-ray tube
   b. Collimator
   c. Added filtration
   d. Protective housing
2. Which component of the x-ray tube is responsible for concentrating the electron cloud?
   a. Anode
   b. Filament
   c. Focusing cup
   d. Focal track

3. The x-ray tube is a part of the:
   a. x-ray circuit primary.
   b. x-ray circuit secondary.
   c. filament circuit.
   d. breaker circuit.
4. A technique of 80 kV, 400 mA, 0.8 seconds is to be used on a 3-phase, 12 pulse machine. How many heat units are produced with a single exposure?
   a. 25,600
   b. 34,560
   c. 36,096
   d. 38,100
5. The intensity of the x-ray beam is less:
   a. in the center of the beam.
   b. at the collimator.
   c. on the cathode side.
   d. on the anode side.
6. Causes of tube failure are most often related to which of the following characteristics?
   a. Electrical
   b. Mechanical
   c. Physical
   d. Thermal
7. What metal is added to the filament to increase thermionic emission and extend tube life?
   a. Thorium
   b. Copper
   c. Rhenium
   d. Tungsten
8. A small anode target angle:
   a. results in an increase in anode heel effect.
   b. results in a decrease in anode heel effect.
   c. results in an equalization of anode heel effect.
   d. does not influence anode heel effect.
9. A dual focus tube refers to a tube with:
   a. two focal tracks.
   b. two filaments.
   c. two focusing cups.
   d. two targets.
10. The purpose of the line focus principle is to create which of the following?
    a. Small actual and effective focal spot size
    b. Large actual and effective focal spot size
    c. Small actual and large effective focal spot size
    d. Large actual and small effective focal spot size
11. A technique of 50 kV, 100 mA, 0.1 seconds is to be used on a 3-phase, 6 pulse machine. How many heat units are produced with a single exposure?
    a. 500
    b. 675
    c. 705
    d. 820

# X-Ray Production

## Outline

## Objectives

- Explain the process of heat production in the x-ray tube.
- Explain the process of characteristic x-ray photon production.
- Explain the process of bremsstrahlung x-ray photon production.
- Determine characteristic and bremsstrahlung photon energy.
- Describe the principles and use of inherent, added, and compensating filters.

- Describe beam quantity and how milliamperage, kilovoltage peak, filtration, and distance affect it.
- Describe beam quality and how kilovoltage peak and filtration affect it.
- Explain half-value layer.
- Interpret the discrete, continuous, and x-ray emission spectrums.
- Explain the effects of milliamperage, kilovoltage peak, filtration, generator type, and target material on the x-ray emission spectrum.

## Key Terms

| | | |
|---|---|---|
| beam quality | characteristic interactions | inverse square law |
| beam quantity | continuous emission spectrum | penetration |
| bremsstrahlung (brems) interactions | discrete emission spectrum | primary beam |
| characteristic cascade | filtration | remnant beam |
| | half-value layer (HVL) | x-ray emission spectrum |

## INTRODUCTION

This chapter examines the anode target interactions at a micro level. To this point, the focus has been on the use of electricity and electrical devices to manipulate the flow of electricity for the purpose of x-ray production. This chapter focuses on the interactions in the anode target that result in x-ray photons and the properties, characteristics, and factors that influence the nature of the x-ray beam. The radiographer's actions at the control panel directly determine the nature and makeup of the x-ray beam, which (in conjunction with patient, image receptor, and processing characteristics) determines image quality. Several complex and overlapping processes result in the radiographic image. The x-ray machine is a tool in this process. An understanding of this tool is one factor that determines the skill of the radiographer.

## PHOTONS (TARGET INTERACTIONS)

Figure 6.1 illustrates the inside of the x-ray tube. Exposure factors have been selected; electricity has traveled to the anode, cathode, and filament; and electrons have been boiled off of the filament and are streaming across to the anode at tremendous speeds. The filament electrons penetrate the face of the target to a depth of approximately 0.5 mm, interacting with the tungsten target atoms in their path. These filament electrons interact with target atoms to produce x-rays in two ways: **characteristic interactions** and **bremsstrahlung (brems) interactions**. Most of the interactions (approximately 99%) do not result in x-rays but produce only heat. Keep in mind also that there are thousands of interactions taking place inside the target at once, but for the sake of explanation we focus on a single event in each case. Refer to the first

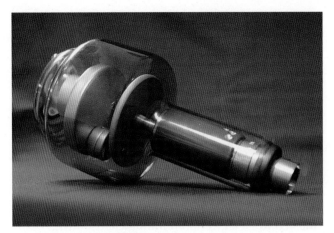

Fig. 6.1 **X-Ray Tube.** A general-purpose x-ray tube.

result in x-ray production, either by characteristic or bremsstrahlung interactions.

> ⚠ **Critical Concept**
>
> **Target Interactions**
>
> There are two interactions in the target that produce x-rays: brems and characteristic. X-rays are produced when filament electrons interact with target atom electrons or nuclei. Ionization of target atom electrons leads to release of characteristic x-ray photons, whereas interactions with target nuclei produce brems photons. During a single exposure, thousands of such events take place. However, most of the interactions in the target result only in heat (approximately 99%).

part of Chapter 2 for a refresher on the general structure of the atom.

## HEAT PRODUCTION

As filament electrons enter the anode target, most interact with outer-shell electrons of the tungsten atoms. They do not transfer enough of their kinetic energy to ionize the atom but rather just enough to raise them to a higher energy level (excitation). This excess energy is immediately given off as infrared radiation (heat) as the outer-shell electron returns to normal. As previously stated, there are thousands of interactions occurring in the anode target during a single exposure, and 99% are causing recurrent excitation and subsequent emission of infrared energy (heat). The end result is that most of the energy from the filament electrons is lost as heat and only 1% will

## CHARACTERISTIC INTERACTIONS

Characteristic interactions involve the filament electron and an orbital electron of a target atom. In general, a filament electron enters a target atom and strikes an orbital electron. If its energy is greater than the binding energy of the orbital electron, it is removed from orbit. Recall from Chapter 2 that orbital shells fill from the shell nearest the nucleus outward, and a vacancy in a shell makes the atom unstable. To correct this situation, outer-shell electrons drop to fill inner-shell vacancies. To do so, the outer-shell electron must expend some of its potential energy. This energy is given off as a characteristic x-ray photon (Fig. 6.2). Note that when the first orbital electron drops to fill the vacancy, it in turn leaves another. This second vacancy is also filled by an outer-shell electron that again must give up some of its energy, producing

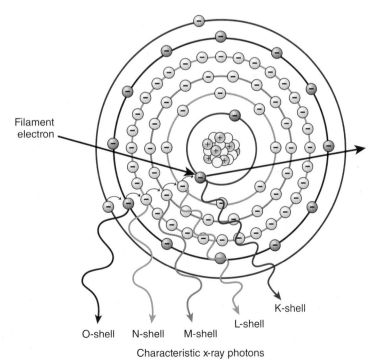

Fig. 6.2 **Characteristic Interaction.** A characteristic interaction event. Note that as outer-shell electrons fill inner-shell vacancies, their excess energy is released as characteristic x-ray photons.

another characteristic photon. This process of outer-shell electrons filling inner-shell vacancies continues down the line, creating a cascading effect called a **characteristic cascade**. Each time an orbital electron moves to a lower orbit, a characteristic photon is produced. This process is not necessarily orderly. If a filament electron removes a K-shell electron from an atom, the most likely electron to fill the vacancy is an L shell because of proximity. However, any outer-shell electron can fill the K-shell vacancy; it is just not as likely that an electron beyond the L shell will do so. Notice that the removal of the orbital electron established the *environment* for x-ray production, and it is the expending of energy during the cascade that produces characteristic x-rays.

 **Critical Concept**

### Characteristic Interactions

Characteristic photons are created when orbital electrons of target atoms are removed from their shell and outer-shell electrons fill inner-shell vacancies. To fill the vacancy, the outer-shell electron releases some of its potential energy as a characteristic photon.

Characteristic photons are so called because their energy is "characteristic" or dependent on the difference in binding energy between the shells involved. The electron shells of each element have specific binding energies. Table 6.1 presents binding energies that can be assumed for tungsten. A tungsten atom has 74 electrons orbiting its nucleus in six different shells. The filament electron may interact with any of them, but medical imaging generally focuses on K-shell (innermost shell) interactions, because they are the highest energy and the most useful for imaging purposes. Recall from Chapter 2 that each orbital electron is held in orbit by a binding energy, and the closer the orbit, the stronger the bond. K-shell electrons in tungsten have the strongest binding energy at 69.5 keV. For a filament electron to remove this orbital electron, it must possess energy equal to or greater than 69.5 keV. For all practical purposes using a general-purpose x-ray machine, if a radiographer selects a kVp less than 70 on the control panel, there will be no photons produced from K-shell interactions.

The characteristic photon is named for the shell being filled in each case. If an outer-shell electron is filling a K shell, regardless of where that filling electron is coming from, the photon produced is called

| Table **6.1** | Binding Energies for Tungsten |
|---|---|
| K shell | 69.5 keV |
| L shell | 12.1 keV |
| M shell | 2.82 keV |
| N shell | 0.6 keV |
| O shell | 0.08 keV |
| P shell | 0.008 keV |

*K characteristic*. If an electron is filling an L shell, the resulting photon is called *L characteristic*, and so on. To find the energy of a characteristic photon, the radiographer needs to know the target element (in this case, tungsten) and the shells involved. Using this information, the radiographer subtracts the binding energy of the farther shell (shell providing electron) from the closer shell (shell with vacancy).

Again, with characteristic interactions, to remove an orbital electron, the filament electron must have kinetic energy equal to or greater than the binding energy of the electron with which it interacts. If, for example, a filament electron has 50 keV of kinetic energy and strikes a tungsten K-shell electron (binding energy = 69.5 keV), it does not have the energy to remove it. The result of this type of interaction is heat production and, as noted earlier, this happens most of the time. The K-shell electron absorbs the kinetic energy from the filament electron and reemits it as heat energy. This also happens with any other orbital electron regardless of shell if the filament electron does not have sufficient energy to remove it. In such cases, the filament electron, having lost all of its kinetic energy, then drifts away to fill a vacancy in another atom or become part of the current through the tube. If, however, that same filament electron had 100 keV of energy, it would easily remove the K-shell orbital electron and be deflected in a new direction. It would still have 30 keV of energy left and with it interact with another atom.

**1₂₃** **Math Application**

### Characteristic Photons

To find the energy of a characteristic photon, one must know the shell-binding energies of the element and the shells involved. The filament electron must possess kinetic energy equal to or greater than the shell-binding energy to remove it from orbit. The photon energy is then equal to the difference in the binding energy of the shells involved.

**EXAMPLE:**
A filament electron removes a K-shell electron, and an
    L-shell electron fills the vacancy:
    K-shell binding energy = 69.5 keV
    L-shell binding energy = 12.1 keV
    69.5 − 12.1 = 57.4 keV
    The energy of the K-characteristic photon produced is
        57.4 keV.
This scenario creates a vacancy in the L shell. An M-shell
    electron fills the L-shell vacancy:
    L-shell binding energy = 12.1 keV
    M-shell binding energy = 2.8 keV
    The energy of the L-characteristic photon produced is
        9.3 keV.
Alternatively, an N shell might fill the original K-shell
    vacancy:
    K-shell binding energy = 69.5 keV
    N-shell binding energy = 0.6 keV
    69.5 − 0.6 = 68.9 keV
    The energy of the K-characteristic photon produced is
        68.9 keV.

## BREMSSTRAHLUNG INTERACTIONS

The second type of interaction in the target that produces x-rays is a brems interaction. *Bremsstrahlung* is a German word roughly meaning braking or slowing down radiation, which is exactly what this interaction involves where the filament electron is concerned. In this interaction, the filament electron misses all of the orbital electrons and interacts with the nucleus of the target atom. Recall that the electron is negatively charged and the nucleus (containing all the protons) is positively charged, and there will be a force of attraction between the two. The strength of this attraction depends on how close the filament electron comes to the nucleus. The attraction causes the filament electron to slow down and change direction and, in doing so, lose kinetic energy. This energy is released as a brems photon (Fig. 6.3). The closer the filament electron passes to the nucleus, the stronger the attraction. The stronger this attraction, the more energy the filament electron loses and the stronger the resultant brems photon. Because of this, the brems photon can vary from the maximum kVp selected (filament electron passes very close and loses all its energy) to near zero (filament electron passes at a distance and loses almost no energy).

### Critical Concept

**Bremsstrahlung Interactions**

Brems photons are produced when filament electrons miss all of the orbital electrons of the target atom and interact with the nucleus. The attraction of the filament electron to the nucleus causes it to slow down and change direction. The resultant loss of energy is given off as a brems photon.

The energy of a brems photon can be found by subtracting the energy that the filament electron leaves the atom with from the energy it had on entering. For example, a filament electron enters an atom with 100 keV of energy, passes very close to the nucleus, and leaves with 30 keV of energy. The brems photon produced is 70 keV (100 keV – 30 keV = 70 keV). If that same filament electron passed at some distance from the nucleus and exited with 80 keV of energy, the brems photon would be 20 keV (100 keV – 80 keV = 20 keV). The average energy of a brems photon is one-third of the kVp selected at the control panel.

In a tungsten target, most of the photons are brems for two reasons. First, with characteristic interactions, only those involving the K shell are of sufficient energy to be useful. All others are too weak to contribute to the radiographic image and are typically filtered out

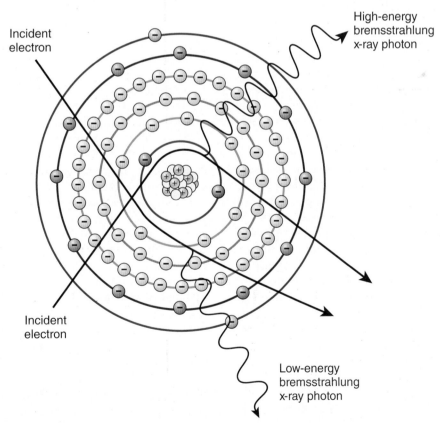

**Fig. 6.3 Bremsstrahlung Interaction.** A bremsstrahlung (brems) interaction event. Note that how close the filament electron passes to the nucleus determines the brems photon energy. Passing very close to the nucleus causes a greater loss of energy, which is released as a high-energy brems photon.

of the beam by the 2.5 mm of total **filtration** (discussed next) that is built into the tube head assembly. Because tungsten has a K-shell binding energy of 69.5 keV, only those kilovoltage peak settings of 70 kVp or greater produce K-characteristic photons. All lower settings result in a beam made up entirely of brems. Second, the filament electron is more likely to miss the orbital electrons of the target atom because they are in constant motion and the atom is mostly empty space.

 **Theory to Practice**

Knowing that the average energy of brems is one-third of the kVp selected and that most of the beam is made up of brems, we can predict the average energy of an x-ray beam to be one-third of the kVp selected.

## PROPERTIES OF THE X-RAY BEAM

Certain properties characterize any given x-ray beam based on how it was produced and how it behaves in its interactions with matter. The interactions with matter are covered in detail in Chapter 7. The properties that the radiographer should be familiar with are **beam quantity** and **beam quality**, and the defining terms of each. But before we get to that, a discussion of filtration is in order. In radiography, filtration refers to the use of a material, usually aluminum (Al) or Al equivalent, to absorb x-ray photons from the x-ray beam. This filtration may be in the form of an inherent, an added, or a compensating filter. In previous chapters the collimator (Chapter 1) and x-ray tube (Chapter 5) were discussed. Filtration is both inherent and added to this design. Inherent filtration is just that, inherent to the tube head assembly (tube and housing). The target window is the primary contributor to inherent filtration and equates to about 0.5 mm Al equivalent. In a general radiography tube head assembly, added filtration comes in the form of another 2.0 mm Al placed between the target window and the top of the collimator. The purpose of this added filtration is to remove low-energy x-ray photons from the beam before they can expose the patient and contribute unnecessarily to radiation dose. So in general-purpose radiography tube head assemblies, a total of 2.5 mm Al equivalent filtration is in place to "clean up" the x-ray beam by removing low-energy photons that would not contribute anything useful to the imaging process. The combination of inherent and added filtration is referred to as *total filtration*. Compensating filters, as their name implies, are used to adjust or "compensate" for variations in patient thickness or density and create a more uniform exposure to the image receptor (IR). Many compensating filter designs are some variation of a wedge shape, with the thin portion of the wedge placed over the thicker anatomic part and the thick part of the wedge placed over the thinner anatomic part. These filters may be designed to attach

to the bottom of the collimator or placed adjacent to or on the anatomic part of interest (Fig. 6.4). The use of compensating filters requires an increase in mAs to maintain overall exposure to the IR and is a tradeoff of increasing patient dose slightly to improve image quality. As with all of radiography, the benefits of exposing a patient to ionizing radiation must outweigh the harm caused by the exposure. The radiographer must always use sound judgment founded in science when incorporating compensating filters.

 **Critical Concept**

**Filtration**

Added and inherent filtration removes low-energy photons before they expose the patient and add to radiation dose unnecessarily. Compensating filters, while requiring an increase in mAs and therefore radiation dose, offset this by balancing exposure to the IR and improving image quality.

### BEAM QUANTITY

*Beam quantity* refers to the total number of x-ray photons in a beam. Beam quantity is affected by mAs, kVp, distance, and filtration. The radiographer should associate quantity with radiation dose. All other factors remaining constant, an increase in quantity increases the radiation dose delivered to the patient. Beam quantity is directly proportional to mAs. Because mAs controls the number of electrons boiled off of the filament and available to produce x-rays, it is considered the primary factor controlling quantity. Doubling the mAs doubles the quantity (output). When adjustments in quantity are desired, mAs is the factor adjusted.

Beam quantity varies as the square of the ratio of the change in kVp. If kVp is doubled, the intensity (quantity) increases by a factor of four. However, because kVp controls both the number and energy of x-rays in the beam, a small change in kVp exerts a large effect on exposure to the image receptor. This is why the 15% rule applies when changing kVp to affect exposure to the image receptor. The 15% rule states that, all other factors remaining constant, the kVp may be increased by 15% and the mAs reduced to 1/2 and still maintain exposure to the IR. A 15% increase in kVp is equivalent to doubling the mAs. Beam quantity is strongly affected by changes in kVp because kVp gives kinetic energy to the filament electrons. That kinetic energy is converted to heat and x-ray photons, and the greater the kinetic energy, the greater the chances for x-ray production. It is less desirable to use kVp to change quantity, because it influences too many other factors (e.g., penetrability, scatter production) related to image production and is less predictable in its imaging effect where quantity is concerned.

Beam quantity varies inversely as the square of the distance. This is the **inverse square law** (introduced

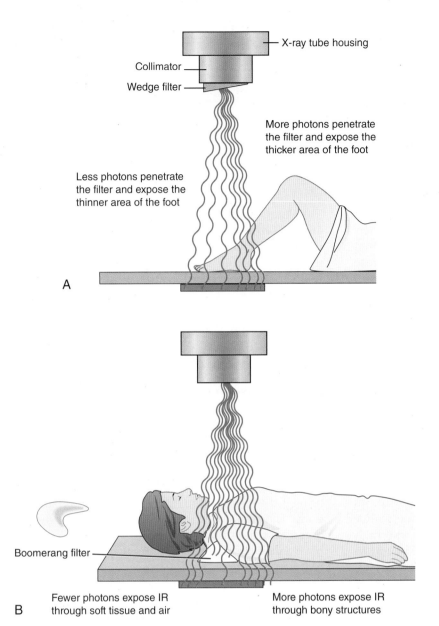

X-ray tube housing

Collimator

Wedge filter

More photons penetrate the filter and expose the thicker area of the foot

Less photons penetrate the filter and expose the thinner area of the foot

A

Boomerang filter

Fewer photons expose IR through soft tissue and air

More photons expose IR through bony structures

B

**Fig. 6.4 Compensating Filters.** Compensating filters may attach to the collimator or be placed adjacent to or on the anatomic area of interest. They serve to filter a portion of the beam to balance exposure to the image receptor (IR) and improve image quality.

in Chapter 3), which states that the intensity of a beam is inversely proportional to the square of the distance from the source. The inverse square law is expressed as $I_1/I_2 = d_2^2/d_1^2$. That is, the intensity (quantity) quadruples if the distance is reduced to one-half of its original value. X-ray photons diverge as they travel away from the source, and if the distance is shorter, they do not have the opportunity to diverge as much and are then concentrated on a smaller area.

### Make the Imaging Connection

#### Chapter 11

To best visualize the anatomic area of interest, the mAs setting selected must produce a sufficient amount of radiation reaching the image receptor, regardless of type. Excessive or insufficient mAs will adversely affect exposure to the image receptor and affect patient radiation exposure.

### 1 2 3 Math Application

#### Inverse Square Law

What will the intensity of a beam be at 40 inches if it is 5 R at 80 inches?

$$5\,R/I_2 = 40^2/80^2$$
$$5/I_2 = 1600/6400$$
$$I_2 = 5 \times 6400/1600$$
$$I_2 = 20\,R$$

If the intensity of a beam is 12 R at 20 inches, at what distance will it be 3 R?

$$12/3 = d_2^2/20^2$$
$$12/3 = d_2^2/400$$
$$12 \times 400/3 = d_2^2$$
$$1600 = d_2^2$$
$$40'' = d_2$$

**Table 6.2    Factors Affecting Beam Quantity**

| INCREASE IN | EFFECT ON QUANTITY |
|---|---|
| mAs | Increases |
| kVp | Increases |
| Distance | Decreases |
| Filtration | Decreases |

*kVp*, Kilovoltage peak; *mAs*, milliamperage/second.

The extent to which use of filtration decreases x-ray quantity depends on the thickness and type of filtration material. Filtration absorbs low-energy photons that do not contribute to the image and would otherwise add to patient radiation dose. Added filtration placed at the collimator serves to reduce patient dose by removing such photons. Table 6.2 presents a summary of the factors affecting beam quantity.

## BEAM QUALITY

*Beam quality* refers to the penetrating power of the x-ray beam. **Penetration** refers to those x-ray photons that are transmitted through the body and reach the image receptor. It is desirable for some of the x-ray photons to penetrate the anatomic area of interest, or no image would result. Photons that reach the image receptor create the dark shades of the image; areas where no photons reach result in the light or clear areas of the image. Both are needed to create the image and provide contrast. Beam quality is affected by kVp and filtration and is controlled mainly by adjusting kVp. As kVp increases, the beam's ability to penetrate matter also increases, and vice versa. X-ray beams with high energy (from high kVp settings) are said to be *high-quality*, or *hard*, beams. X-ray beams with low energy (from low kVp settings) are said to be *low-quality*, or *soft*, beams.

Beam quality is also affected by filtration. Filtration serves to remove the lower-energy photons, making the average energy (quality) higher. Think of this as the instructor dropping a student's two lowest test grades. Doing so will increase the student's average. Table 6.3 provides a summary of the factors affecting beam quality.

Beam quality is measured by the **half-value layer (HVL)**. HVL is defined as the thickness of absorbing material (Al or Al equivalent filtration) necessary to reduce the energy of the beam to one-half its original intensity. It is found by first measuring the intensity of the beam with a radiation detector, then placing Al filters of known thicknesses between the tube and detector until the intensity reading is reduced to one-half

**Table 6.3    Factors Affecting Beam Quality**

| INCREASE IN | EFFECT ON QUALITY |
|---|---|
| kVp | Increases |
| Filtration | Increases |

*kVp*, Kilovoltage peak.

the original value. Normal HVL of general diagnostic beams is 3 to 5 mm Al.

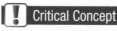 **Critical Concept**

**Beam Quantity and Quality**

*Beam quantity* refers to the intensity or number of photons, and *beam quality* refers to the energy or penetrating power of a given x-ray beam.

Related to this discussion of quantity and quality are the terms **primary beam** and **remnant beam**. *Primary beam* refers to the x-ray beam as it is on exiting the collimator and exposing the patient. *Remnant beam* refers to the x-ray beam that remains after interaction with the patient and is exiting the patient to expose the image receptor. The remnant beam is composed of transmitted photons (those exiting the patient without having interacted with anatomic structures) and scattered photons (those that have lost energy and have been redirected after interacting with anatomic structures). Both of these are discussed in detail in Chapter 7.

## EMISSION SPECTRUM

The emission spectrum graphically illustrates the x-ray beam (Fig. 6.5). As previously discussed, the x-ray beam is the result of two different anode target interactions. The emission spectrum for each looks different because of the nature of each. Characteristic photons have a **discrete emission spectrum** and brems photons have a **continuous emission spectrum**. We combine the essential parts of each to create the **x-ray emission spectrum**. These graphs are handy visuals of the nature of the beam and are useful for illustrating the effects of different influencing factors on them.

The discrete emission spectrum illustrates characteristic x-ray production. The x-axis is the x-ray energy, and the y-axis is the number of each type of

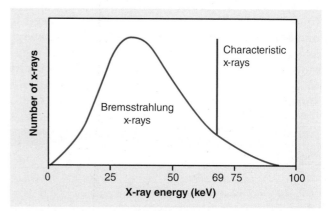

**Fig. 6.5    X-Ray Emission Spectrum.** The x-ray emission spectrum is a graphic representation of the important parts of an x-ray beam (i.e., brems photons and K-characteristic photons). *keV*, Kiloelectron volt.

x-ray photon. It is called *discrete* because the photon energies are limited to just a few exact values. Characteristic photons are produced when outer-shell electrons fill inner-shell vacancies in atoms, and the energy is determined by the difference in the shells involved. Recall that characteristic photons are named for the shell being filled. There are a number of bars at each level (K, L, M, etc.) representing the energy variations depending on the shells involved. For example, there is a bar for K-characteristic photons produced when L electrons fill K, and a bar for when M electrons fill K, and so on. The bars are at different points along the x-axis according to their energy, but all are K characteristic. The same is true for L-characteristic photons and each of the others. The lowest-energy bars (those representing the lowest energy interactions) may not be labeled because they are of no diagnostic value. The height of the bars relative to the y-axis indicates the number of photons of that type. Figure 6.6 demonstrates a spectrum for a tungsten target; other target materials are similar, but the energy range on the x-axis is different.

With tungsten targets, K-characteristic x-rays are of the greatest importance because they contribute to the radiographic image. Beginning on the right side of the graph, K-characteristic photons have an energy range of approximately 57 keV (if an L electron fills the K-shell vacancy) to 69 keV (if the O or P shell fills the K-shell vacancy). Then, moving down the x-axis, L-characteristic x-ray energies are plotted. They have an energy range of approximately 9 keV (if an M-shell electron fills the L-shell vacancy) to 12 keV (if an O- or P-shell electron fills the L-shell vacancy). Beyond L-characteristic, there is really no point in plotting the energies because they are so low that they are filtered out of the beam and are of no consequence.

The continuous emission spectrum illustrates brems x-ray production. Again, the x-axis represents the energy and the y-axis the number of photons. Because brems photons are the result of the filament electrons' attraction to the nucleus, their energy depends on the

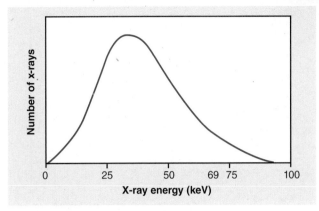

Fig. 6.7 **Continuous Emission Spectrum.** Continuous emission spectrum for a tungsten target. *keV*, Kiloelectron volt.

strength of this attraction, ranging from just above zero to the maximum kVp selected on the control panel. Unlike the finite characteristic photon energies, brems photons have a range of energy, with most being one-third of the kVp selected. A graph of brems photons creates a bell-shaped continuum. The left side of the curve is just above zero and the right side of the curve touches the x-axis at the kVp selected. The peak of the curve is approximately one-third of the kVp indicated. Figure 6.7 illustrates a tungsten target spectrum; other target materials are similar, but the energy range on the x-axis is different.

To graphically represent the x-ray beam as a whole, we combine the two spectra (see Fig. 6.5). As with the other two graphs, the x-axis represents the energy and the y-axis the quantity of each type of photon. The continuous portion is used as is because it represents most of the beam. The discrete line is reduced to the highest-energy K-characteristic bar. For a tungsten target, it is positioned at approximately 69 keV. As previously stated, the other discrete lines are omitted because they represent photons that are generally filtered out of the beam and are of no consequence to imaging. The x-ray emission spectrum is used to graphically represent the energies of the x-ray beam. It can also be used to reflect the effects of different factors on the x-ray beam. Changes in the spectrum with respect to the y-axis indicate changes in quantity. Changes in the spectrum with respect to the x-axis indicate changes in quality. Five factors change the appearance of the x-ray emission spectrum: mA, kVp, tube filtration, generator type, and target material.

Changes in mA affect beam quantity. All other factors remaining constant, an increase in mA increases the amplitude of both the continuous and discrete portions of the spectrum. Remember that when mA is increased on the control panel, more electrons are boiled off of the filament and are available for x-ray production. This increases the quantity of x-rays produced. Because the kVp setting controls energy, the spectrum does not move along the x-axis with

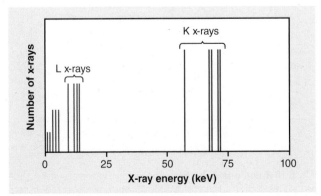

Fig. 6.6 **Discrete Emission Spectrum.** Discrete emission spectrum for a tungsten target. *keV*, Kiloelectron volt.

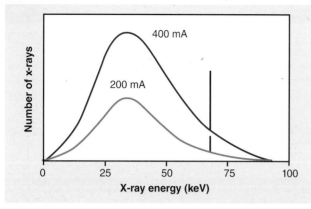

Fig. 6.8 **Change in Milliamperage.** Two emission spectra illustrating the result of an increase in mA *(purple curve)*. Increases in mA increase the quantity of radiation. *keV*, Kiloelectron volt; *mA*, milliampere.

changes in mA, nor does the discrete line move because it is related specifically to the target material (Fig. 6.8).

## Critical Concept

**Milliamperage and Emission Spectrum**

Increasing milliamperage increases x-ray beam quantity but has no effect on quality and does not change the position of the discrete line.

Changes in kVp affect beam quality and quantity. All other factors remaining constant, an increase in kVp increases the amplitude of both continuous and discrete portions of the spectrum and shifts the right side of the curve to the right along the x-axis. When kVp is increased at the control panel, a larger potential difference occurs in the x-ray tube, giving more electrons the kinetic energy to produce x-rays and increasing the kinetic energy overall. The result is more photons (quantity), which increases the amplitude of the spectrum and higher-energy photons (quality), which shifts the right side of the curve farther to the right. The discrete line does not move because it is related specifically to the target material (Fig. 6.9).

## Critical Concept

**Kilovoltage Peak and Emission Spectrum**

Increasing kVp increases the x-ray beam quantity and quality but does not change the position of the discrete line.

The addition of tube filtration or introducing a more efficient filtration material into the tube head assembly removes photons from the beam. All other factors remaining constant, an increase in tube filtration causes a decrease in quantity and an increase in quality. The removal of photons causes a decrease in quantity

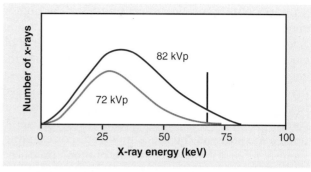

Fig. 6.9 **Change in Kilovoltage Peak.** Two emission spectra illustrating the result of an increase in kVp *(purple curve)*. Increases in kVp increase the quantity and quality of radiation. *keV*, Kiloelectron volt; *kVp*, kilovoltage peak.

reflected by a decrease in amplitude of both the continuous and discrete portions of the curve. Because it removes more low-energy photons than high-energy photons, there is a greater decrease on the left side of the continuous portion and there is a shift in the peak of the curve to the right. Remember that with the low-energy photons removed, the average energy is higher. Again, the discrete line does not move because it is related specifically to the target material (Fig. 6.10).

## Critical Concept

**Tube Filtration and Emission Spectrum**

An increase in tube filtration causes a decrease in x-ray beam quantity and an increase in quality, but the discrete line is unaffected.

Changes in generator type change the x-ray production efficiency of the machine. High-frequency units are much more efficient in producing x-rays than single-phase units. This means that with the same amount of electricity (power), a high-frequency unit produces more x-rays. In the x-ray emission spectrum, this is represented by an increase in amplitude and average

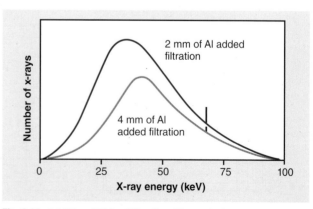

Fig. 6.10 **Additional Tube Filtration.** Two emission spectra illustrating the result of an addition of filtration *(green curve)*. Increases in filtration decrease the quantity and increase quality of radiation. *Al*, Aluminum; *keV*, kiloelectron volt.

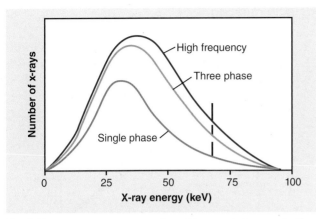

Fig. 6.11 **Change in Generator Type.** Three emission spectra illustrating the result of a change in generator type. Note that as the efficiency of the generator type increases, so does x-ray quantity given the same amount of electricity used. *keV,* Kiloelectron volt.

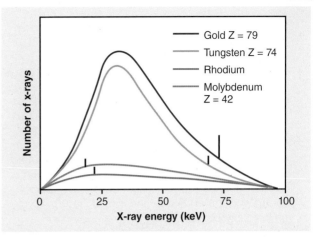

Fig. 6.12 **Change in Target Material.** Four emission spectra illustrating the effect of changes in target material. Note that as the atomic number of the material increases, so does the average energy and quantity of the x-rays and the position of the discrete line changes. *keV,* Kiloelectron volt.

energy. If a generator operates more efficiently, more filament electrons have the energy to produce x-rays, increasing quantity (amplitude of the curve). There are also a greater number of higher-energy photons, increasing the average energy and shifting the peak to the right (Fig. 6.11).

### Critical Concept

**Generator Efficiency and Emission Spectrum**

Improving the efficiency of the generator increases x-ray beam quantity and quality, but the discrete line is unaffected.

The general radiographer does not have the ability to select the target material used, except in mammography. Although virtually all radiographic x-ray tubes employ tungsten targets, it is instructive to consider how altering the target material might affect the emission spectrum. As the atomic number (Z number) of the target material goes up, so does the average energy, quantity of photons, and the position of the discrete line of the spectrum (Fig. 6.12). With increases in atomic number, each atom is more complex, representing a bigger "target" for filament electrons to interact with. This increases the likelihood of interaction and the number of photons produced. As quantity increases, the number of higher-energy photons increases, as well as the average energy. In Fig. 6.12, the discrete lines represent K-characteristic photons. The energy of these photons depends on the K-shell binding energy and which outer shell fills the vacancy. As the binding energy of the target material increases, the discrete line shifts to the right. Note that low atomic number targets such as molybdenum and rhodium are currently used in mammography because their lower K-characteristic x-rays are better suited to the lower energies used in that modality. On the other hand, gold is never suitable as a

target material because of its low melting point and high cost. Table 6.4 provides a summary of the factors affecting the emission spectrum.

| Table **6.4** Factors Affecting Emission Spectrum | | |
| --- | --- | --- |
| **INCREASE (IMPROVEMENT) IN** | **EFFECT ON QUANTITY** | **EFFECT ON QUALITY** |
| mA | Increases | No effect |
| kVp | Increases | Increases |
| Tube filtration | Decreases | Increases |
| Generator type | Increases | Increases |
| Target material | Increase | Increases |

*kVp,* Kilovoltage peak; *mA,* milliampere.

### Critical Concept

**Target Material and Emission Spectrum**

Improvement (increasing atomic number) of the target material increases x-ray beam quality and quantity and shifts the discrete line to the right.

### On the Spot

- When filament electrons interact with atoms of the target, one of three things happen: characteristic interactions, brems interactions, and heat production.
- Most of the filament electrons entering the target interact with outer-shell electrons of the tungsten atoms but do not ionize them; rather, they cause excitation and release of infrared radiation (heat).
- Characteristic interactions involve the removal of orbital electrons of target atoms by filament electrons. This vacancy makes the atom unstable, and outer-shell electrons fill inner-shell vacancies, giving up some of their potential energy in the process as characteristic photons.

- The energy of characteristic photons depends on the shells involved and is named for the shell being filled. In a tungsten target, the filament electron must have 69.5 keV of energy or more to remove a K-shell electron.
- Brems interactions are the result of filament electrons interacting with the nucleus of a target atom. The filament electron is attracted to the nucleus, which causes it to slow down and change direction, resulting in a loss of energy. This loss of energy is given off as a brems photon.
- The energy of a brems photon can be found by subtracting the energy the electron leaves the atom with from the energy it had upon entering the atom. The average energy of brems is equal to one-third of the kVp selected on the control panel.
- Filtration is used in two forms in radiography. Total filtration (inherent plus added) filters are designed into the x-ray tube head assembly to filter low-energy photons from the beam. Compensating filters are used to balance exposure to the IR by filtering x-rays from the thinner or less dense areas of the anatomic area of interest.
- *Beam quantity* refers to the total number of x-ray photons in the beam and is affected by mAs, kVp, distance, and filtration.
- Beam quantity is directly proportional to mAs. Doubling the mAs doubles the output.
- Beam quantity varies as the square of the change in kVp. Doubling the kVp increases quantity by a factor of four.
- Beam quantity varies inversely as the square of the distance (inverse square law).
- *Beam quality* refers to the penetrating power of the beam and is affected by kVp and filtration.
- Beam quality varies directly with changes in kVp.
- Beam quality is measured by its HVL and is defined as "the thickness of absorbing material (aluminum or aluminum equivalent filtration) necessary to reduce the energy of the beam to one-half its original intensity."
- Characteristic photons are graphically represented by a discrete emission spectrum and brems by a continuous emission spectrum. The two are combined to create the x-ray emission spectrum, which incorporates the K-characteristic line and the continuous curve of brems.
- Five factors will change the appearance of the x-ray emission spectrum: mA (changes beam quantity), kVp (changes beam quantity and quality), filtration (changes beam quantity and quality), generator type (changes quantity and quality), and target material (changes beam quantity, quality, and position of discrete line).

## CRITICAL THINKING QUESTIONS

1. Describe the x-ray beams produced with 80 kVp and 40 mAs versus 60 kVp and 160 mAs in terms of bremsstrahlung photon presence, characteristic photon presence, beam quantity, and quality.
2. How would a radiographer use their knowledge of the factors affecting beam quality and quantity to optimize exposure factors to minimize radiation dose and maximize image quality?

## REVIEW QUESTIONS

1. What is the most likely cause of the change in the emission spectrum represented by the green line?

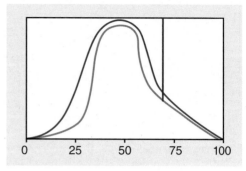

  a. Added filtration
  b. Increase in kVp
  c. Increase in mA
  d. Single phase to three phase

2. Which of the following is the most likely cause of the change in the emission spectrum represented by the purple line?

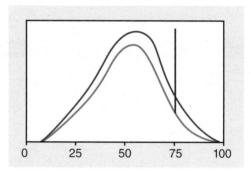

  a. Increase in kVp
  b. Increase in mA
  c. Added filtration
  d. Single phase to three phase

3. Which of the following is the most likely cause of the change in the emission spectrum represented by the purple line?

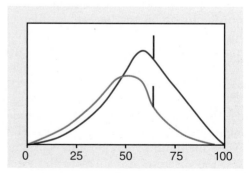

  a. Added filtration
  b. Increase in kVp
  c. Increase in mA
  d. Single phase to three phase

4. A filament electron interacts with an outer-shell electron of a tungsten but does not remove it. Which of the following is produced?
   a. 50 keV photon
   b. 70 keV photon
   c. Heat
   d. Brems photon

5. At what point in the interaction chain of events is a characteristic photon produced?
   a. Filament electron entering a target atom
   b. Collision of two electrons
   c. Removal of an orbital electron
   d. Outer-shell electron filling inner-shell vacancy

6. A filament electron enters a tungsten target atom with an energy of 70 kVp. It interacts first with an L-shell electron, then with a K-shell electron. Which of the following are produced?
   1. K-characteristic x-ray photon
   2. L-characteristic x-ray photon
   3. Heat
   a. 1 and 2 only
   b. 1 and 3 only
   c. 2 and 3 only
   d. 1, 2, and 3

7. What is the energy of an x-ray photon produced when an O-shell electron fills a K-shell vacancy?
   a. 69.42 KeV
   b. 69.58 KeV
   c. 67.42 KeV
   d. 68.58 KeV

8. What is the energy of an x-ray photon produced when an L-shell electron fills a K-shell vacancy?
   a. 81.9 KeV
   b. 65 KeV
   c. 66.68 KeV
   d. 57.4 KeV

9. What is the energy of an x-ray photon produced when an M-shell electron fills an L-shell vacancy?
   a. 14.92 KeV
   b. 9.28 KeV
   c. 11.5 KeV
   d. 57.4 KeV

10. What is the energy of an x-ray photon produced when an O-shell electron fills an L-shell vacancy?
   a. 12.02 KeV
   b. 12.18 KeV
   c. 11.5 KeV
   d. 10.2 KeV

# 7 X-Ray Interactions With Matter

## Outline

Introduction
Classical Interactions
Compton Interactions
Photoelectric Interactions

Pair Production
Photodisintegration
Differential Absorption
Macrolevel Interactions

## Objectives

- Explain classical interactions, including production, energy, effects on patient dose, and effects on image quality.
- Explain Compton interactions, including production, energy, effects on patient dose, and effects on image quality.
- Explain photoelectric interactions, including production, energy, effects on patient dose, and effects on image quality.

- Explain pair production.
- Explain photodisintegration.
- Relate differential absorption to x-ray beam interactions with the human body and image formation.
- Describe broadly x-ray interactions with macromolecules and cells.

## Key Terms

| | | |
|---|---|---|
| absorption | main-chain scission | photoelectron |
| classical interaction | occupational exposure | radiolucent |
| Compton electron | pair production | radiopaque |
| Compton scattering | photodisintegration | secondary photons |
| differential absorption | photoelectric interaction | transmission |

## INTRODUCTION

It is helpful for the radiographer to understand the way x-ray photons interact with matter for two important reasons (Fig. 7.1). First, it allows the radiographer to minimize the physical effects of x-ray photons on the patient that result in radiation dose and biologic harm. Second, an understanding of x-ray photon-body tissue interaction allows the radiographer to better manipulate how the particular anatomic area of interest appears radiographically. Minimizing harm to the patient and producing a quality radiographic image are both integral to the role and responsibility of the radiographer. X-rays may interact with matter in five different ways, depending on their energy. This chapter discusses all five, but keep in mind that only the first three occur within the range of energy used in diagnostic radiography. The chapter concludes with a discussion of differential absorption and other terms related to how the x-ray beam interacts in general with body tissues.

 **Critical Concept**

**Understanding X-Ray Interactions**

Interactions between x-ray photons and human tissues determine how anatomic structures are imaged and the patient's radiation dose.

## CLASSICAL INTERACTIONS

**Classical interactions** are also commonly known as *coherent scattering* or *Thomson scattering*. In this scattering event, the incident x-ray photon interacts with an orbital electron of a tissue atom and changes direction. In this particular interaction, the incident x-ray photon is of a rather low energy (generally less than 10 keV). When such low-energy incident photons interact with tissue atoms, they are not likely to ionize (remove orbital electrons from their shell). Instead, the atom absorbs the energy of this x-ray photon, causing excitation of the atom, and then immediately releases the energy in

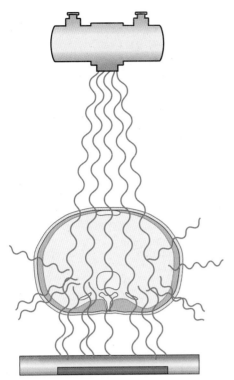

Fig. 7.1 **X-Ray Interactions.** When x-rays interact with the body, some are absorbed, some are scattered, and some penetrate to expose the image receptor.

a new direction (Fig. 7.2). Because the energy is reemitted in a new direction, it is now a scatter photon. It is of equal energy to the incident photon but travels in a new direction. Because of its low energy, most classical scatter photons are absorbed in the body through other interactions and do not contribute significantly to the image but do add slightly to patient dose.

> **! Critical Concept**
>
> **Classical Interactions**
>
> Classical interactions do not involve ionization of the atom. They are scattering events that do not contribute significantly to the image but contribute slightly to patient dose.

## COMPTON INTERACTIONS

**Compton scattering** occurs throughout the diagnostic range but generally involves moderate-energy x-ray photons (e.g., 20-40 keV). In this interaction, an incident x-ray photon enters a tissue atom, interacts with an orbital electron (generally a middle- or outer-shell electron), and removes it from its shell. In doing so, the incident photon loses up to one-third of its energy and is usually deflected in a new direction (Fig. 7.3). This interaction does three things. First, it ionizes the atom, making it unstable. Ionization in the body is significant because the atom is changed and may bond differently to other atoms, potentially causing biologic damage. If one of the "middle" orbital shells is involved, a characteristic cascade (outer-shell electrons filling inner-shell vacancies and emitting x-ray photons) also results, creating characteristic photons just as in the tube target. But here they are called **secondary photons**. These secondary photons are x-ray photons but of a rather low-energy variety. Such photons generally contribute only to patient dose. Second, the ejected electron, called a **Compton electron**, or *secondary electron*, leaves the atom with enough energy to go through interactions of its own in adjacent atoms. The type of interaction the Compton electron undergoes depends on the energy it has and the type of atom with which it interacts. Third, the incident photon is deflected in a new direction and is now a Compton scatter photon. It, too, has enough energy to go through other interactions in the tissues or exit the patient and interact with the image receptor. The problem with Compton scatter interacting with the image receptor is that it is not following its original path through the body and strikes the image receptor in the wrong area. In so doing, it contributes no useful information to the image and only results in image fog. Because most scattered photons are still directed toward the image receptor and result in image fog, it is desirable to minimize Compton scattering as much as possible.

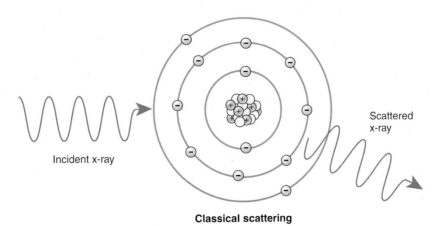

**Classical scattering**

Fig. 7.2 **Classical Interaction.** A classical scattering event. Note that no electron is removed; the atom absorbs the energy and then releases it in a new direction.

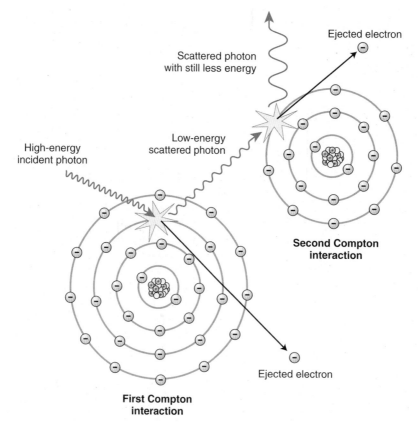

**Second Compton interaction**

Scattered photon with still less energy

Ejected electron

High-energy incident photon

Low-energy scattered photon

Ejected electron

**First Compton interaction**

Fig. 7.3 **Compton Interaction.** A Compton scattering event. Note that two events are illustrated, stemming from the initial high-energy incident photon.

Compton scattering is one of the most prevalent interactions between x-ray photons and the human body in general diagnostic imaging and is responsible for most of the scatter that fogs the image. The probability of Compton scattering does not depend on the atomic number of atoms involved. Compton scattering may occur in both soft tissue and bone. The probability of Compton scattering is related to the energy of the photon. As x-ray photon energy increases, the probability of that photon penetrating a given tissue without interaction increases. However, with this increase in photon energy, the likelihood of Compton interactions relative to photoelectric interactions also increases.

Compton scatter photons may travel in any direction from their point of scattering. A deflection of zero degrees means no energy is transferred. Those photons scattered at 180 degrees represent maximum deflection and energy transfer. But keep in mind that the scattered photon still retains about two-thirds of its energy. This is one reason the radiographer should never stand near the patient during exposure. Some Compton scatter photons exit the patient and would expose the radiographer. This is why shielding (lead aprons, lead gloves, etc.) is necessary during fluoroscopy or any procedure in which the radiographer or other health care worker may be near the patient and x-ray tube during exposure. It is important for the radiographer to remember that Compton scattering is the major source of **occupational exposure**.

 **Critical Concept**

**Compton Interactions**

Compton interactions are scattering events that ionize the atom. They may contribute negatively to the radiographic image as fog and add to patient and occupational radiation dose.

## PHOTOELECTRIC INTERACTIONS

**Photoelectric interactions** occur throughout the diagnostic range (e.g., 20-120 kVp) and involve inner-shell orbital electrons of tissue atoms. For photoelectric events to occur, the incident x-ray photon energy must be equal to or greater than the orbital shell binding energy. In these events the incident x-ray photon interacts with the inner-shell electron of a tissue atom and removes it from orbit. In the process, the incident x-ray photon expends all of its energy and is totally absorbed (Fig. 7.4). The resulting ejected electron is called a **photoelectron**. The energy transfer between the incident photon and inner-shell electron is equal to the incident photon energy minus the binding energy of the orbital electron. This energy transfer constitutes the energy of the photoelectron. In soft-tissue atoms, the energy of the photoelectron is nearly equal to that of the incident x-ray photon because the binding energy of the soft-tissue atom is very low and more is left over as kinetic energy for the photoelectron. In

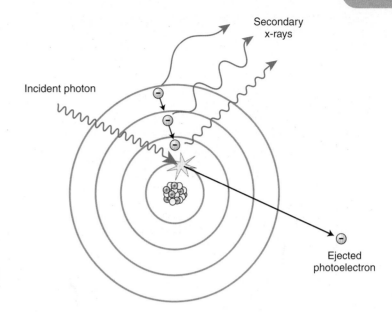

**Fig. 7.4 Photoelectric Interaction.** A photoelectric event. Note the total absorption of the incident photon and the characteristic cascade creating secondary x-rays.

bone, the energy of the photoelectron is less because the orbital electron-binding energy of bone atoms is greater and the incident x-ray photon has to expend more energy to remove it, leaving less as kinetic energy for the photoelectron. In either case, the photoelectron has enough kinetic energy to undergo interactions of its own before filling a vacancy in another atom elsewhere.

Note that this absorption that constitutes photoelectric interactions contributes significantly to patient dose accrued with each diagnostic image. Although some absorption is necessary to create an x-ray image, it is the radiographer's responsibility to select technical factors that strike a balance between image quality (absorption and transmission of x-ray photons needed to produce a good image) and patient dose.

In photoelectric interactions, as with Compton interactions, the tissue atom is ionized. In the case of photoelectric interactions, the inner-shell vacancy makes the atom unstable; to regain stability a characteristic cascade occurs, producing secondary x-ray photons. This cascade is the same phenomenon that occurs with Compton interactions that produce secondary photons. Again, these secondary photons are of low energy and are absorbed by the body in other photoelectric events. Note that the absorption of these secondary photons also contributes to patient dose.

## Critical Concept

### Photoelectric Interactions

Photoelectric events result in the total absorption of the incident photon. For this to occur, the incident photon energy must be equal to or greater than the orbital shell binding energy. In this process the atom is ionized, a characteristic cascade producing secondary photons results, and an ejected photoelectron exits the atom with enough energy to undergo many more interactions.

The probability of photoelectric interaction depends on the energy of the incident photons and the atomic number of the tissue atoms with which they interact. For photoelectric interactions to occur, the incident x-ray photon energy must be greater than or equal to the inner-shell binding energy of the tissue atoms involved. The greatest number of photoelectric interactions occurs when the incident x-ray photon energy is equal to or slightly greater than the inner-shell binding energy of the tissue atom. As the incident photon energy begins to exceed the inner-shell binding energy of the tissue atom, the chances of photoelectric interaction begin to decline and the chances increase that it will penetrate the tissue being examined. This function is a cubic relationship. That is, the probability of a photoelectric event is inversely proportional to the third power of the x-ray energy. What this means to the radiographer is that if a kVp range is too high for the anatomic part of interest, less absorption takes place, and some absorption is necessary for image formation.

The probability of photoelectric events is directly proportional to the third power of the atomic number of the absorber. What this cubic relationship means to the radiographer is that when they make small changes in the kVp setting or there are small changes in the atomic number of the tissue (from anatomic variations or a pathologic condition), large changes in the probability of photoelectric events will result. With tissues, the higher the atomic number of the tissue atom, the greater the number of photoelectric events. Such atoms are more complex; that is, they have more electrons and stronger binding energies and are more likely to absorb the incident x-ray photon. This is why bone shows up as lighter shades on radiographic images. In bone, more photons are absorbed, which means fewer photons are exposing the image receptor, resulting in the lighter shades of the image.

If more photoelectric events are needed to make a particular structure visible on a radiographic image (when, for example, the tissues to be examined do not have high atomic-number atoms), contrast agents such as barium or iodine are added. These agents have high atomic numbers and thereby increase the number of photoelectric events in these tissues. Protective shielding is another way of using photoelectric interactions. Lead has a very high atomic number and is used as a shielding material because the odds are great that photons will be absorbed by it.

 Critical Concept

**Photoelectric Probability**

Photoelectric probability depends on the energy of the incident photon and the atomic number of the tissue being irradiated. The energy must be equal to or greater than the orbital shell binding energy, and the greater the atomic number of the tissue atom, the greater the probability of photoelectric interactions.

## PAIR PRODUCTION

**Pair production** occurs only with very high-energy photons of 1.02 MeV or greater. The interaction occurs when the incident x-ray photon has enough energy to escape interaction with the orbital electrons and interact with the nucleus of the tissue atom. In this interaction, two particles are produced: a positron (positively charged electron) and an electron (may also be called a negatron) (Fig. 7.5). For these particles to exist, they must each have energy of 0.51 MeV (the energy equivalent of an electron). If the photon has energy greater than 1.02 MeV, it is shared between the two as kinetic energy.

Both particles travel out of the atom. The electron undergoes many interactions before coming to rest in another atom. The positron is an "unnatural particle" and, as such, travels until it strikes an electron, causing an annihilation event. In this annihilation event, the positron and the electron it interacts with are destroyed and their energy is converted into two x-ray photons that radiate out of the atom. Pair production does not occur in radiography because the energy levels required exceed the range used in diagnostic x-ray production.

## PHOTODISINTEGRATION

The last type of interaction between x-rays and matter is called **photodisintegration**. Photons with extremely high energies of more than 10 MeV may strike the nucleus of the atom and make it unstable. In photodisintegration, the nucleus of the atom involved regains stability by ejecting a nuclear particle such as a proton, neutron, or alpha particle (Fig. 7.6). Like pair production, photodisintegration does not occur in radiography because the energy levels required far exceed the kVp range used in diagnostic x-ray production.

## DIFFERENTIAL ABSORPTION

**Differential absorption** is the difference between the x-ray photons that are absorbed photoelectrically and those that penetrate the body (Fig. 7.7). It is called *differential* because different body structures absorb x-ray photons to different extents. Anatomic structures such as bone are denser and absorb more x-ray photons than structures filled with air, such as the lungs.

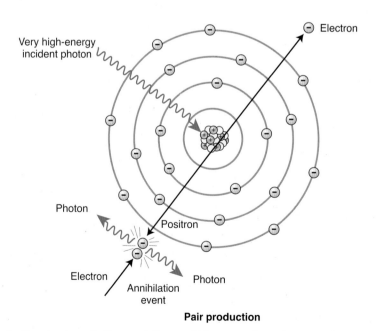

**Fig. 7.5 Pair Production.** A pair production event. The very high-energy photon interacts with the nucleus, causing the release of a positron and an electron.

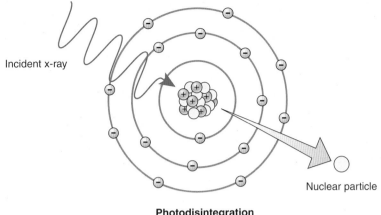

**Photodisintegration**

**Fig. 7.6 Photodisintegration.** A photodisintegration event. The very high-energy photon interacts with the nucleus, causing the release of a nuclear particle to regain stability.

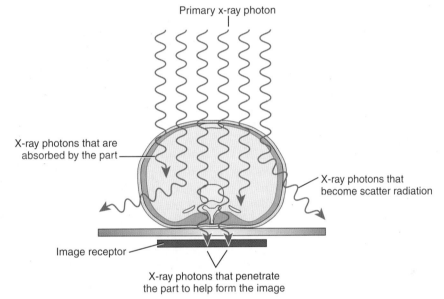

**Fig. 7.7 Differential Absorption.** X-rays interact with the body in one of three ways: They penetrate to the receptor, scatter in a new direction, or are absorbed in the body.

 **Make the Imaging Connection**

**Chapter 8**

The process of image formation is the result of differential absorption of the x-ray beam as it interacts with anatomic tissue. Differential absorption of the primary beam creates an image that structurally represents the anatomic area of interest.

 **Critical Concept**

**Differential Absorption**

Differential absorption is the difference between x-ray photons that are absorbed photoelectrically and those that penetrate the body. Denser tissue such as bone has greater absorption.

When radiographers speak broadly about differential absorption—how the x-ray beam interacts with the tissues of the body—they may speak of transmission versus absorption. *Transmission* refers to those x-ray photons that pass through the body and reach the image receptor. It is desirable for some of the x-ray photons to pass through the body area of interest; otherwise, no image would result. X-ray photons reaching the image receptor create the dark (less bright) shades of the image. *Absorption* refers to those photons that are attenuated by the body and do not reach the image receptor. Absorption has the opposite effect on the image as penetration. Recall that these photons are absorbed photoelectrically and will not reach the image receptor. This "lack" of exposure to the image receptor results in the lighter (brighter) shades of the image. It is also desirable to have some absorption or the image would be uniformly dark.

Again, absorption depends on the density of body tissues through which the x-ray photons are passing. Denser tissue, such as bone, increases the probability of x-ray photons being absorbed in photoelectric interactions. The result is that fewer x-ray photons pass through these areas of the body to reach the image receptor, and those structures appear lighter. Body structures that readily absorb x-rays are called **radiopaque**. Less dense structures have a much lower probability of absorption and are said to be **radiolucent**.

## MACROLEVEL INTERACTIONS

Throughout this chapter, x-ray interactions with matter have been discussed at the atomic level where they occur. It is important for the radiographer to understand these atomic-level interactions, but it is also important to relate these transfers of energy to a macrolevel where radiation dose and damage is more apparent. Although this subject will be covered thoroughly in the radiography student's radiobiology course, a brief discussion is offered here to complete the concepts and subject of this chapter.

Macromolecules are large molecules made up of thousands of atoms. When an x-ray photon interacts with one of these atoms as previously described, the energy transfer may manifest as a change to the structure of the macromolecule. The three most common effects are main-chain scission, cross-linking, and point lesions (Fig. 7.8). Main-chain scission refers to a breakage of the major structure, the framework if you will, of the macromolecule itself. Cross-linking is the result of the formation of "limbs" as a result of irradiation (although these exist naturally in some macromolecules) that "stick" to adjacent parts of the macromolecule or neighboring molecules, creating

an unnatural framework. Point lesions are the result of damage to a single chemical bond. Think of these as a "wound" to the macromolecule that may cause a malfunction of the macromolecule and damage to the cell overall. Among the contents of the human cell are two types of nucleic acids: deoxyribonucleic acid (DNA) and ribonucleic acid (RNA). The most sensitive of molecules is DNA. You may recall that DNA has a coiled helix shape created by its configuration of two sugar phosphate chains connected by pairs of nitrogenous bases, like a twisted ladder. DNA is the essential ingredient of our chromosomes (tiny rod-shaped structures segmented into genes). Genes contain the "instructions" for every cell (heredity). Damage similar to that previously described may occur in DNA as a result of radiation exposure and manifest as a range of responses from minor damage that is reversible by the actions of repair enzymes to malignant responses and permanent damage. This is a critical reason for the radiographer to be mindful of radiation dose and make every effort to limit that dose to the patient and others. X-ray photons interacting with a cell may cause a range of damage from cell membrane rupture to damage to one of the internal structures. As noted previously, some of this damage may be reparable and some may result in cell death. X-ray photons may also interact with water molecules within the body. This interaction is called radiolysis of water. The x-ray photon ionizes the water molecule, creating an ion pair. Both the positively charged water molecule (HOH+) and the negatively charged freed electron are unstable and will undergo interactions or events to regain stability. Finally, because the human body is about 80% water, radiolysis of water can create harmful free radicals that then indirectly damage molecules and cells.

### Theory to Practice

It is important to remember that absorption equates to patient dose. Because of the strong inverse dependence of photoelectric absorption on x-ray energy, patient dose increases as kVp decreases. When there is too much absorption resulting from a kVp setting that is too low, the patient experiences an increased radiation dose. Patient dose is a result of the radiation absorbed by the body, not the radiation that passes through it.

### Critical Concept

#### Differential Absorption and Clinical Practice

In the clinical setting, some absorption and some penetration of x-ray photons through the anatomic area of interest are necessary for image production. But keep in mind that absorption equates to patient dose, and it is the radiographer's responsibility to maintain a balance of absorption and penetration so that the risk of exposure outweighs the biologic harm to the tissues and so that the resulting image benefits the patient.

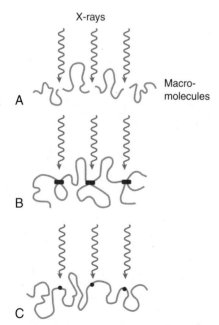

**Fig. 7.8 Damage to Macromolecules.** The three most common effects of x-ray photon damage to macromolecules are **(A)** main-chain scission, **(B)** cross-linking, and **(C)** point lesions.

## On the Spot

- Classical interactions are scattering events in which the atom involved is not ionized. They do not significantly affect the radiographic image but contribute slightly to patient dose.
- Compton interactions are scattering events in which the atom is ionized and a characteristic cascade may result. The incident photon is deflected in a new direction, becoming a scatter photon, and this photon and the ejected Compton electron both have sufficient energy to undergo many other interactions.
- Compton interactions are one of the most prevalent interactions and may contribute negatively to the radiographic image as fog and add to patient and occupational radiation dose.
- Photoelectric events result in the total absorption of the incident photon. For this to occur, the incident photon energy must be equal to or greater than the orbital shell binding energy.
- Photoelectric events result in ionization of the atom, a characteristic cascade producing secondary photons, and an ejected photoelectron capable of many more interactions.
- Photoelectric probability depends on the energy of the incident photon and the atomic number of the tissue being irradiated.
- Pair production involves very high-energy photon interactions with the nucleus of the tissue atom producing a positron and an electron. This event occurs outside of the energy range of diagnostic radiography.
- Photodisintegration is a very high-energy photon interaction with the nucleus of a tissue atom, resulting in the nucleus emitting a nuclear particle to regain stability. This event occurs outside of the energy range of diagnostic radiography.
- Differential absorption is the difference between x-ray photons that are absorbed photoelectrically and those that penetrate the body.
- Some absorption and some transmission of x-ray photons through the anatomic area of interest are necessary for image production. But keep in mind that absorption equates to patient dose, and a balance of absorption and penetration must be kept so that the benefit of exposure outweighs the biologic harm to the tissues.
- X-ray photons interact at an atomic level (classical, Compton, photoelectric, pair production, and photodisintegration), but the damage they may cause manifests at the macrolevel through changes or damage sustained by the macromolecules. This may occur directly when x-ray photons interact with atoms composing the macromolecule or indirectly through irradiation of water that creates harmful free radicals that then damage macromolecular structures.

## CRITICAL THINKING QUESTIONS

1. How would a radiographer use their knowledge of x-ray interactions with human tissue to describe to a patient how an image is formed?
2. Imagine you are testifying before Congress on the need for regulation of professionals who dispense ionizing radiation for medical imaging, and a committee member wants to know what happens inside the body when it is exposed to x-rays. Use material from this chapter to formulate a response that a layperson would understand.

## REVIEW QUESTIONS

1. Which of the following is a major source of occupational exposure?
   a. Photodisintegration
   b. Pair production
   c. Photoelectric interactions
   d. Compton interactions
2. Which interaction, within the diagnostic range, does not involve the removal of an orbital electron?
   a. Pair production
   b. Photoelectric effect
   c. Compton effect
   d. Classical scattering
3. Which interaction requires 1.02 MeV of energy?
   a. Pair production
   b. Photodisintegration
   c. Compton effect
   d. Photoelectric effect
4. A photon of 10 MeV colliding with a nucleus will likely result in what type of interaction?
   a. Photoelectric
   b. Photodisintegration
   c. Thompson
   d. Compton
5. Which technique will produce the greatest number of photodisintegration events in an average abdomen?
   a. 120 kV and 5 mAs
   b. 108 kV and 10 mAs
   c. 98 kV and 20 mAs
   d. none of the above
6. Which of the following events will not occur in the diagnostic range of x-ray energies?
   a. Classical
   b. Compton
   c. Photoelectric
   d. Photodisintegration
7. Positive-contrast media is administered to increase what type of interactions?
   a. Photoelectric
   b. Pair production
   c. Classical
   d. Compton
8. Which of the following contributes most to image fog?
   a. Classical
   b. Photoelectric
   c. Pair production
   d. Compton

9. Which interaction in the diagnostic range involves the total absorption of the incident photon?
   a. Pair production
   b. Photodisintegration
   c. Compton effect
   d. Photoelectric effect

10. When the kV selected is equal to or slightly greater than the inner-shell binding energy of a target tissue atom, which interaction predominates?
    a. Photoelectric
    b. Thompson
    c. Pair production
    d. Photodisintegration

# Image Production

## Outline

## Objectives

- Describe the process of radiographic image formation.
- Explain the process of beam attenuation.
- Identify the factors that affect beam attenuation.
- Describe the x-ray interactions termed *photoelectric effect* and *Compton effect*.
- Define the term *ionization*.
- State the composition of exit radiation.
- State the effect of scatter radiation on the radiographic image.

- Explain the process of creating the various shades of gray in the image.
- Recognize the relationship between matrix and pixel size and digital image quality.
- Define pixel bit depth and its relationship to contrast resolution.
- State the benefits of digital imaging.
- Differentiate radiographic from fluoroscopic imaging.

## Key Terms

absorption
attenuation
coherent scattering
Compton effect
Compton electron
contrast resolution
differential absorption
dynamic range
exit radiation

fluoroscopy
fog
image receptor
ionization
latent image
manifest image
matrix
photoelectric effect
photoelectron

pixel
pixel bit depth
remnant radiation
scattering
secondary electron
tissue density
transmission

## INTRODUCTION

To produce a radiographic image, x-ray photons must pass through tissue and interact with an **image receptor** (a device that receives the radiation leaving the patient) such as a digital imaging system. Both the quantity and quality of the primary x-ray beam affect its interaction within the various tissues that make up the anatomic part. In addition, the composition of the anatomic tissues affects the x-ray beam interaction. The **absorption** characteristics of the anatomic part are determined by its composition, such as thickness, atomic number, and **tissue density** (compactness of the cellular structures). Finally, the radiation that exits the patient is composed of varying energies and interacts with the image receptor to form the latent or invisible image.

## DIFFERENTIAL ABSORPTION

The process of image formation is a result of **differential absorption** of the x-ray beam as it interacts with the anatomic tissue.

**Make the Physics Connection**

**Chapter 7**

Differential absorption is the difference between the x-ray photons that are absorbed photoelectrically and those that penetrate the body.

The term *differential* is used because varying anatomic parts do not absorb the primary beam to the same degree. Anatomic parts composed of bone absorb more x-ray photons than parts comprising soft tissue or filled with air. Differential absorption of the primary x-ray beam creates an image that structurally represents the anatomic area of interest (Fig. 8.1).

**Critical Concept**

**Differential Absorption and Image Formation**

A radiographic image is created by passing an x-ray beam through the patient and interacting with an image receptor, such as a digital imaging system. The variations in absorption and transmission of the exiting x-ray beam structurally represent the anatomic area of interest.

## BEAM ATTENUATION

As the primary x-ray beam passes through anatomic tissue, it loses some of its energy. Fewer x-ray photons remain in the beam after it interacts with anatomic tissue. This reduction in the energy or number of photons in the primary x-ray beam is known as **attenuation**. Beam attenuation occurs because of the photon interactions with the atomic structures that compose the tissues. Two distinct processes occur during beam attenuation in the diagnostic range: absorption and scattering.

## ABSORPTION

When the energy of the primary x-ray beam is deposited within the atoms composing the tissue, some x-ray photons are completely absorbed. Complete absorption of the incoming x-ray photon occurs when it has enough energy to remove (eject) an inner-shell electron. The ejected electron, called a **photoelectron**, quickly loses energy by interacting with nearby tissues.

The ability to remove (eject) electrons, known as **ionization**, is one of the characteristics of x-rays. In the diagnostic range, this x-ray interaction with matter, is known as the **photoelectric effect**.

**Make the Physics Connection**

**Chapter 7**

Photoelectric interactions occur throughout the diagnostic range (i.e., 20 kVp–120 kVp) and involve inner-shell orbital electrons of tissue atoms. For photoelectric events to occur, the incident x-ray photon energy must be equal to or greater than the orbital shell binding energy. In these events, the incident x-ray photon interacts with the inner-shell electron of a tissue atom and removes it from orbit. In this process, the incident x-ray photon expends all its energy and is totally absorbed.

With the photoelectric effect, the ionized atom has a vacancy, or electron hole, in its inner shell. An electron from an outer shell moves to fill the vacancy. Because of the difference in binding energies between the two electron shells, a secondary x-ray photon is emitted (Fig. 8.2). This secondary x-ray photon typically has very low energy and is therefore unlikely to exit the patient.

**Critical Concept**

**X-Ray Photon Absorption**

During attenuation of the x-ray beam, the photoelectric effect is responsible for total absorption of the incoming x-ray photon.

The probability of total photon absorption during the photoelectric effect depends on the energy of the incoming x-ray photon and the atomic number of the anatomic tissue. The energy of the incoming x-ray photon must be at least equal to the binding energy of the inner-shell electron. After absorption of some of the x-ray photons, the overall energy or quantity of the primary beam decreases as it passes through the anatomic part.

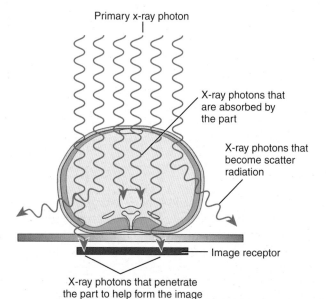

Primary x-ray photon

X-ray photons that are absorbed by the part

X-ray photons that become scatter radiation

Image receptor

X-ray photons that penetrate the part to help form the image

**Fig. 8.1 Differential Absorption.** As the primary beam interacts with the anatomic part, x-ray photons are transmitted, absorbed, and scattered based on the tissue's composition. Differential absorption of the primary x-ray beam creates an image that structurally represents the anatomic area of interest.

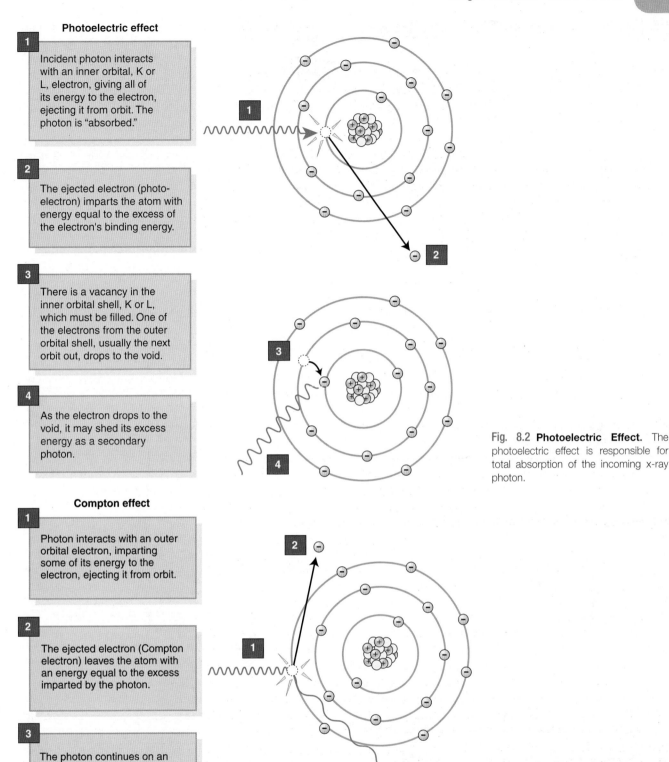

**Photoelectric effect**

**1** Incident photon interacts with an inner orbital, K or L, electron, giving all of its energy to the electron, ejecting it from orbit. The photon is "absorbed."

**2** The ejected electron (photo-electron) imparts the atom with energy equal to the excess of the electron's binding energy.

**3** There is a vacancy in the inner orbital shell, K or L, which must be filled. One of the electrons from the outer orbital shell, usually the next orbit out, drops to the void.

**4** As the electron drops to the void, it may shed its excess energy as a secondary photon.

Fig. 8.2 **Photoelectric Effect.** The photoelectric effect is responsible for total absorption of the incoming x-ray photon.

**Compton effect**

**1** Photon interacts with an outer orbital electron, imparting some of its energy to the electron, ejecting it from orbit.

**2** The ejected electron (Compton electron) leaves the atom with an energy equal to the excess imparted by the photon.

**3** The photon continues on an altered path, scattered, with less energy (longer wavelength) than before the collision.

Fig. 8.3 **Compton Effect.** During the Compton effect, the incoming x-ray photon loses energy and changes its direction.

## SCATTERING

Some incoming photons are not absorbed but instead lose energy during interactions with the atoms composing the tissue. This process is called **scattering**. It results from the diagnostic x-ray interaction with matter, known as the **Compton effect**. The loss of some energy of the incoming photon occurs when it ejects an outer-shell electron from a tissue atom. The ejected electron is called a **Compton electron** or **secondary electron**. The remaining lower-energy x-ray photon changes direction and may leave the anatomic part to interact with the image receptor (Fig. 8.3).

## Critical Concept
### X-Ray Beam Scattering

During attenuation of the x-ray beam, the incoming x-ray photon may lose energy and change direction because of the Compton effect.

Compton interactions can occur within all diagnostic x-ray energies and are therefore an important interaction in radiography. The probability of a Compton interaction occurring depends on the energy of the incoming photon. It does not depend on the atomic number of the anatomic tissue. For example, a Compton interaction is just as likely to occur in soft tissue as in tissue composed of bone. However, if the tissue has more complex atoms, there are more opportunities for interaction. With higher atomic number particles, such as bone, if the energy of the incoming photon is appropriate (high enough), more scatter will occur; otherwise, more absorption will take place. For Compton interactions to occur, the energy of the photon is more important, whereas the atomic number of the tissue is just the opportunity for x-ray interactions.

At higher kilovoltages within the diagnostic range, the percentage of photoelectric interactions generally decreases whereas the percentage of Compton interactions is likely to increase. Box 8.1 compares photoelectric and Compton interactions. Scattered and secondary radiations provide no useful information and must be controlled during radiographic imaging.

## Make the Physics Connection
### Chapter 7

The problem with Compton scatter interacting with the image receptor is that it is not following its original path through the body and strikes the image receptor in the wrong area. In so doing, it contributes no useful information to the image and results only in image fog. Because most scattered photons are still directed toward the image receptor and result in image fog, it is desirable to minimize Compton scattering as much as possible.

Coherent scattering is an interaction that occurs with low-energy x-rays, typically below the diagnostic range. The incoming photon interacts with the atom, causing it to become excited. The x-ray does not lose energy but changes direction. Coherent scattering could occur within the diagnostic range of x-rays and may interact with the image receptor, but it is not considered an important interaction in radiography.

If a scattered photon strikes the image receptor, it does not contribute any useful information about the anatomic area of interest. If scattered photons are absorbed within the anatomic tissue, they contribute to the radiation exposure to the patient. In addition, if the scattered photon leaves the patient and does not strike the image receptor, it could contribute to the radiation exposure of anyone near the patient.

## TRANSMISSION

If the incoming x-ray photon passes through the anatomic part without any interaction with the atomic structures, it is called transmission (Fig. 8.4). The combination of absorption and transmission of the x-ray beam provides an image that structurally represents

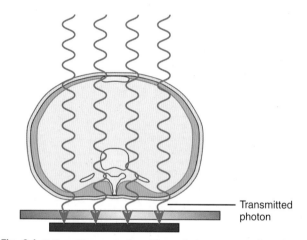
Transmitted photon

Fig. 8.4 X-Ray Transmission. Transmission occurs when the incoming x-ray photon passes through the anatomic part without any interaction.

| Box 8.1 Comparing Photoelectric and Compton Effects | |
|---|---|
| PHOTOELECTRIC EFFECT | COMPTON EFFECT |
| An incoming photon has sufficient energy to eject an inner-shell electron and be completely absorbed. | An incoming photon loses energy when it ejects an outer-shell electron and changes direction. |
| An electron from an outer-shell fills the electron hole or vacancy. | The scattered photon may be absorbed within the patient tissues, leave the anatomic part, interact with the image receptor, or expose anyone near the patient. |
| A secondary photon is created because of the difference in the electrons' binding energies. | Scattered photons that strike the image receptor provide no useful information. |
| The probability of this effect depends on the energy of the incoming x-ray photon and the composition of the anatomic tissue. | The probability of this effect depends on the energy of incoming x-ray photon but not the composition of the anatomic tissue. |
| Fewer photon interactions occur at higher kVp, but of those interactions, a smaller percentage are photoelectric interactions. | Fewer photon interactions occur at higher kVp, but of those interactions, a greater percentage are Compton interactions. |

kVp, Kilovoltage peak.

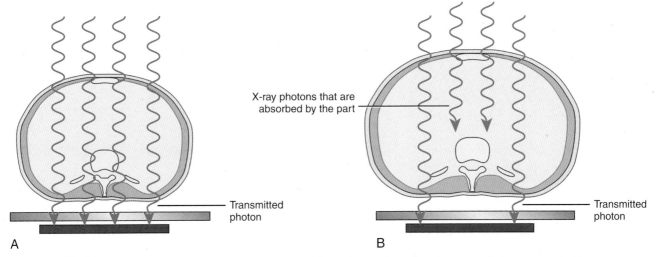

Fig. 8.5 **Tissue Thickness and X-Ray Absorption. (A)** A thinner patient transmits more radiation compared with a thicker patient. **(B)** A thicker patient absorbs more radiation than a thinner patient.

the anatomic part. Because scatter radiation is also a process that occurs during interaction of the x-ray beam and anatomic part, the quality of the image created is compromised if the scattered photon strikes the image receptor.

The preceding discussion focused on photon interactions that occur in radiography when using x-ray energies within the moderate or diagnostic range. Very high-energy x-rays, beyond the diagnostic range, result in other interactions, such as pair production and photodisintegration. X-ray interactions beyond the diagnostic range are important in radiation therapy.

## FACTORS AFFECTING BEAM ATTENUATION

The amount of x-ray beam attenuation is affected by the thickness of the anatomic part, its tissue atomic number and tissue density, and the energy of the x-ray beam.

### Tissue Thickness

For a given anatomic tissue, increasing its thickness increases beam attenuation by either absorption (see Fig. 8.5) or scattering. X-rays are attenuated exponentially and generally reduced by approximately 50% for each 4 to 5 cm of tissue thickness (Fig. 8.6). The thicker the anatomic part, the more x-rays are needed to produce a radiographic image. The thinner the anatomic part, the fewer x-rays are needed to produce a radiographic image.

### Type of Tissue

Tissue composed of a higher atomic number, such as bone, attenuates the x-ray beam more than tissue composed of a lower atomic number, such as fat. The higher atomic number indicates there are more atomic particles for interaction with the x-ray photons. X-ray absorption is more likely to occur in tissues composed of a higher atomic number compared with tissues composed of a lower atomic number (Fig. 8.7). Tissues that

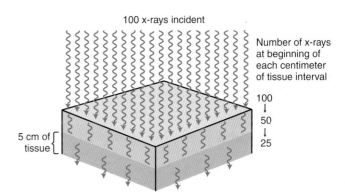

Fig. 8.6 **Tissue Beam Attenuation.** X-rays are attenuated exponentially and generally reduced by approximately 50% for each 4 to 5 cm of tissue thickness.

absorb more x-rays demonstrate increased brightness in a digital image. Tissues that transmit more x-rays (and absorb fewer x-rays) demonstrate decreased brightness in the digital image.

### Tissue Density

Matter per unit volume—or the compactness of the atomic particles composing the anatomic part—also affects the amount of beam attenuation. For example, muscle (effective atomic number 7.4) and fat (effective atomic number 6.3) tissue are similar in composition; however, their atomic particles differ in compactness, and therefore tissue density varies. Muscle tissue has atomic particles that are more dense or compact and therefore attenuate the x-ray beam more than fat cells. Bone is composed of tissue with a higher atomic number (effective atomic number 13.8), and the atomic particles are more compacted or dense. Four substances account for most of the beam attenuation in the human body: bone, muscle, fat, and air. Bone attenuates the x-ray beam more than muscle, muscle attenuates the x-ray beam more than fat, and fat attenuates the x-ray beam more than the air. The atomic number of

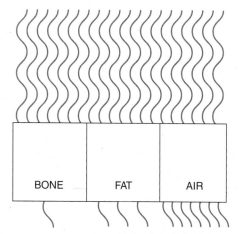

Fig. 8.7 **Type of Tissue and X-Ray Absorption.** Bone absorbs more radiation than fat and air. Air transmits more radiation than fat and bone.

Table 8.1 **Effective Atomic Number and Tissue Density**

| HUMAN TISSUE | EFFECTIVE ATOMIC NUMBER | TISSUE DENSITY (KG/M³) |
|---|---|---|
| Bone | 13.8 | 1850 |
| Muscle | 7.4 | 1000 |
| Fat | 6.3 | 910 |

kg/m³, Kilograms per cubic meter.

Table 8.2 **Factors Affecting Attenuation**

| FACTOR | BEAM ATTENUATION | ABSORPTION | TRANSMISSION |
|---|---|---|---|
| **Tissue Thickness** | | | |
| Increasing thickness | ↑ | ↑ | ↓ |
| Decreasing thickness | ↓ | ↓ | ↑ |
| **Tissue Atomicnumber** | | | |
| Increasing atomic number | ↑ | ↑ | ↓ |
| Decreasing atomic number | ↓ | ↓ | ↑ |
| **Tissue Density** | | | |
| Increasing tissue density | ↑ | ↑ | ↓ |
| Decreasing tissue density | ↓ | ↓ | ↑ |
| **X-Ray Beam Quality** | | | |
| Increasing beam quality | ↓ | ↓ | ↑ |
| Decreasing beam quality | ↑ | ↑ | ↓ |

the anatomic part and its tissue density affect x-ray beam attenuation (see Table 8.1).

## X-Ray Beam Quality

The quality of the x-ray beam or its penetrating ability affects its interaction with anatomic tissue. Higher-penetrating x-rays (shorter wavelength with higher frequency) are more likely to be transmitted through anatomic tissue without interacting with the tissues' atomic structures. Lower-penetrating x-rays (longer wavelength with lower frequency) are more likely to interact with the atomic structures and be absorbed. The kilovoltage selected during x-ray production determines the energy or penetrability of the x-ray photons and this affects its attenuation in anatomic tissue (Fig. 8.8). Beam attenuation is decreased with a higher-energy x-ray beam and increased with a lower-energy x-ray beam (Table 8.2).

**! Critical Concept**

**Factors Affecting Beam Attenuation**

Increasing tissue thickness, atomic number, and tissue density increases x-ray beam attenuation because the tissue absorbs more x-rays. Increasing the quality of the x-ray beam decreases beam attenuation because the higher-energy x-rays penetrate the tissue.

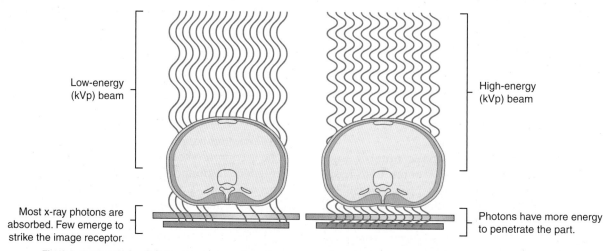

Low-energy (kVp) beam

High-energy (kVp) beam

Most x-ray photons are absorbed. Few emerge to strike the image receptor.

Photons have more energy to penetrate the part.

Fig. 8.8 **X-Ray Beam Quality.** The energy of the x-ray beam affects its interaction within the anatomic tissues. Lower kVp results in more absorption in the tissue. Higher kVp results in more transmission through the tissue.

## Imaging Effect

When the attenuated x-ray beam leaves the patient, the remaining x-ray beam, referred to as **exit radiation** or **remnant radiation**, is composed of both transmitted and scattered radiation (Fig. 8.9). The varying amounts of transmitted and absorbed radiation (differential absorption) create an image that structurally represents the anatomic area of interest. Scatter exit radiation (Compton interactions) that reaches the image receptor does not provide any diagnostic information about the anatomic area. Scatter radiation creates unwanted exposure on the image called **fog**. Methods used to decrease the amount of scatter radiation reaching the image receptor are discussed in later chapters.

The areas within the anatomic tissue that absorb incoming x-ray photons (photoelectric effect) create the white or clear areas (increased brightness) on the displayed image. The incoming x-ray photons that are transmitted create the dark areas (decreased brightness) on the displayed image. Anatomic tissues that vary in absorption and transmission create a range of dark and light areas (shades of gray) (Fig. 8.10). The various shades of gray or brightness displayed in the radiographic image make anatomic tissue visible. Skeletal bones are differentiated from the air-filled lungs because of their differences in absorption and transmission.

> ### ⚠ Critical Concept
>
> #### Image Brightness
>
> The range of brightness levels visible after image processing is a result of the variation in x-ray absorption and transmission as the x-ray beam passes through anatomic tissues. In addition, the radiographer can manipulate the quality of the primary x-ray beam to affect its attenuation and modify the visibility of anatomic structures.

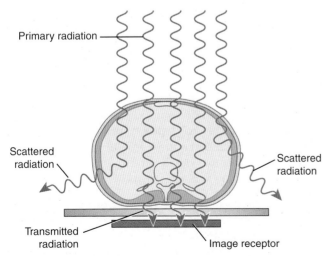

**Fig. 8.9** **Exit Radiation.** When the attenuated x-ray beam leaves the patient, the remnant x-ray beam is composed of both transmitted and scattered radiation.

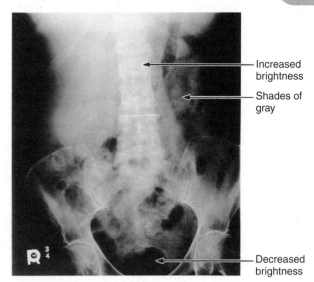

**Fig. 8.10** **Radiographic Image.** Anatomic tissues vary in their absorption and transmission of x-ray photons to create the range of brightness or gray levels that structurally represents the anatomic area of interest. Increased brightness represents absorbed radiation, whereas decreased brightness represents transmitted radiation. (Courtesy Fauber TL: *Radiographic imaging and exposure*, ed 3, St Louis, 2009, Mosby.)

Image characteristics and exposure techniques are discussed in more detail in later chapters.

## IMAGE RECEPTORS

Less than 5% of the primary x-ray beam interacting with the anatomic part reaches the image receptor, and an even lower percentage is used to create the radiographic image. The exit or remnant radiation leaving the patient interacts with an image receptor to create the latent (invisible) image. This **latent image** is not visible until processed to produce the **manifest** (visible) **image**.

### DIGITAL IMAGE RECEPTORS

Digital imaging is the common method used in radiography and can be accomplished by using a specialized image receptor that acquires the latent image from which the computer processes the latent image for display on a monitor. There are several types of digital image receptors used in diagnostic imaging. Regardless of the type of digital imaging receptor, the radiographic image is composed of digital data and can then be altered in a variety of ways. A more detailed discussion of digital image receptors can be found in Chapter 10.

> ### ⚠ Critical Concept
>
> #### Differential Absorption and Image Receptor
>
> The process of differential absorption for image formation remains the same regardless of the type of image receptor. The varying x-ray intensities exit the anatomic area of interest to form the latent image.

# THE DIGITAL IMAGE

Digital image receptors can respond to a wide range of x-ray exposures (wide dynamic range). The **dynamic range** of an imaging system refers to the range of exposure intensities an image receptor can accurately detect. Anatomic areas of widely different attenuation such as soft tissues and bony structures can be more easily visualized because of the wider dynamic range in digital imaging. In addition, because of computer processing, moderately underexposed or overexposed images may still be of acceptable diagnostic quality.

 **Critical Concept**

**Dynamic Range and Digital Imaging**

The range of exposure intensities an image receptor can accurately detect determines its dynamic range. Digital image receptors have a wide dynamic range and can accurately detect very low exposure intensities and very high exposure intensities.

Digital images are composed of numerical data that can be easily manipulated by a computer. When displayed on a computer monitor, this allows tremendous flexibility in terms of altering in real time the brightness and contrast of a digital image. The practical advantage of such capability is that, regardless of the original exposure parameters (within reason), any anatomic structure can be independently and optimally visualized. Computers can also perform various postprocessing image manipulations to further improve visibility of the anatomic region.

A digital image is displayed as a **matrix**, or combination of rows and columns (termed an array), of small, usually square "picture elements" called pixels. Each **pixel** is displayed as a single numerical value, which is represented as a single brightness level on a computer monitor. The location of the pixel within the image matrix corresponds to an area within the patient or volume of tissue (Fig. 8.11).

Given the dimensions of an anatomic area, or field of view (FOV), a matrix size of 1024 × 1024 has 1,048,576 individual pixels; a matrix size of 2048 × 2048 has 4,194,304 pixels. Digital image quality is improved with a larger matrix size that includes a greater number of smaller pixels (Fig. 8.12 and Box 8.2). Although image quality is improved for a larger matrix size and smaller pixels, it is important to understand that computer processing time, network transmission time, and digital storage space increase as the matrix size increases.

 **Critical Concept**

**Matrix and Pixel Size and Image Quality**

For a given FOV, increasing the matrix size will decrease the pixel size and increase image quality. Decreasing the matrix size will increase the pixel size and decrease image quality.

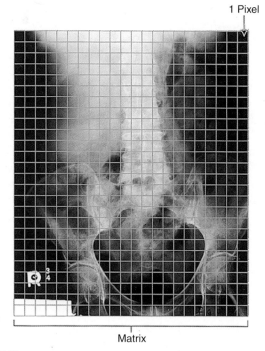

**Fig. 8.11 Image Matrix.** Location of the pixel within the image matrix corresponds to an area within the patient or volume of tissue. Note: Pixel size is not to scale and used for illustration only. (Courtesy Fauber TL: *Radiographic imaging and exposure*, ed 3, St Louis, 2009, Mosby.)

The numerical value assigned to each pixel is determined by the relative attenuation of x-rays passing through the corresponding volume of tissue. Pixels representing highly attenuating tissues (increased absorption), such as bone, are assigned a different value for higher brightness than pixels representing tissues of low x-ray attenuation (decreased absorption) (Fig. 8.13). Each pixel also has a **bit depth**, or number of bits (Box 8.3), that determines the amount of precision in digitizing the analog signal and therefore the number of shades of gray that can be displayed in the image. Bit depth is determined by the analog-to-digital converter, which is an integral component of every digital imaging system. Because the binary system is used, bit depth is expressed as 2 to the power of n, or the number of bits ($2^n$). A larger bit depth allows a greater number of shades of gray to be displayed on a computer monitor. For example, a 12-bit depth ($2^{12}$) can display 4096 shades of gray, a 14-bit depth can display 16,384 shades of gray, and a 16-bit depth can display 65,536 shades of gray. A system that can digitize and display a greater number of shades of gray has better contrast resolution. An image with increased contrast resolution increases the visibility of anatomic details and the ability to distinguish among small anatomic areas of interest (Fig. 8.14).

**Critical Concept**

**Pixel Bit Depth and Image Quality**

A digital imaging system that has pixels with a larger bit depth will display a greater number of shades of gray and have increased image quality.

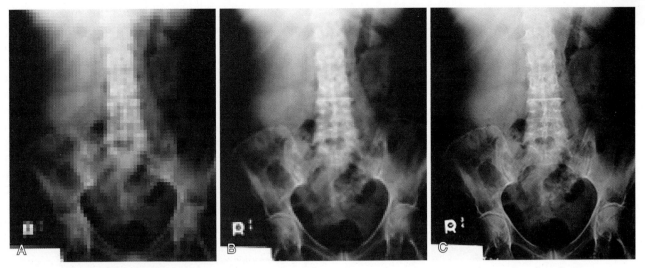

**Fig. 8.12 Matrix Size.** For a given field of view (FOV), the larger the matrix size, the greater the number of smaller individual pixels. Increasing the number of pixels improves the quality of the image. **(A)** Matrix size is 64 × 64. **(B)** Matrix size is 215 × 215. **(C)** Matrix size is 2048 × 2048. (Courtesy Fauber TL: *Radiographic imaging and exposure*, ed 3, St Louis, 2009, Mosby.)

---

| Box 8.2 | Digital Imaging Terminology |
|---------|------------------------------|

Matrix: Image displayed as a combination of rows and columns (array); for a given field of view (FOV), a larger matrix size improves spatial resolution.

Pixel: Smallest component of the matrix; a greater number of smaller pixels improves spatial resolution.

Pixel bit depth: The number of bits that determines the amount of precision in digitizing the analog signal and therefore the number of shades of gray that can be displayed in the image.

Digital image quality and characteristics will be discussed in more detail in Chapter 9.

Digital radiographic images can be acquired and displayed quickly and can be efficiently transmitted, processed, interpreted on a display monitor, stored, and retrieved via electronic means. Digital image receptors exhibit excellent dynamic range and contrast resolution.

Radiography creates a static image of the anatomic area of interests whereas dynamic imaging, or **fluoroscopy**, provides imaging of the movement of internal structures.

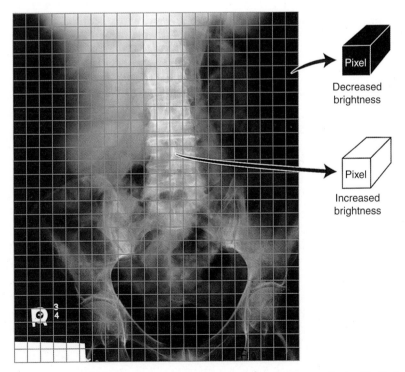

**Fig. 8.13 Pixel Value.** Each pixel value represents a volume of tissue imaged. (Courtesy Fauber TL: *Radiographic imaging and exposure*, ed 3, St Louis, 2009, Mosby.)

### Digital image pixel bit depth

Bits per pixel

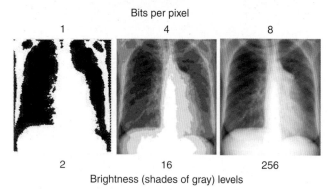

Brightness (shades of gray) levels

**Fig. 8.14 Pixel Bit Depth.** Pixel bit depth determines the shades of gray displayed on the monitor. The greater the pixel depth a digital system can display, the greater the contrast resolution displayed in the image. (Courtesy Sprawls P: *The physical principles of medical imaging online*, ed 2, http://www.sprawls.org/ppmi2/.)

## DYNAMIC IMAGING: FLUOROSCOPY

Fluoroscopy (Fig. 8.15) differs from static imaging by its use of a continuous beam of x-rays to create images of moving internal structures that can be viewed on a display monitor. Internal structures, such as the vascular or gastrointestinal systems, can be visualized in their normal state of motion with the aid of special liquid or gas substances (contrast media) that are either injected or instilled. The equipment used in fluoroscopy has undergone major changes over the past few years. Image-intensified fluoroscopy is rapidly being replaced with flat-panel detector fluoroscopy. Regardless of the type of fluoroscopic equipment, the x-ray tube is usually positioned underneath the table, and the x-rays pass through the patient to interact with a device that converts the x-rays into either light intensities (image-intensified) or digital data (flat-panel detector).

### ⚠ Critical Concept

**Fluoroscopy**

Dynamic imaging of internal anatomic structures can be visualized with the use of a flat panel detector or image intensifier. The exit radiation interacts with the acquisition device, is processed or converted, and then transmitted to the display monitor for viewing.

Fluoroscopy will be discussed in detail in Chapter 15.

Regardless of the type of imaging system (digital or fluoroscopic), the process of differential absorption for image formation remains the same. The varying x-ray intensities exiting the anatomic area of interest form the image.

Several important steps in creating a radiographic image have been discussed in this and the previous chapters. Further discussion of radiographic image characteristics, exposure technique selection, image receptors, control of scatter radiation, and problem solving are included in subsequent chapters.

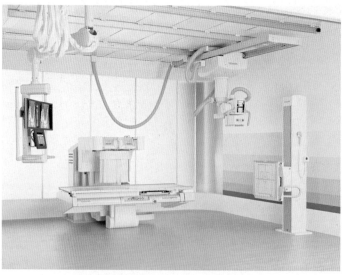

**Fig. 8.15 Fluoroscopy.** Digital fluoroscopy using flat-panel detector technology. (Courtesy Fauber TL: *Radiographic imaging and exposure*, ed 5, St Louis, 2016, Mosby.)

**Critical Concept**

**Image Formation**

The process of differential absorption for image formation remains the same regardless of the type of imaging system, digital or fluoroscopic. The varying x-ray intensities exiting the anatomic area of interest form the image, which is displayed on a monitor.

**On the Spot**

- A radiographic image is a result of the differential absorption of the primary x-rays that interact with the varying tissue composition of the anatomic area of interest.
- Beam attenuation occurs when the primary x-ray beam loses energy as it interacts with anatomic tissues.
- Beam attenuation is affected by tissue thickness, atomic number, tissue density, and x-ray beam quality.
- X-rays can eject electrons (ionization) from atoms within anatomic tissue.
- Three primary processes occur during x-ray interaction with anatomic tissues: absorption, transmission, and scattering.
- Total absorption of the incoming x-ray photon is a result of the photoelectric effect.
- Scattering of the incoming x-ray photon is a result of the Compton effect.
- Scatter radiation reaching the image receptor provides no useful information and creates unwanted exposure or fog on the radiographic image.
- A radiographic image is composed of varying brightness levels that structurally represent the anatomic area of interest.
- Digital image receptors receive the exit radiation from the area of interest to record the latent image.
- A digital image with a larger matrix and smaller-sized pixels has improved quality.
- A pixel's bit depth determines the available shades of gray to display the digital image or its contrast resolution.
- Digital image receptors have a wide dynamic range.
- Fluoroscopy allows imaging of the movement of internal structures for viewing on a display monitor.
- The process of differential absorption remains the same for image formation regardless of the type of imaging system: digital imaging or fluoroscopy.

## CRITICAL THINKING QUESTIONS

1. During beam attenuation, what occurs at the molecular level of anatomic tissues to affect the radiation exiting the patient?
2. Why is scatter radiation detrimental to the radiographic image, patient, and personnel in the vicinity?
3. How does radiographic and fluoroscopic imaging differ?

## REVIEW QUESTIONS

1. Which of the following describes the process of radiographic image formation?
   a. Beam attenuation
   b. Differential absorption
   c. Dynamic imaging
   d. Ionization
2. X-rays can eject electrons from atoms. This is known as:
   a. beam attenuation.
   b. differential absorption.
   c. dynamic imaging.
   d. ionization.
3. The x-ray interaction with anatomic tissue that is responsible for scattering is:
   a. ionization.
   b. photoelectric.
   c. Compton.
   d. absorption.
4. Which of the following will increase beam attenuation?
   a. Higher kilovoltage
   b. Decreasing tissue density
   c. Thicker anatomic part
   d. Lower atomic number
5. Factors that decrease x-ray absorption include:
   a. increased tissue density.
   b. increased x-ray beam quality.
   c. increased tissue thickness.
   d. increased atomic number.
6. The range of exposure intensities an image receptor can accurately detect defines:
   a. pixel bit depth.
   b. dynamic range.
   c. ionization.
   d. attenuation.
7. Digital image quality is improved with:
   a. larger pixel sizes.
   b. smaller pixel bit depths.
   c. increased tissue density.
   d. larger matrix size.
8. Increasing the pixel bit depth will:
   a. decrease scattering.
   b. increase contrast resolution.
   c. decrease image quality.
   d. increase pixel size.
9. Dynamic imaging of internal structures can be visualized with a/an:
   a. image intensifier.
   b. flat-panel detector.
   c. x-ray tube.
   d. a and b.
10. The process of differential absorption to form an image is the same for digital imaging and fluoroscopy.
    a. True
    b. False

# Image Quality and Characteristics

## Outline

## Objectives

- Describe the necessary components of radiographic image quality.
- Differentiate between the visibility and sharpness factors of radiographic images.
- Recognize and describe the image characteristics of brightness, radiographic contrast, spatial resolution, and distortion.
- Differentiate between tissues that have high and low subject contrast.
- Explain how adjusting the window level and window width affect digital image quality.
- Differentiate between high- and low-contrast radiographic images.

- State the relationship between spatial frequency and spatial resolution.
- Explain the relationship among display field of view (FOV), matrix, and pixel size.
- Define the concepts modulation transfer function (MTF), detective quantum efficiency (DQE), signal-to-noise ratio (SNR), and contrast-to-noise ratio (CNR) and state their relationship to image quality.
- Differentiate between size and shape distortion.
- Recognize the effect of quantum noise and scatter on digital image quality.
- Discuss the effects of image artifacts on radiographic quality.

## Key Terms

| | | |
|---|---|---|
| artifact | foreshortening | radiographic contrast |
| brightness | grayscale | resolution |
| contrast | high subject contrast | saturation |
| contrast resolution | low subject contrast | sharpness factors |
| contrast-to-noise ratio (CNR) | magnification | signal-to-noise ratio (SNR) |
| detective quantum efficiency | matrix | size distortion |
| distortion | modulation transfer function (MTF) | spatial resolution |
| dynamic range | pixel bit depth | subject contrast |
| elongation | pixel density | visibility factors |
| exposure indicator | pixel pitch | window level |
| field of view | quantum noise | window width |

## INTRODUCTION

A quality radiographic image accurately represents the anatomic area of interest, and information is well visualized for diagnosis. It is important to identify the characteristics of a quality radiographic image before comprehending all the factors that affect its quality.

As stated in Chapter 8, the latent image is created by the process of differential absorption. Once the digital image has been acquired, it must then be processed before it can be displayed on a computer monitor.

## Make the Physics Connection

### Chapter 7

*Transmission* refers to those x-ray photons that pass through the body and reach the image receptor. It is desirable for some of the x-ray photons to pass through the anatomic area of interest; otherwise, no image would result. X-ray photons reaching the image receptor create the dark shades of the image. *Absorption* refers to those photons that are attenuated by the body and do not reach the image receptor. Absorption has the opposite effect on the image as transmission. Recall that these photons are absorbed photoelectrically and do not reach the image receptor. This lack of exposure to the image receptor results in the lighter shades of the image. It is also desirable to have some absorption; otherwise, the image would be uniformly dark.

This chapter will focus on the characteristics of a quality image displayed on a computer monitor. We will first describe the **visibility** and **sharpness factors** that compose a quality radiographic image and then differentiate among the characteristics that are used to evaluate image quality. Information about the construction of image receptors and how the image is acquired, processed, and displayed is discussed in detail in subsequent chapters.

## IMAGE QUALITY AND CHARACTERISTICS

The *visibility* of anatomic structures and the *accuracy* of their structural lines displayed *(sharpness)* determine the overall quality of the radiographic image (Fig. 9.1). Visibility of the anatomic structures of interest refers to the brightness and radiographic contrast of the image. The accuracy of the structural lines displayed (sharpness) is achieved by maximizing the amount of spatial resolution and minimizing the amount of distortion. Visibility of anatomic tissues is achieved by the proper balance of image brightness and radiographic contrast.

### BRIGHTNESS

Because the image is composed of numerical data, the brightness level displayed on the computer monitor can be easily altered to visualize the range of anatomic structures recorded. **Brightness** is the amount of luminance (light emission) of a display monitor.

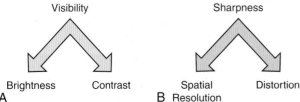

Fig. 9.1 **Radiographic Quality.** Factors affecting radiographic image quality. **(A)** Visibility factors. **(B)** Sharpness factors.

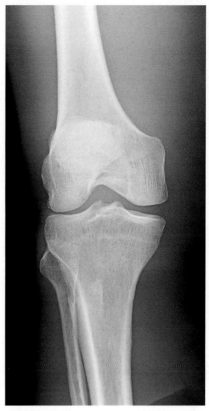

Fig. 9.2 **Brightness.** Radiographic image with sufficient brightness.

A radiographic image must have sufficient brightness to make visible the anatomic structures of interest (Fig. 9.2). A radiographic image that is too light has too much brightness to allow visualization of the structures of the anatomic part (Fig. 9.3). Conversely, a radiographic image that is too dark has insufficient brightness and the anatomic part cannot be well visualized (Fig. 9.4). The radiographer must evaluate the overall brightness on the image to determine whether it is sufficient to visualize the anatomic area of interest. They then decide whether the radiographic image is diagnostic or unacceptable.

### Critical Concept

**Brightness and Radiographic Quality**

A radiographic image must have sufficient brightness to visualize the anatomic structures of interest.

The x-ray beam that exits the patient contains a wide range of x-ray intensities (often varying by more than 1000-fold). To adequately capture these intensity extremes, a receptor with a wide dynamic range is required. Because digital imaging provides a wide dynamic range the computer can adjust for exposure errors, a greater margin of error exists for exposure techniques to yield acceptable brightness levels.

Because digital image processing can compensate for exposure errors, the image may display the appropriate level of brightness, yet also have been over- or underexposed. As a result, the radiographer may be unaware of the exposure error. However, extreme

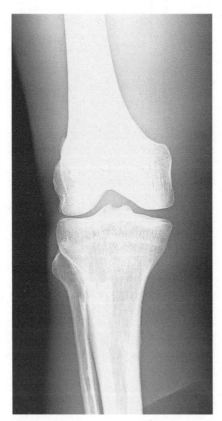

Fig. 9.3 **Brightness.** Radiographic image with excessive brightness. Brightness altered with postprocessing.

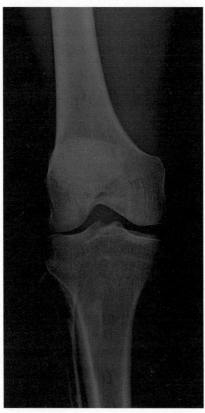

Fig. 9.4 **Brightness.** Radiographic image with insufficient brightness. Brightness altered with postprocessing.

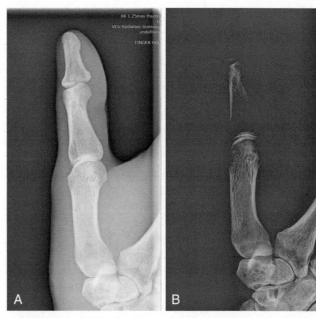

Fig. 9.5 **Saturation. (A)** Radiographic image with sufficient exposure. **(B)** Radiographic image with extreme overexposure and severely degraded quality.

exposure errors can affect image quality and be visible to the radiographer. When exposure to the digital image receptor is too low for the anatomic area, excessive quantum noise may be visible. When the image receptor is extremely overexposed, **saturation** may occur when the image cannot be properly processed and the quality is severely degraded (Fig. 9.5).

An important feature of digital imaging systems is the **exposure indicator**. The exposure indicator provides a numeric value indicating the level of radiation exposure to the digital image receptor. The radiographer should evaluate the exposure indicator value along with the quality of the digital image before determining whether a repeat image is warranted. Radiographers should evaluate the exposure indicator for every exposure and use it to improving their knowledge of exposure techniques and the quality of their future images.

A wide dynamic range is only useful, however, if the displayed image brightness can be optimized for human perception. This adjustment is accomplished using the windowing function. The **window level** (or center) sets the midpoint of the range of brightness levels visible in the image. Changing the window level on the display monitor allows the image brightness to be increased or decreased throughout the entire range of brightness levels. When the range of brightness levels displayed is less than the maximum, the processed image presents only a small sample of the total information contained within the computer (Fig. 9.6 and Fig. 9.7).

### ! Critical Concept

**Window Level and Image Brightness**

A relationship exists between window level and image brightness displayed on the monitor. Increasing or decreasing the window level will increase or decrease the image brightness.

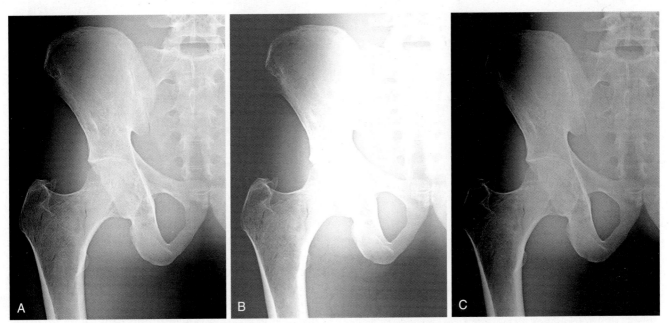

Fig. 9.6 **Window Level.** Changing the window level increases or decreases the image brightness throughout the range of brightness levels in the displayed image. (Courtesy Kuni C: *Introduction to computers and digital processing in medical imaging*, Chicago, 1988, Year Book Medical Publishers.)

To evaluate other attributes of radiographic quality, such as radiographic contrast and sharpness, the image must have sufficient brightness to visualize the anatomic area of interest.

## RADIOGRAPHIC CONTRAST

In addition to sufficient brightness, the radiograph must exhibit differences in the brightness levels (radiographic **contrast**) to differentiate among the anatomic tissues. The range of brightness levels is a result of tissues' differential absorption of the x-ray photons. An image that has sufficient brightness but no differences appears as a homogeneous object (Fig. 9.8).

This appearance indicates that the absorption characteristics of the object are equal. When the absorption characteristics of an object differ, the image has varying levels of brightness (Fig. 9.9). The anatomic tissues are easily differentiated because of these differences in brightness levels (i.e., radiographic contrast). Tissues that attenuate the x-ray beam equally are more difficult to visualize because the brightness levels are too similar to differentiate. To differentiate among the anatomic tissues, there must be differences in the brightness levels.

Radiographic contrast is the combined result of multiple factors associated with the anatomic structure, quality of the radiation, capabilities of the image receptor, and, in digital imaging, computer processing and display. **Subject contrast** refers to the absorption characteristics of the anatomic tissue radiographed and the quality of the x-ray beam. Differences in tissue thickness, tissue density, and effective atomic number contribute to subject contrast. For example, the chest is composed of tissues that vary greatly in x-ray lucency, such as the air-filled lungs, the heart, and the bony thorax. This anatomic region creates **high subject contrast** because the tissues attenuate the x-ray beam very differently compared with the abdomen for the same beam quality (Fig. 9.10 and Fig. 9.11). When the thorax is imaged, great differences in brightness levels are displayed for the varying tissues. The abdomen is composed of tissues that attenuate the x-ray beam similarly and is a region of **low subject contrast**. The brightness levels representing the soft-tissue organs in the abdomen are more similar (Fig. 9.12 and Fig. 9.13); therefore, it is difficult to distinguish the stomach from the kidneys.

Fig. 9.7 **Window Level.** **(A)** Image of the hip as originally processed. Because of the variation in tissue thickness in the hip, the lateral edge of the greater trochanter is displayed with less brightness compared with the femoral head. **(B)** Changing the window level to increase the brightness in the overall image shows increased brightness in the greater trochanter and improved visualization of the trabecular patterns. **(C)** Changing the window level to decrease brightness in the overall image shows decreased brightness in the femoral head and improved visualization of the trabecular patterns.

**Fig. 9.8 Homogeneous.** Radiographic image of a homogeneous object having no differences in brightness levels. (Courtesy Fauber TL: *Radiographic imaging and exposure*, ed 3, St Louis, 2009, Mosby.)

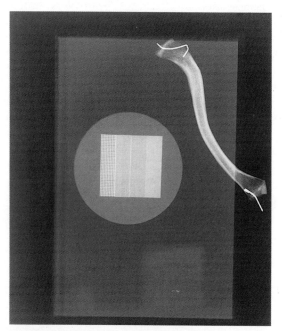

**Fig. 9.9 Differential Absorption.** Object with different absorption characteristics produces an image with varying brightness levels. (Courtesy Fauber TL: *Radiographic imaging and exposure*, ed 3, St Louis, 2009, Mosby.)

### Make the Physics Connection

#### Chapter 7

Differential absorption is the difference between the x-ray photons that are absorbed photoelectrically and those that penetrate the body. It is called *differential* because different body structures absorb x-ray photons to different extents. Anatomic structures such as bone are denser and absorb more x-ray photons than structures filled with air, such as the lungs.

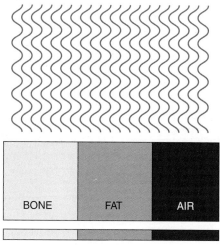

**Fig. 9.10 High Subject Contrast.** Higher subject contrast resulting from great differences in radiation absorption for tissues that have greater variation in composition.

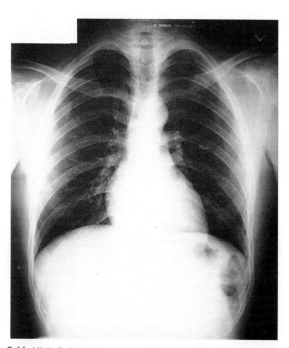

**Fig. 9.11 High Subject Contrast.** The chest is an area of high subject contrast because there is great variation in tissue composition. (Courtesy Fauber TL: *Radiographic imaging and exposure*, ed 3, St Louis, 2009, Mosby.)

As discussed previously, the quality of the x-ray beam also affects its attenuation in tissues, which alters subject contrast. Increasing the penetrating power of the x-ray beam decreases attenuation, reduces absorption, and increases x-ray transmission—resulting in fewer differences in brightness levels displayed in the radiographic image (Fig. 9.14). However, decreasing the penetrating power of the x-ray beam increases attenuation and absorption and decreases x-ray transmission—resulting in greater differences in the brightness levels displayed in the radiographic image (Fig. 9.15).

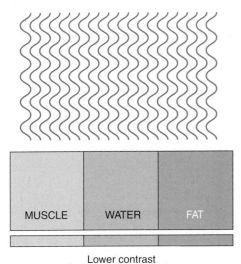

MUSCLE    WATER    FAT

Lower contrast

**Fig. 9.12 Low Subject Contrast.** Lower subject contrast resulting from fewer differences in radiation absorption for tissues that are more similarly composed.

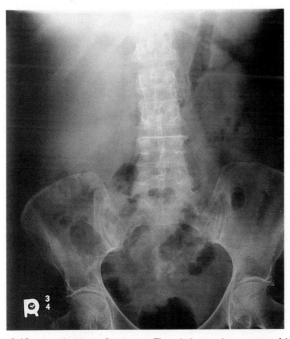

**Fig. 9.13 Low Subject Contrast.** The abdomen is an area of low subject contrast because it is made up of similar tissue types. (Courtesy Fauber TL: *Radiographic imaging and exposure*, ed 3, St Louis, 2009, Mosby.)

Brightness is easily measurable; however, radiographic contrast is a more complex attribute. Evaluating radiographic quality in terms of contrast is more subjective (it is affected by individual preferences). The level of radiographic contrast desired in an image is determined by the composition of the anatomic tissue to be radiographed and the amount of information needed to visualize the tissue for an accurate diagnosis. For example, the level of contrast desired in a chest image is different from the level of contrast required in an extremity or abdominopelvic image.

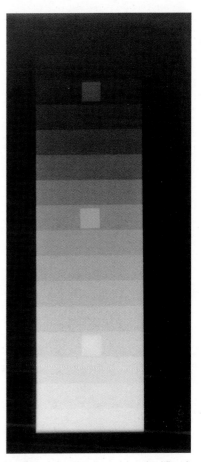

**Fig. 9.14 X-Ray Beam Quality.** Increasing the kilovoltage creates a low-contrast step wedge image showing many gray tones and little difference between individual brightness levels. (Courtesy Fauber TL: *Radiographic imaging and exposure*, ed 3, St Louis, 2009, Mosby.)

In digital imaging, the number of different shades of gray that can be stored and displayed by a computer system is termed **grayscale**. **Contrast resolution** is a term associated with digital imaging and is used to describe the ability of the imaging system to distinguish between small objects that attenuate the x-ray beam similarly. The contrast resolution of the imaging system determines the level of visibility of small objects having similar brightness levels or shades of gray. As mentioned previously, the **pixel bit depth** or number of bits (e.g., 12, 14, 16) affects the number of shades of gray available for image display. Increasing the number of shades of gray increases the contrast resolution within the image. An image with increased contrast resolution increases the visibility of anatomic structures and the ability to distinguish among small anatomic areas of interest.

> ### ! Critical Concept
>
> **Pixel Bit Depth and Contrast Resolution**
>
> The greater the pixel bit depth (e.g., 16-bit), the greater the number of shades of gray available for image display. Increasing the number of shades of gray available to display on a digital image improves its contrast resolution.

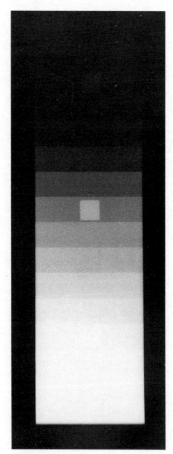

Fig. 9.15 **X-Ray Beam Quality.** Decreasing the kilovoltage creates a high-contrast step wedge image showing fewer gray tones and greater differences between individual brightness levels. (Courtesy Fauber TL: *Radiographic imaging and exposure*, ed 3, St Louis, 2009, Mosby.)

Once the digital image is processed, contrast can be adjusted to vary visualization of the area of interest. This is necessary because the contrast resolution of the human eye is limited. The **window width** is a control that adjusts the contrast. Because the digital image can display grayscale levels ranging from black to white, the display monitor can vary the range or number of brightness levels visible on the image to show all the anatomy. Adjusting the range of brightness levels visible varies the image contrast (Fig. 9.16). When the entire range of brightness levels is displayed (wide window width), the image has lower contrast, or more shades of gray; when a smaller range of brightness levels is displayed (narrow window width), the image has higher contrast, or fewer shades of gray (Fig. 9.17).

The center or midpoint of the window level and the width of the window determine the brightness and contrast of the displayed image (Fig. 9.18).

It is also important to display digital images on a monitor with high luminance to optimally visualize the wide range of gray levels contained within the image.

---

### ! Critical Concept

**Window Width and Image Contrast**

A narrow (decreased) window width increases image contrast, whereas a wider (increased) window width decreases image contrast.

---

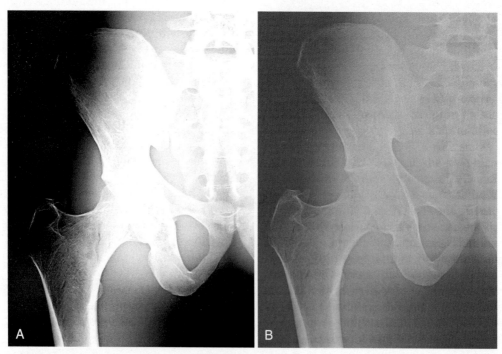

Fig. 9.16 **Contrast Altered by Changing the Window Width. (A)** Radiographic image demonstrating high radiographic contrast (narrow window width). **(B)** Radiographic image demonstrating low radiographic contrast (wide window width).

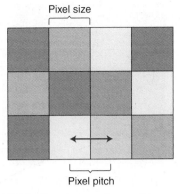

Fig. 9.19 **Pixel Pitch.** The pixel spacing or distance measured from the center of a pixel to an adjacent pixel (pixel pitch) affects the spatial resolution of the digital image.

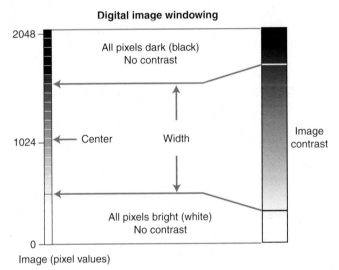

Fig. 9.17 **Window Width.** Changing the window width increases or decreases the range of brightness levels displayed. A narrow window width decreases the range of brightness levels and increases contrast. Wider window width increases the range of brightness levels and reduces radiographic contrast. (Courtesy Kuni C: *Introduction to computers and digital processing in medical imaging*, Chicago, 1988, Year Book Medical Publishers.)

Fig. 9.18 **Windowing.** The level or center of window and the window width changes the visual display of the digital image. (Courtesy Sprawls P: *The physical principles of medical imaging online*, ed 2, http://www.sprawls.org/ppmi2/.)

## SPATIAL RESOLUTION

The quality of a radiographic image depends on both the visibility and the accuracy of the anatomic structural lines (sharpness). Adequate visualization of the anatomic area of interest (brightness and contrast) is just one component of image quality. To produce a quality image, the anatomic structures must be accurately displayed and with the greatest amount of sharpness. **Spatial resolution** is a term used to evaluate accuracy of the anatomic structural lines. A digital image is composed of discrete information in the form of pixels that display various brightness levels. The size of the pixel is measured in microns (100 μm = 0.1 mm). As mentioned previously, the greater the number of pixels in a matrix, the smaller their size. A typical digital radiography (DR) image comprises millions of pixels

with a pixel size of less than 200 μm. For example, a DR image comprising 5 million pixels with a pixel size of 175 μm would produce a spatial resolution of 3 line pairs (Lp)/mm. An image consisting of a greater number of pixels per unit area, or **pixel density**, provides improved spatial resolution. In addition to its size, the pixel spacing, or distance measured from the center of a pixel to an adjacent pixel, determines the **pixel pitch** (Fig. 9.19). A typical DR image may have a pixel pitch of 100 to 150 μm. As matrix size increases, the number of pixels increases, pixel size decreases, and pixel pitch decreases, all of which increases spatial resolution. Characteristics of the digital image receptor affect spatial resolution similarly. As detector element (DEL) matrix size increases, the number of DELs increases, DEL size decreases, and DEL pitch decreases, all of which increases spatial resolution of the displayed image.

Different types of digital image receptors use varying methods of transforming the continuous exit radiation intensities into the array of discrete pixels for image display. Some digital image receptors use a sampling technique, whereas others have fixed detector elements that are used to capture the exit radiation intensities. Regardless of the type used, a major determinant of spatial resolution of digital images is the pixel size and its spacing (Fig. 9.20).

### ! Critical Concept

**Pixel Density and Pitch and Spatial Resolution**

Increasing the pixel density and decreasing the pixel pitch increases spatial resolution. Decreasing pixel density and increasing pixel pitch decreases spatial resolution.

The device used for digital image display also affects the ability to view anatomic structures. High-resolution monitors are required to maximize the amount of spatial resolution viewed in the digital image.

There is a relationship among pixel size, **field of view** (FOV, the dimensions of an anatomic area displayed on

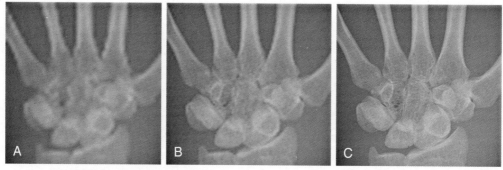

Fig. 9.20 **Images Showing How Pixel Size Affects Spatial Resolution.** **(A)** Image with 20 pixels per cm; therefore, the pixel size is larger and the spatial resolution is poor. **(B)** Image with 40 pixels per cm. **(C)** Image with 100 pixels per cm; therefore, the pixel size is smaller than that in images **(A)** and **(B)** and the spatial resolution is improved. (Courtesy Andrew Woodward.)

the monitor), and matrix size, as demonstrated in the following formula:

$$Pixel\ size = \frac{FOV}{Matrix\ size}$$

This relationship demonstrates that if the FOV displayed on the monitor is increased for a fixed matrix size, then the pixel size is also increased (direct relationship). However, if the matrix size is increased for a fixed FOV, then the pixel size is decreased (inverse relationship).

### 1 2 3 Mathematical Application

**Pixel Size and FOV**

FOV = 17 inches (431.8 mm) and matrix size = 1024:

$$\frac{431.8}{1024} = 0.42\ mm\ pixel\ size$$

If the FOV was decreased to 12 inches (304.8 mm) for the same matrix size of 1024:

$$\frac{304.8}{1024} = 0.30\ mm\ pixel\ size$$

Decreasing the displayed FOV for a given matrix size will decrease the size of the pixels and increase spatial resolution.

### 1 2 3 Mathematical Application

**Pixel Size and Matrix Size**

FOV = 17 inches (431.8 mm) and matrix size = 1024:

$$\frac{431.8}{1024} = 0.42\ mm\ pixel\ size$$

If the matrix size was increased to 2048 for the same FOV:

$$\frac{431.8}{2048} = 0.21\ mm\ pixel\ size$$

Increasing the matrix size for a given FOV displayed will decrease the size of the pixels and increase spatial resolution.

### ! Critical Concept

**Pixel Size, FOV, and Matrix Size**

The pixel size is directly related to the FOV displayed on the monitor and inversely related to matrix size. Increasing the FOV for the same matrix size will increase the size of the pixel and decrease the spatial resolution, whereas increasing the matrix size for the same FOV will decrease the pixel size and increase spatial resolution.

## SPATIAL FREQUENCY AND SPATIAL RESOLUTION

Spatial resolution in digital imaging is primarily limited to the size of the pixel; however, when measuring an imaging system's ability to resolve small objects, it is important to understand the concept of spatial frequency and its relationship with spatial resolution. Anatomic structures are composed of large and small objects, and radiographic images display those structures as variations from white-to-black brightness levels. Small objects have higher spatial frequency and large objects have lower spatial frequency. It is more difficult to accurately image small anatomic objects (high spatial frequency) compared with imaging large ones (low spatial frequency). **Spatial frequency** can be defined by the unit of Lp/mm. A resolution test pattern is a device used to image and measure line pairs (Fig. 9.21). In the space of 1 mm, the number of line pairs resolved determines the amount of sharpness. Each line pair is made up of a line and a space. If 5 Lp/mm were resolved, each line or space measures 0.1 mm and a line pair measures 0.2 mm (Fig. 9.22).

An imaging system that can resolve a greater number of line pairs per millimeter (higher spatial frequency) has increased spatial resolution (Fig. 9.23).

The ability to discern small changes in spatial resolution when viewing radiographic images depends on the viewer's visual acuity and distance from the image.

The imaging process makes it impossible to produce a radiographic image without some degree of unsharpness. A radiographic image that has a greater

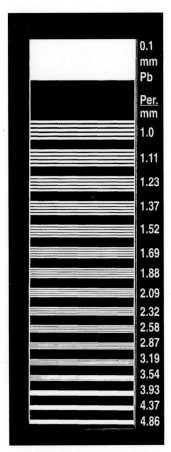

**Fig. 9.21 Resolution Test Pattern.** A resolution test pattern that measures line pairs per millimeter. (Courtesy Fluke Biomedical.)

amount of spatial resolution minimizes the amount of unsharpness of the anatomic structural lines.

Sharpness and visibility of anatomic structures have typically been discussed as two separate qualities of the radiographic image. Generally, this separation remains true except when imaging small anatomic structures. A small anatomic structure is best visualized when its brightness varies significantly from the background. If unsharpness is increased, the visibility of small anatomic structures is compromised. An increase in the amount of unsharpness displayed on the image decreases the contrast of small anatomic structures, reducing the overall visibility of the structural lines. The spreading of the structural lines with increased unsharpness decreases the differences in brightness between the structural lines of the area of interest and the background. As a result, the difference in brightness between the area of interest and the background becomes less (low contrast) and the visibility of the anatomic structure is reduced (Fig. 9.24).

## MODULATION TRANSFER FUNCTION

A radiographic image displays a range of brightness levels (grayscale) based on the variation in radiation intensities exiting the tissue. Anatomic structures are best visualized when the brightness level of the object is different than its surrounding tissue (high radiographic contrast). Larger-sized objects (low spatial frequency) are more easily visualized. As the size of the object decreases, it attains higher spatial frequency and becomes more difficult to visualize in a radiographic image. **Modulation transfer function (MTF)** is a measure of the imaging system's ability to display the radiographic contrast of anatomic objects varying in size, and the value will be between 0 (no difference in brightness levels) and 1.0 (maximum difference in brightness levels). The formula for MTF is as follows:

$$MTF = \frac{(maximum\,intensity - minimum\,intensity)}{(maximum\,intensity + minimum\,intensity)}$$

An MTF of 1 (100% difference) would signify the difference between maximum and minimum brightness. An MTF of 1 is easier to achieve when large objects have low spatial frequency. It is more difficult to visualize smaller objects having high frequency; therefore, most digital imaging systems' MTFs would measure much lower than 1.0.

> **! Critical Concept**
>
> **Modulation Transfer Function (MTF) and Anatomic Structures**
>
> MTF is a measure of the imaging system's ability to accurately display small anatomic objects having high spatial frequency. An imaging system that has a high MTF can display anatomic structures with improved visibility.

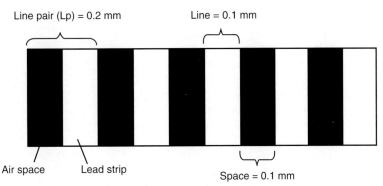

**Fig. 9.22 Line Pairs per Millimeter.** Five line pairs in the space of 1 mm (5 Lp/mm). A line pair includes a line and a space. If 5 Lp/mm are visualized, a line pair measures 0.2 mm, and each line measures 0.1 mm.

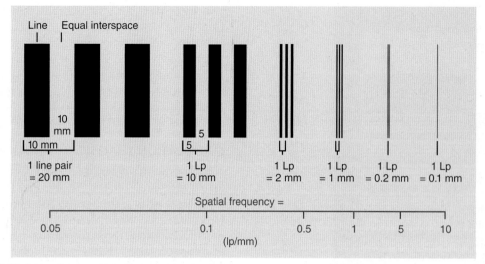

Fig. 9.23 **A Line Pair is a High-Contrast Line Separated by an Interspace of Equal Width.** The spatial frequency is shown for each of the line pairs. (Courtesy Bushong SC: *Radiologic science for technologists,* ed 10, St Louis, 2013, Mosby.)

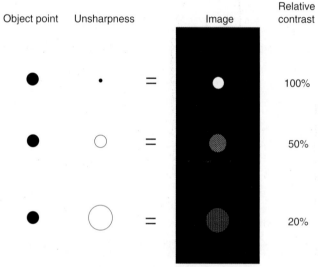

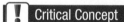

Fig. 9.24 **Unsharpness and Image Contrast.** Increasing the amount of unsharpness decreased the brightness difference (radiographic contrast) between the area of interest and its surrounding background. (Courtesy of Sprawls. *Physical principles of medical imaging online,* ed 2, http://www.sprawls.rg/ppmi2/.)

## DETECTIVE QUANTUM EFFICIENCY

**Detective quantum efficiency** (DQE) is a measurement of the efficiency of an image receptor in converting the x-ray exposure it receives to a quality radiographic image. If an image receptor system is able to convert x-ray exposure into a quality image with 100% efficiency (meaning no information loss), the DQE would measure 100% or 1.0. However, no imaging system has 100% conversion efficiency. Nevertheless, the higher the DQE of a system, the lower the radiation exposure required to produce a quality image, thereby decreasing patient exposure. The system's DQE value is affected by both the type of material used in the image receptor to capture the exit radiation and the energy of the x-ray.

### Critical Concept

**Detective Quantum Efficiency (DQE) and X-Ray Exposure**

An image receptor with a higher DQE requires less x-ray exposure to produce a quality radiographic image compared with an image receptor with a lower DQE value.

A radiographic image cannot be an exact reconstruction of the anatomic structure. Some information is always lost during the process of image formation. In addition, factors such as patient motion increase the amount of unsharpness displayed in the image (Fig. 9.25). Eliminating motion unsharpness is an important skill required of the radiographer. Voluntary

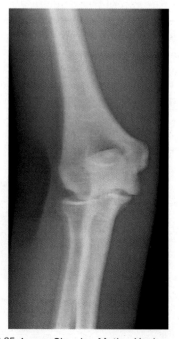

Fig. 9.25 Image Showing Motion Unsharpness.

motion, under the control of the patient, is best alleviated by effective communication. However, some pediatric and elderly patients may have difficulty controlling voluntary motion. Reducing the exposure time and using immobilization devices may be needed in addition to effective communication. Reducing exposure time is the best method to eliminate motion unsharpness for involuntary motion (not under the control of the patient). A less common type of motion unsharpness is a result of equipment malfunction and is more difficult to identify.

It is the radiographer's responsibility to minimize the amount of information lost by manipulating the factors that affect the sharpness of the displayed image. Diagnostic quality is achieved by maximizing the amount of spatial resolution and minimizing the amount of image distortion.

## DISTORTION

**Distortion** results from the radiographic misrepresentation of either the size (magnification) or the shape of the anatomic part. When the image is distorted, spatial resolution is also reduced.

### Size Distortion (Magnification)

The term **size distortion** (or **magnification**) refers to an increase in the image size of an object compared with its true, or actual, size. Radiographic images of objects are always magnified in terms of the true object size. The source-to-image receptor distance (SID) and object-to-image receptor distance (OID) have a geometric relationship and play an important role in minimizing the amount of size distortion of the radiographic image.

Because radiographers produce two-dimensional images of three-dimensional objects, some size distortion always occurs as a result of OID. The parts of the object that are farther away from the image receptor are represented radiographically with more size distortion than parts of the object that are closer to the image receptor. Even if the object is in close contact with the image receptor, some part of the object is farther away from the image receptor than other parts. SID also influences the total amount of magnification on the image. As SID increases, size distortion (magnification) decreases; as SID decreases, size distortion (magnification) increases.

### Shape Distortion

In addition to size distortion, objects that are being imaged can be misrepresented radiographically by distortion of their shape. Shape distortion can appear in two different ways radiographically: elongation or foreshortening. **Elongation** refers to images of objects that appear longer than the true objects. **Foreshortening** refers to images that appear shorter than the true objects. Examples of elongation and foreshortening can be seen in Fig. 9.26.

Shape distortion can occur from inaccurate central ray (CR) alignment of the tube, the part being radiographed, or the image receptor. Any misalignment of

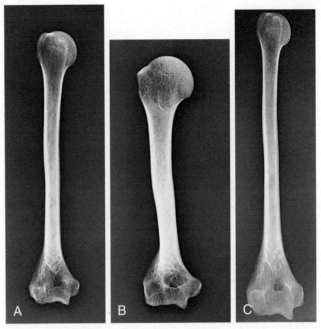

**Fig. 9.26 Shape Distortion. (A)** No distortion. **(B)** Foreshortened. **(C)** Elongated. (Courtesy Mosby's *Instructional radiographic series: radiographic imaging*, St Louis, 1998, Mosby.)

the CR among these three factors—tube, part, or image receptor—alters the shape of the part displayed in the image.

Sometimes shape distortion is used to an advantage, in particular with projections or positions. For example, CR angulation is sometimes required to elongate a curved part so that a particular anatomic structure can be better visualized (for example, an anteroposterior projection of the sacrum). Also, rotating the part (and therefore creating shape distortion) is sometimes required to eliminate superimposition of objects that normally obstruct visualization of the area of interest (for example, the internal rotation oblique projection of the foot). In general, shape distortion is not a necessary or desirable characteristic of radiographic images.

Both SID and OID determine the amount of magnification of the anatomic structures on the image. In addition, improper alignment of the CR, anatomic part, image receptor, or a combination of these components distorts the shape of the image. The factors that affect size and shape distortion are discussed in more detail in Chapter 11.

## SCATTER

Scatter radiation, as described previously, can add unwanted exposure to the radiographic image as a result of Compton interactions. Unwanted exposure or fog on the image does not provide information about the anatomic area of interest. Scatter degrades or decreases the visibility of the anatomic structures. The scatter or unwanted exposure displayed on the image decreases radiographic contrast by masking the desired brightness on the image and changing the degree of differences (Fig. 9.27).

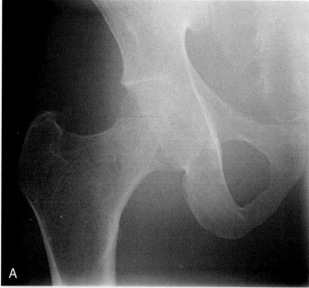

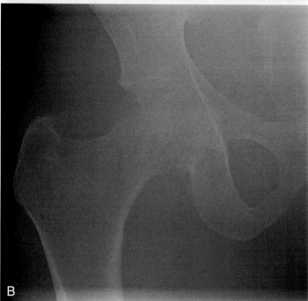

Fig. 9.27 **Scatter.** Scatter degrades or decreases the visibility of the anatomic structures. **(A)** Image created with less scatter compared with image **(B)**, created with increased scatter. (Courtesy Johnston JN, Fauber TL: *Essentials of radiographic physics and imaging*, ed 3, St Louis, 2020, Elsevier, Inc.)

### Make the Physics Connection

#### Chapter 7

Compton scattering is one of the most prevalent interactions between x-ray photons and the human body in general diagnostic imaging and is responsible for most of the scatter that fogs the image. The probability of Compton scattering does not depend on the atomic number of atoms involved. Compton scattering may occur in both soft tissue and bone. The probability of Compton scattering is related to the energy of the photon. As x-ray photon energy increases, the probability of that photon penetrating a given tissue without interaction increases. However, with this increase in photon energy, the likelihood of Compton interactions relative to photoelectric interactions also increases.

Fog produced because of scatter reaching the image receptor can be visualized on a digital image. Even though the computer can change the radiographic contrast or gray levels displayed in the digital image, scatter radiation reaching the image receptor does not provide any information about the area of interest. Because digital image receptors can detect low levels of radiation intensity, they are more sensitive to scatter radiation.

 **Critical Concept**

**Scatter and Digital Image Receptors**

Because digital image receptors can detect low levels of radiation intensity, they are sensitive to scatter radiation's effect (fog) on the digital image.

There are multiple factors that affect the amount of scatter reaching the image receptor. These factors along with controlling scatter are discussed more thoroughly in Chapter 12.

### NOISE

Image noise contributes no useful diagnostic information and serves only to detract from the quality of the image. Quantum noise (mottle), a concern in digital imaging, is photon-dependent. **Quantum noise** is visible as brightness fluctuations (graininess) on the image Fig. 9.28. The fewer the photons reaching the image receptor to form the image, the greater the quantum noise visible on the digital image. It is important to minimize the amount of quantum noise (mottle) on a radiographic image.

### SIGNAL-TO-NOISE RATIO

**Signal-to-noise ratio (SNR)** is a method of describing the strength or amount of the radiation exposure compared with the amount of noise apparent in a digital image. Image noise is a concern with any electronic digital image. Because the photon intensities are converted to an electronic signal that is digitized, the term *signal* refers to the strength or amount of radiation exposure captured by the image receptor (IR) to create the image. Increasing the SNR improves the quality of the digital image; this means that the strength of the signal is high in comparison with the amount of noise, and therefore image quality is improved. However, when the signal (amount of radiation exposure) is increased to improve image quality, patient exposure is also increased. Radiographers usually increase mAs to increase SNR, and mAs has a direct effect on patient exposure. Decreasing the SNR means there is increased noise compared with the strength of the signal, and therefore, the quality of the radiographic image is degraded. Quantum noise results when there are too few x-ray photons captured by the IR to create a latent image. In addition to quantum noise, sources of noise

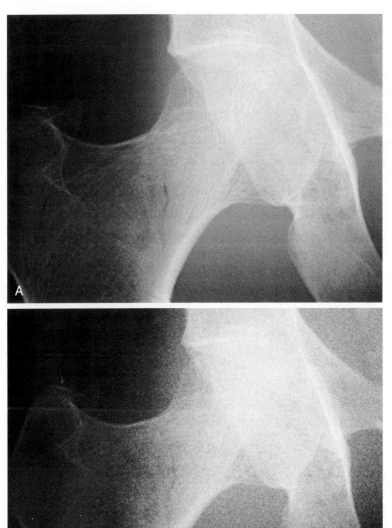

Fig. 9.28 **Quantum Noise. (A)** Image created using an appropriate x-ray exposure technique. **(B)** Image shows increased quantum noise as a result of insufficient x-ray exposure to the image receptor. (Courtesy Fauber TL: *Radiographic imaging and exposure*, ed 3, St Louis, 2009, Mosby.)

include the electronics that capture, process, and display the digital image.

The SNR affects the ability to visualize anatomic structures. Noise interferes with the signal strength just as background static would interfere with the clarity of music heard. When the digital image displays increased noise, regardless of the source, anatomic structures have decreased visibility.

> **! Critical Concept**
>
> **Signal-to-Noise Ratio, Image Quality, and Patient Exposure**
>
> Increasing the SNR increases the visibility of anatomic structures (improved image quality) but with increased patient exposure, whereas decreasing the SNR decreases the visibility of anatomic structures (decreased image quality) with decreased patient exposure.

## CONTRAST-TO-NOISE RATIO

**Contrast-to-noise ratio (CNR)** is a method of describing the contrast resolution compared with the amount of noise apparent in a digital image. Just as increased noise affects SNR and the visibility of anatomic structures, it also affects the radiographic contrast displayed within the digital image. Brightness differences in the digital image are a result of varying exit-radiation intensities from the attenuation of the x-ray beam in anatomic tissue (differential absorption). As previously stated, digital imaging systems have higher contrast resolution. A system with higher contrast resolution means that anatomic tissues that attenuate the x-ray beam similarly (low subject contrast) can be better visualized. However, if the image has increased noise, the low subject contrast tissues will not be as well visualized. Digital

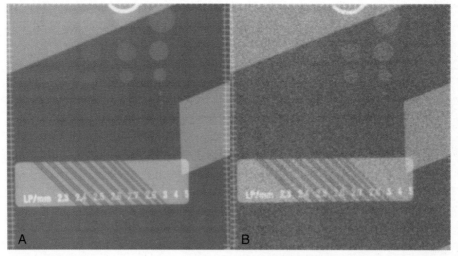

Fig. 9.29 **Contrast-to-Noise Ratio. (A)** Image of a contrast detail phantom showing an increased contrast-to-noise ratio. Phantom objects are more visible. **(B)** Image of contrast detail phantom showing a decreased contrast-to-noise ratio. Phantom objects are less visible. (Courtesy Andrew Woodward.)

images with a higher CNR will increase the visibility of anatomic tissues (see Fig. 9.29).

 **Critical Concept**

**Contrast-to-Noise Ratio and Image Quality**

Increasing the CNR increases the visibility of anatomic structures, whereas decreasing the CNR decreases the visibility of anatomic structures.

## IMAGE ARTIFACTS

An **artifact** is any unwanted brightness level on a radiographic image. Artifacts are detrimental to images because they can make visibility of anatomy, a pathologic condition, or patient identification information difficult or even impossible. They decrease the overall quality of the radiographic image.

Errors such as double exposing an image receptor, or the improper use of equipment, can result in image artifacts and must be avoided. Foreign bodies are a source of artifacts imaged within the patient's body. Variation in exposure techniques may be necessary when imaging for a suspected foreign body, including a decrease in mAs or kVp.

Artifacts from patient clothing and items imaged that are not a part of the area of interest are handled the same regardless of the type of imaging system. The radiographer must be diligent in removing clothing or items that could obstruct visibility of the anatomic area of interest (Fig. 9.30). Scatter radiation (or fog) and image noise have also been classified as radiographic artifacts because they add unwanted information on the displayed image.

Digital imaging artifacts occur for various reasons and generally have a bright or dark appearance. The complexity of the electronics involved in creating the digital image often make it difficult to isolate the cause of the problem. Digital image artifacts can be a result of errors during extraction of the latent image from the image receptor,

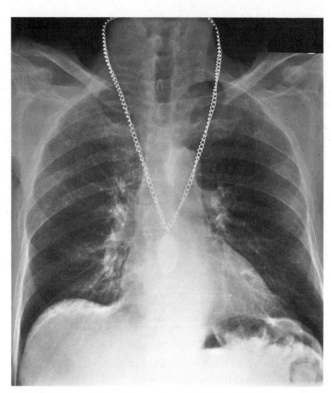

Fig. 9.30 **Image Artifact.** (From Long B, Rollins J, Smith B: *Merrill's Atlas of Radiographic Positioning and Procedures*, ed 13, St Louis, 2016, Mosby.)

inadequate IR erasure, or performance of the electronic detectors. Fig. 9.31 shows examples of image artifacts.

Regardless of the image receptor type, the radiographer must select the required exposure factors to produce a quality radiographic image. In addition, accurate positioning of the patient for a variety of projections remains a critical part of the imaging process. Various accessory devices such as grids and collimators are used to improve the quality of the image. Exposure technique factors and selection as well as accessory devices will be discussed in more detail in subsequent chapters.

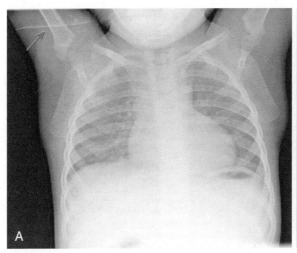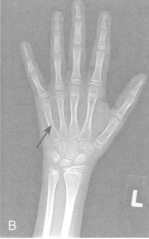

**Fig. 9.31  Digital Image Artifacts. (A)** Bright lines in the shoulder region as a result of scratches on the imaging plate. **(B)** Bright specks between the fourth and fifth metacarpals as a result of dirt on the image plate. (Courtesy Andrew Woodward.)

## On the Spot

- A good-quality radiographic image accurately represents the anatomic area of interest, and its information is well visualized for diagnosis.
- *Visibility factors* refer to the visibility of the anatomic structures, and *sharpness factors* refer to the accuracy of their structural lines displayed in the radiographic image.
- A radiographic image must have sufficient brightness to permit visualization of the anatomic structures of interest.
- Digital image receptors have a wide dynamic range and can accurately detect very low-exposure intensities and very high-exposure intensities.
- The exposure indicator provides a numeric value indicating the level of radiation exposure to the digital image receptor.
- Digital imaging systems can adjust for exposure technique errors, but poor image quality or increased patient exposure may result.
- The window level controls image brightness by manipulating the midpoint of the range of brightness levels visible in the image.
- Image contrast is a result of tissue differential absorption of the x-ray beam and makes anatomic structures visible.
- The pixel bit depth determines the number of shades of gray the digital image can display.
- The larger the bit depth, the greater the number of shades of gray displayed to improve image quality.
- Contrast resolution determines the level of visibility of small objects having similar shades of gray.
- The window width adjusts the grayscale to display the level of contrast. Increasing the (wider) window width will decrease the contrast displayed in the digital image. Decreasing the (narrow) window width will increase the contrast displayed in the digital image.
- Differences in tissue thickness, tissue density, and effective atomic number, along with the quality of the x-ray beam, contribute to subject contrast.
- A digital image consisting of a greater number of smaller pixels (with a smaller pixel pitch) will improve spatial resolution.
- Spatial resolution is an expression of the imaging system's ability to distinguish between two adjacent structures and can be measured in line pairs per millimeter.
- Small objects have higher spatial frequency and large objects have lower spatial frequency.
- Modulation transfer function (MTF) is a measure of the imaging system's ability to accurately display small anatomic objects having high spatial frequency. An imaging system with a high MTF can display anatomic structures with improved visibility.
- Detective quantum efficiency (DQE) is a measurement of the efficiency of an image receptor in converting the x-ray exposure it receives to a quality radiographic image. The higher the DQE of a system, the lower the radiation exposure required to produce a quality image; therefore, patient exposure is decreased.
- Distortion results from the misrepresentation of either the size (magnification) or shape of the anatomic part and should be minimized to improve radiographic quality.
- Reducing image unsharpness is achieved by maximizing the amount of spatial resolution and minimizing the amount of distortion of the image.
- Shape distortion can appear radiographically as elongation or foreshortening.
- Scatter radiation provides unwanted exposure or fog on the image and does not provide information about the anatomic area of interest.
- Quantum noise is visible as brightness fluctuations on the image and contributes no useful information.
- SNR is a method of describing the strength of the radiation exposure compared with the amount of noise apparent in a digital image. When the digital image displays increased noise, regardless of the source, anatomic structures will have decreased visibility.
- CNR is a method of describing the contrast resolution compared with the amount of noise apparent in a digital image. Digital images with a higher CNR will increase the visibility of anatomic tissues.
- Image artifacts are detrimental to radiographs and should be avoided.

## CRITICAL THINKING QUESTIONS

1. Why does the visibility of anatomic tissue depend on the image's brightness and radiographic contrast?
2. How does anatomic tissue composition affect beam attenuation and subsequently the radiographic contrast produced after processing?
3. Why does a good-quality radiographic image also depend on its spatial resolution and distortion?
4. How do the effects of quantum noise, scatter, and artifacts affect the quality of radiographic images?

## REVIEW QUESTIONS

1. A quality radiograph must include:
   a. accuracy of structural lines displayed.
   b. minimal unsharpness.
   c. visibility of anatomic structures.
   d. all of the above.
2. Visibility factors of a quality radiograph include:
   a. brightness.
   b. spatial resolution.
   c. contrast.
   d. a and c.
3. Which of the following results in a poor-quality digital image because of improper processing due to extreme over exposure to the image receptor?
   a. Distortion
   b. Saturation
   c. Quantum noise
   d. Modulation transfer function
4. What feature provides a numeric value indicating the level of radiation exposure to the digital image receptor?
   a. Exposure indicator
   b. Saturation
   c. Pixel density
   d. Grayscale
5. Anatomic tissues that attenuate the x-ray beam equally are said to have:
   a. quantum noise.
   b. high contrast.
   c. low subject contrast.
   d. less unsharpness.
6. An imaging system that can resolve 10 Lp/mm instead of 6 Lp/mm is said to have:
   a. less distortion.
   b. more unsharpness.
   c. more distortion.
   d. improved sharpness.
7. Unwanted scatter exposure to the image receptor will likely increase:
   a. unsharpness.
   b. brightness.
   c. fog.
   d. saturation.
8. What is defined as "The range of exposure intensities an image receptor can accurately detect"?
   a. Resolution
   b. Contrast
   c. Window level
   d. Dynamic range
9. For a given field of view (FOV), a _____ matrix size will result in _____ pixels.
   a. large, fewer
   b. large, more
   c. small, more
   d. none of the above
10. In digital imaging, which of the following determines the range of grayscale available for display?
    a. Pixel density
    b. Matrix size
    c. Pixel bit depth
    d. Exposure indicator
11. During digital image display, the contrast can be lowered (decreased) by increasing _____.
    a. pixel density
    b. grayscale
    c. window level
    d. window width
12. The ability of the imaging system to distinguish between small objects that attenuate the x-ray beam similarly defines:
    a. dynamic range.
    b. grayscale.
    c. insufficient detective quantum efficiency.
    d. contrast resolution.
13. Increasing the displayed field of view (FOV) for a fixed matrix size will result in:
    a. decreased pixel pitch.
    b. increased pixel size.
    c. decreased pixel size.
    d. increased pixel bit depth.
14. The visibility of anatomic structures is increased with:
    a. increased contrast-to-noise ratio (CNR).
    b. increased quantum noise.
    c. increased signal-to-noise ratio (SNR)
    d. a and c only.
15. An imaging system with a higher detective quantum efficiency (DQE):
    a. is more efficient in converting x-ray exposure to a quality image.
    b. produces images with decreased spatial resolution.
    c. can display anatomic structures with less distortion.
    d. produces images with decreased contrast resolution.
16. Double exposing an image receptor will likely result in:
    a. pixel pitch.
    b. foreshortening.
    c. increased quantum noise.
    d. image artifact.

# Digital Image Receptors

## Outline

## Objectives

- Describe the design of computed radiography detectors.
- Describe the design of direct radiography detectors.
- Explain the process of image acquisition using computed radiography detectors.
- Explain the process of image acquisition using the three general types of direct radiography detectors.
- Explain the process of image extraction and processing for computed radiography and direct radiography systems.

- Describe digital image display and postprocessing functions.
- Explain the use of exposure indicators for computed radiography systems and dose-area products for direct radiography systems.
- Identify quality control tests and test patterns used with digital systems.
- Describe the Picture Archiving and Communication System, including its role, principal systems, and challenges.

## Key Terms

bit depth
cassette
charge-coupled device (CCD)
complementary metal oxide semiconductor (CMOS)
computed radiography (CR)
detective quantum efficiency (DQE)
detector array
diffusion
Digital Imaging and Communications
   in Medicine (DICOM)
digital radiography (DR)

direct radiography (DR)
dose-area product (DAP)
dynamic range
exposure indicator
exposure latitude
histogram analysis
latent image
luminescence
manifest image
modulation transfer function (MTF)
photoconductor
photodetector

photostimulable luminescence
photostimulable phosphor (PSP)
   plate
Picture Archiving and Communication
   System (PACS)
plate reader
teleradiology
thin-film transistor (TFT)
values of interest (VOI)
x-ray scintillator

## INTRODUCTION

This chapter covers digital detectors as image receptors. Radiography is the last of the medical imaging modalities to make this transition to digital technology.

As digital radiography advances, new and experienced radiographers alike must learn a few new concepts and practices. But it is equally important they learn what remains the same. Digital receptors bring many benefits to medical imaging, but they also bring challenges as to how to use them in the best interest of the patient and the profession.

## DIGITAL RECEPTORS

Digital imaging is not a new concept. Computed tomography, sonography, nuclear medicine, and magnetic resonance imaging, for example, have been digital for some time in that they display the initial image on a computer monitor. Digital radiography may be divided into two groups by the digital receptor type. Digital receptors may either be **computed radiography (CR)** or **digital radiography (DR)**. Computed radiography systems are those that use storage phosphors to temporarily store energy representing the image

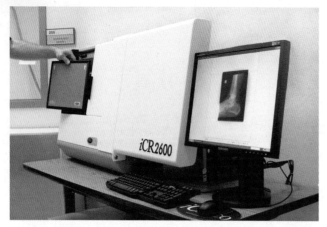

Fig. 10.1 **Computed Radiography Reader, Cassette, and Viewing Station.** Desktop computed radiography reader and viewing station. The cassette is placed in the reader, which removes and scans the plate, clears it, and returns it to the cassette.

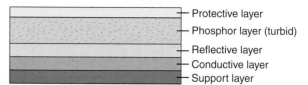

Fig. 10.2 **Cross-Section of a PSP Plate.**

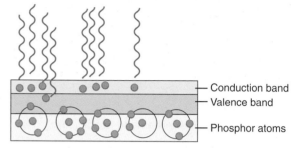

Fig. 10.3 **Phosphor Layers of a PSP Plate During Exposure.**

signal. The phosphor then undergoes a process to extract the latent image. Digital radiography systems have detectors that capture (directly or indirectly) and read out an electronic image signal. Generally, CR systems use a cassette as a container for the **photostimulable phosphor (PSP) plate** and a reader and will be described fully here. Broadly speaking, internally contained digital systems may be CR or DR technology. The radiographer should be aware of the type of equipment they are working with to fully understand the piece of equipment and image formation process to use it to its best advantage.

## DETECTOR TYPES

### Computed Radiography Systems

When first introduced, CR systems (Fig. 10.1) were attractive because they could be integrated with existing radiographic equipment without physical modification of the x-ray unit itself. The primary components of a typical CR system are the cassette, the PSP plate that goes inside the cassette, the **plate reader**, and a computer workstation. PSP technology may also be built into a larger device and incorporated into the Bucky system. The PSP and image extraction process described in the following paragraphs is essentially the same for all versions of CR. The difference is how the plate is moved from the exposure area to the processing area.

The **cassette**, made of a lightweight plastic, is simply a container for the PSP plate. The inside of the cassette is lined with a felt material to prevent static buildup and dust collection. The backing, a sheet of aluminum to absorb x-rays that penetrate the plate, reduces the amount of backscatter radiation that strikes the plate.

The PSP plate is made up of several layers as follows (Fig. 10.2). The protective layer is a thin layer of plastic to protect the phosphor layer. The phosphor layer is the heart of the plate and contains the phosphor, which is usually of the barium fluorohalide family and europium activated. The phosphor may be either a turbid or

structured phosphor layer. A turbid phosphor has a random distribution of phosphor crystals within the active layer and can be used with both CR and DR systems. A structured phosphor layer has columnar phosphor crystals within the active layer that resemble needles standing on end and packed together. The reflective layer reflects light released during the reading phase toward the photodetector. The conductive layer reduces and conducts away static electricity. The color layer may be in some newer plates to absorb stimulating light and reflect emitted light. The support layer is a sturdy material to give some rigidity to the plate. Finally, the soft backing layer protects the back of the plate.

An understanding of how the plate responds to x-ray exposure is necessary before the reader can be described. When the PSP plate is exposed to x-rays, some electrons are removed from the phosphor atoms, and approximately 50% of those liberated are trapped in the conduction band (Fig. 10.3). The conduction band is an energy level just beyond the valence band (the outermost energy band of an atom). The remainder returns immediately and emits the excess energy as light (stimulated light). Europium is a silvery rare earth metal used as an activator for the phosphor. The role of europium is to capture some of the energy in the interaction process. The europium-activated barium fluorohalide of the phosphor layer emits some light immediately in response to x-ray stimulus. But because of the presence of europium, it will also store some of the x-ray energy as the latent image. The quantity and distribution of the liberated electrons are proportional to the x-ray exposure received in each particular area of the plate. The liberated electrons remain trapped in the conduction band for hours (although deterioration begins immediately); these trapped electrons represent the **latent image**. At the time of processing, the energy of these trapped electrons is released by exposure to a laser in a process called **photostimulable luminescence**. The reader processes the PSP plate.

### Photostimulable Phosphor Plate Response

When the PSP plate is exposed to x-rays, phosphor atoms are ionized. Approximately half of the removed electrons are "trapped" in the conduction band. The quantity and distribution are proportional to exposure and represent the latent image. When the PSP plate is exposed to the laser of the reader, the energy is released and converted to a digital signal, becoming a visible image.

The reader design may vary somewhat from one vendor to the next but generally has the same major components. A drive mechanism moves the plate through the laser-scanning process. An optical system comprising a laser, beam-shaping optics, light-collecting optics, and optical filters is designed to project and guide a precisely controlled laser beam back and forth across the plate as the plate moves through the scan area. (In some systems, the plate is stationary and the laser and optical system move.) A **photodetector** is used to sense the light released from the PSP plate during scanning. The photodetector amplifies this light, but it is in an analog electronic signal form. To make it digital, this amplified signal is sent to an analog-to-digital converter (ADC) that converts it to a digital electronic signal. Finally, a computer is used to process and display the image.

To summarize this process, the PSP plate is exposed to x-ray energy and many electrons are trapped in the

conduction bands as a latent image. When the cassette is inserted into the reader, the plate is removed and fed into the scanning area at a controlled and precise speed. As the plate moves forward, a laser beam is projected onto the phosphor layer. The laser energy releases the trapped electrons from the conduction band. As these electrons return to their respective valence shells, the excess energy is given off as spontaneous light energy. This light energy is directed to the photodetector via a fiber-optic bundle or a solid, light-conducting material. The photodetector sends this light to the ADC, where it is converted to a digital electronic signal that is sent to the computer for processing and display. The computer's role in this process is discussed later in this chapter.

### Direct Radiography Systems

With **DR**, a **detector array** (Fig. 10.4) replaces what historically was the Bucky assembly. With these systems, the image-forming radiation is captured and transferred to a computer from the detector array for almost instant viewing at the control panel. The two general categories of DR systems are referred to as *indirect capture* and *direct capture*.

Currently, there are two forms of indirect capture. One uses a **charge-coupled device (CCD)** (Fig. 10.5), an **x-ray scintillator**, and optics. The CCD is a light-sensitive device first developed by the military that has since been incorporated into digital cameras and other applications. The CCD is very light sensitive and can respond to very low light intensities. It also has a wide dynamic range and can respond to a wide range of light intensities. The scintillator for this form of indirect capture is a cesium iodide phosphor plate. A scintillator is a material that absorbs x-ray energy and emits visible light in response. Cesium iodide is a hygroscopic material (it readily absorbs moisture) that must be hermetically sealed to avoid water absorption and prevent rapid degradation but is otherwise a high-efficiency scintillation material. The cesium iodide phosphor plate may be coupled to the CCD using either a fiber-optic bundle or an optical lens system.

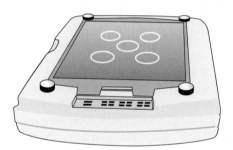

**Fig. 10.4 Digital Radiography System Detector Assembly.** The detector assembly replaces the Bucky tray and cassettes and serves as the image receptor.

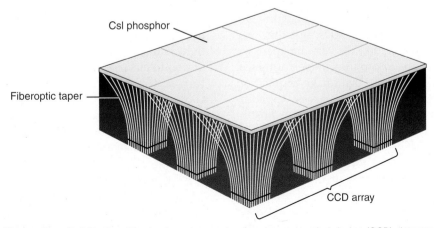

**Fig. 10.5 Charge-Coupled Device.** The basic components of a charge-coupled device (CCD) detector array. The cesium iodide (CsI) phosphor plate is connected to the CCD array using fiber-optic bundles.

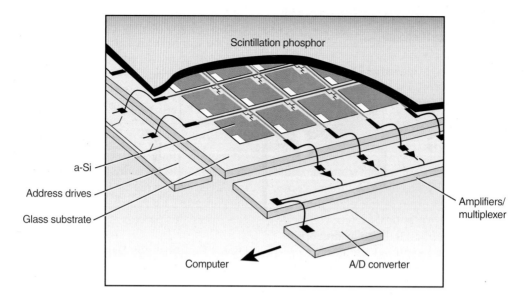

**Fig. 10.6 Thin-Film Transistor Array.** This cutaway view of the thin-film transistor (TFT) array reveals the detector elements, consisting of a photodetector and a TFT layered on a glass substrate.

With this form of indirect capture, x-rays are absorbed by the scintillator and converted to light. This light energy is then transmitted to the CCD, where it is converted to an electronic signal and sent to the computer workstation for processing and display. Because there are currently technical limits to how large a single CCD device can be, an x-ray receptor may consist of an array of closely spaced CCDs. One challenge of this design is the seams at which the CCDs are joined (called *tiling* or *tiled*). Tiling is a process in which several CCD detectors abut to create one larger detector. This process results in seams with unequal response. This is addressed with computer correction software that interpolates (averages) the pixel values along the seams (termed flat-field correction), in effect making the seams disappear.

Serving a similar purpose as the CCD is the **complementary metal oxide semiconductor (CMOS).** CMOS devices are scintillators made up of a crystalline silicon matrix. Each detector element has its own amplifier, photodiode, and storage capacitor and is surrounded by transistors. CMOS devices do not have quite the light sensitivity or resolution of CCDs, but they use a fraction of the power to run, are very inexpensive to manufacture, and are improving in performance. The newest versions have very fast image acquisition times because of their random pixel access capabilities. This feature also makes for automatic exposure control functions that are not as easy to achieve with CCDs. Creation of CMOS detectors of sufficient size for general radiography have not been available, but this is changing. Recent advances in CMOS technology, particularly the creation of crystal light tubes that prevent light spread and methods for increasing their size, make them future possibilities. They are currently options for mammography and dental radiography machines, and their quality and performance continues to improve.

The other indirect capture method also uses a scintillator with cesium iodide or gadolinium oxysulfide as the phosphor, photodetectors, and a **thin-film transistor (TFT)** array. As a scintillator, gadolinium oxysulfide is also a high-efficiency material but with significantly more light spread than cesium iodide. The photodetector is generally an amorphous silicon photodiode. Amorphous silicon, a liquid that can be painted onto a substrate (the foundation or underlying layer), is the material that makes flat-panel detectors possible. Earlier semiconductor technology required a single-crystal structure, which limited the size of the electrical component to the size of the crystal. The final component is the TFT array. TFTs are electronic components layered onto a glass substrate that include the readout, charge collector, and light-sensitive elements. The panel is configured into a network of pixels (or detector elements [DELs]) covered by the scintillator plate, with each pixel containing a photodetector and a TFT (Fig. 10.6). With this form of indirect capture, x-ray energy is absorbed by the scintillator and converted to light energy. This light is then absorbed by the photodetectors and converted to electric charges. These electric charges are in turn captured and transmitted by the TFT array to the computer workstation for processing and display.

> ## ! Critical Concept
>
> ### DR Indirect-Capture Methods
>
> DR indirect-capture methods capture the remnant beam through a detector array and transfer it to a computer for almost immediate processing and viewing. The DR indirect-capture methods both involve the use of a scintillator that converts x-rays to light and then to an electronic signal. This process results in some loss of resolution.

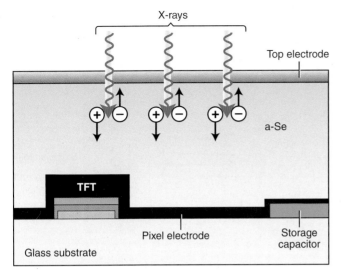

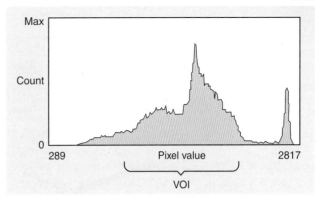

Fig. 10.8 **Histogram.** Example of a histogram representing an image data set. The x-axis represents the amount of exposure and the y-axis the incidence of pixels for each exposure level. Note that the values of interest are indicated by the bracket.

Fig. 10.7 **Direct-Capture Array.** Cross-section of the components of a direct-capture array.

One problem with the indirect-capture methods is that there is an extra step during which x-rays are converted to light and then to electrons, which causes a loss of resolution. The direct-capture method avoids the extra step and the problem by not using a scintillator. Instead it uses a **photoconductor** and a TFT array (Fig. 10.7). The photoconductor is amorphous selenium, and the TFT is the same as described previously. Amorphous selenium layers have the same single-crystal layer structure across short distances but are less ordered across larger distances, thereby providing uniform x-ray detection ability across the large surface areas needed by flat-panel detectors. This detector design is also layered. The top layer is a bias electrode (with a dielectric layer), followed by the amorphous selenium, and then the TFTs connected to storage capacitors. Before exposure, an electric field is applied through the bias electrode across the surface of the amorphous selenium layer. Once exposure begins, x-rays are absorbed by the amorphous selenium and electric charges are created in proportion to the x-ray exposure received. Under the influence of the electric field, the charges migrate toward the TFT array. These charges are stored in the storage capacitors, where they are amplified and converted to digital code by the underlying electronics. The TFTs then read the signal and transmit it to the computer workstation for processing and display.

 **Critical Concept**

**DR Direct-Capture Method**

The DR direct-capture method does not use a scintillator. Rather, it uses a photoconductor and TFT array, thereby avoiding the loss of resolution caused by indirect capture.

## IMAGE ACQUISITION, EXTRACTION AND PROCESSING, AND DISPLAY

### ACQUISITION

During image acquisition the computer creates a histogram (Fig. 10.8). A histogram is a graphic representation

of a data set. This graph represents the number of digital pixel values versus the relative prevalence of those values in the image. The x-axis represents the amount of exposure and the y-axis the incidence of pixels for each exposure level. The computer then analyzes the histogram using processing algorithms and compares it to a preestablished histogram specific to the anatomic part being imaged. This process is called **histogram analysis.** The computer software has histogram models for all menu choices. These stored histogram models have **values of interest (VOI)** and determine what section of the histogram data set should be included in the displayed image. During this process of "recognition," the computer identifies the exposure field and the edges of the image, and all exposure data outside this field are excluded from the histogram. Ideally, all four edges of a collimated field are recognized. If at least three edges are not identified, then all data, including raw exposure or scatter outside the field, may be included in the histogram, resulting in a histogram analysis error. This is discussed in greater detail shortly. More specifically, this is a description of the *a priori* model of histogram analysis. The other method of analysis is the neural analysis model, which determines optimal minimum and maximum VOI locations. The method used affects how the image displays.

 **Critical Concept**

**Digital Image Acquisition**

With digital systems, the computer creates a histogram of the data set. The data set is the exposure received to the pixel elements and the prevalence of those exposures within the image. This created histogram is compared with a stored histogram model for that anatomic part; VOI are identified and the image is displayed.

### EXTRACTION AND PROCESSING

Image extraction for CR systems is discussed first. Recall that when the PSP plate is exposed to x-rays, phosphor atoms are ionized and the liberated electrons are trapped in the conduction band and represent the

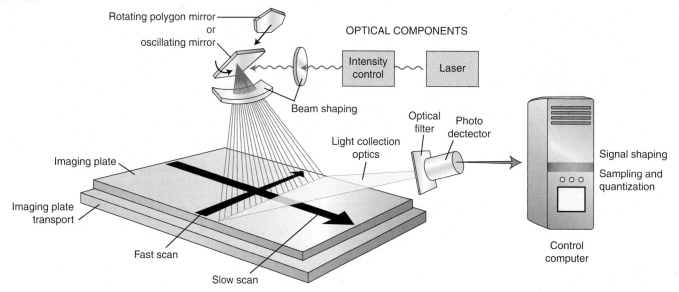

Fig. 10.9 **Cassette Reader Operation.** The general steps of a computed radiographic scanning process.

latent image. When the plate is processed, it is removed from the cassette by the reader and moved through the scanning area at a very precise speed by the drive system (Fig. 10.9). This movement through the reader is called a "slow scan." As the plate moves through the reader, it is exposed to a laser that sweeps back and forth across the plate, releasing the trapped electrons. The laser is deflected back and forth by a rotating polygon or oscillating mirrors and blanked on each retrace. This scanning movement by the laser is called a "fast scan." The scanning of the plate must be very precise to avoid image artifacts. The tolerance is a fraction of a pixel.

As the electrons that have been liberated by the laser return to their shells, they release excess energy as light. This light is directed to the photodetector via a fiber-optic bundle or a solid, light-conducting material. The photodetector then amplifies the light energy and converts it to an electronic analog signal. This signal is then passed through an ADC, where it is digitized. As the analog signal is digitized, it is divided into a matrix or series of squares; each square is a picture element called a *pixel*. The distance between the center of one pixel and the center of an adjacent pixel is called *pixel pitch* and is measured in microns. The *detector size* or *field of view* describes the useful imaging area of the digital receptor. The size of the matrix determines the resolution: the larger the matrix, the greater the number of pixels (because each pixel is smaller), the smaller the pixel pitch, and the greater the resolution. Sampling is a time-based event of the signal that is being sent from the photodetector to the ADC. The scanning of the plate results in a continuous signal being sent to the photodetector and onto the ADC for sampling and quantization. The sampling occurs along the extracted signal. The closer the samples are to each other, the greater the sampling frequency. The *sampling frequency* is the frequency at which a data sample is acquired from the

detector and is expressed as sampling pitch. *Sampling pitch* describes how digital detectors sample the x-ray exposure. They do so discretely—that is, at specific locations separated by specific intervals. For CR systems, the sampling pitch is the distance between laser beam positions during processing of the plate, and for DR systems it is the distance between adjacent DELs.

The image is digitized by both location (spatial resolution) and intensity (grayscale) of each part of the signal. Grayscale is assigned during the process of digitizing the image. **Bit depth**, or number of bits, is the available grayscale and refers to the number of shades of gray that can be displayed within a pixel. Bit depth is determined by the analog-to-digital converter, which is an integral component of every digital imaging system. DR and CR systems have bit depths of up to $2^{14}$ or 16,384 shades of gray. The number of photons detected within a given pixel determines the shade of gray it displays; the greater the number of photons, the darker the shade of gray. In addition, the greater the bit depth of the digital system, the more shades of gray available to display the attenuated anatomic tissue. The computer of the CR reader is in control of the entire process and transmits the image data through a series of steps to create the displayed image.

> ### ! Critical Concept
>
> #### CR Image Extraction
>
> In CR systems, the image is stored in the plate and "extracted" when the plate is exposed to the laser of the reader. The energy liberated by the reader is passed through an ADC, in which it is digitized. The digitized signal is converted to a matrix and assigned grayscale values.

In DR systems, there are two indirect capture methods and one direct capture method. One indirect method uses a cesium iodide phosphor plate as the scintillator coupled to a CCD by a fiber-optic bundle or by optical lenses. The x-ray energy is absorbed by the scintillator and converted to light. The light is transmitted to the CCD, and an electronic signal is created. This analog signal is passed through an ADC, in which it is digitized in the manner described previously. The use of a CMOS system follows the same steps and would be used in place of the CCD. The other indirect method uses either a cesium iodide or gadolinium oxysulfide scintillator, which is coupled to a photodetector, usually an amorphous silicon photodiode, and a TFT. The panel is configured as a network of pixels, with each pixel containing a photodetector and a TFT. With this system, the x-rays are absorbed by the scintillator and converted to light. The light is absorbed by the photodetectors and converted to an analog electronic signal that is collected by the DELs and then digitized by an ADC, as described previously.

The direct capture method does not use a scintillator. With this approach, an amorphous selenium photoconductor and a TFT array are used. Before exposure, an electric field is applied via the bias electrode across the surface of the amorphous selenium layer. During exposure, x-rays are absorbed by the amorphous selenium, and electric charges are created in proportion to the x-ray exposure received. These charges are stored in the storage capacitors attached to the TFTs, where they are amplified and converted to digital code by the underlying electronics. The TFTs first read the signal and then pass it through an ADC, as described previously.

From this point, all three DR systems go through the same basic image-forming steps previously described: A histogram is created and analyzed, the exposure field is recognized and the histogram analysis occurs, and finally automatic rescaling takes place. During automatic rescaling, the computer adjusts the image based on the comparison of the histograms, which is actually a process of mapping the grayscale to the VOI to present a specific display of brightness. This process is what the radiographer would recognize as the system automatically correcting for over- or underexposure. With these systems, only those detector pixels that received x-ray exposure contribute to the image.

## DISPLAY

The display of a digital image illustrates perhaps the profound advancement of radiography. Image display begins with understanding exposure latitude and dynamic range. Exposure latitude represents the digital receptor's ability to record a wide range of exposure values. Also, recall that with digital systems, the brightness is a separate function of display. Brightness levels can be changed by adjusting window width and window level as a postprocessing function. With digital receptors, the response to exposure is linear and the range of exposures is very wide. This may be described as **dynamic range**. *Dynamic range* is the range of exposure intensities that an image receptor can respond to and use to acquire image data. Ultimately, this means

that digital receptors can respond to very low and very high exposure levels and process them to display as visible shades of gray. The result is that more anatomic information can be captured and displayed.

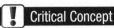

### Critical Concept

#### Digital Image

The digital image has a linear response to x-ray exposure and can respond to a wider range of x-ray energy.

Display workstation guidelines apply to primary display workstations (those used for official interpretation of the images). Secondary workstations do not have to adhere to the established guidelines as long as they are not used for interpretation. Among these guidelines are maximum luminance levels of at least 171 candelas per $m^2$, contrast response that meets the requirements of the American Association of Physicists in Medicine (AAPM) Task Group 18, a minimum of eight-bit luminance resolution, minimal veiling glare, and minimal reflections from and levels of ambient light sources. Some of the test patterns used are discussed later, as is information for obtaining a complete list of quality-control requirements that the medical physicist follows in evaluation of the equipment.

One great advantage of digital radiography is that it is possible to preprocess and postprocess the image. Preprocessing is generally an automatic function of the system and occurs before the image is displayed. In addition to the histogram analysis and automatic rescaling, the system corrects for variations in pixel, row, and column responses. Other automatic calibration functions may be performed by the system to make the receptor response more uniform.

Postprocessing functions are computer software operations available to the radiographer and radiologist that allow manual manipulation of the displayed image. These functions allow the operator to manually adjust many presentation features of the image to enhance the diagnostic value. Box 10.1 presents some of the most common functions. Window width and window level are discussed further here because they are particularly valuable tools. Recall that window width is a control that adjusts radiographic contrast by determining the range of pixel values incorporated into image display. Window level sets the midpoint of the range of brightness levels visible in the image. Digital radiography uses a 14-bit dynamic range, which equates to 16,384 distinct shades of gray. However, the human eye can only appreciate approximately 30 shades of gray at any level. Think of the 16,384 shades of gray as a continuum scale viewed through a window and stretched out from left to right. This window allows the viewer to look only at a small segment of the continuum directly in front but expands that segment to a visible black and white scale. The window may move from left to right as far as the viewer likes but

---

**Box 10.1  Postprocessing Functions**

- **Window width and window level:** A technique to take advantage of the more than 16,000 shades of gray. *Windowing* refers to the shade of gray displayed (radiographic contrast of the image); *leveling* refers to where on the scale the window is set (brightness of the image).
- **Annotation:** Allows text to be added to the image to identify areas of interest or add information important for diagnosis. This should *not* be routinely used in place of anatomic side markers.
- **Image flip:** Allows for the flipping of the image so that it is oriented properly for interpretation.
- **Image inversion:** Allows for the changing of the image from negative (bone is white, surrounding tissues are dark) to positive (bone is dark, surrounding tissues are light). Some pathologic conditions are better identified this way.
- **Magnification:** An electronic magnifying glass is available for use with digital images. With very high-resolution monitors, such as those used by the radiologist, magnification to see fine detail is possible.
- **Edge enhancement:** Increases the radiographic contrast along the edge of a structure through a sophisticated software function. The part must have been sufficiently exposed and have a low signal-to-noise ratio because noise is also enhanced.
- **Smoothing:** A software function to suppress noise. Image noise is considered a high-frequency variation in the histogram, and postprocessing adjustment of these high frequencies can reduce noise.
- **Equalization:** Software-weighted processing function whereby underexposed areas (light areas) are made darker and overexposed areas (dark areas) are made lighter. The effect is an image that appears to have lower radiographic contrast so that dense and lucent structures are better seen within the same image.
- **Region of interest:** A quantitative function of digital imaging that allows for the pixel value of a selected area of interest to be calculated. This value can then help characterize disease.

---

the window allows the viewer to see and expand only what is directly in front. Leveling "moves the window" to the place specified on the continuum, and windowing expands that portion of the grayscale to a visible black and white scale. Increasing the level reduces image brightness while decreasing the level increases brightness. Adjusting window width "expands" or "reduces" the width of the window. Thus, increasing window width increases the number of shades of gray available to the viewer, resulting in lower radiographic contrast. Decreasing window width decreases the number of shades of gray, resulting in higher radiographic contrast.

A word of caution regarding postprocessing: Overuse of these functions can drastically and negatively alter the data set that is the digital image. Doing so reduces the diagnostic and archival quality of the data. One should also keep in mind that in many facilities the radiographer's workstations use monitors of significantly lower quality and viewing conditions that are very different than the radiologist's workstations. How an image appears on the radiographer's workstation in a brightly lit work area may be very different from the way it appears on the radiologist's high-resolution monitor in a darkened reading room. Care should be taken in the postprocessing of an image before forwarding it for interpretation.

## USING DIGITAL RECEPTORS

The use of digital receptors requires an understanding of **exposure indicators**. In CR systems, the exposure indicator value represents the exposure level to the PSP plate and the values are vendor-specific. Fuji, Philips, and Konica use sensitivity (S) numbers, and the value is inversely related to the exposure to the plate (Philips also has an exposure index [EI] value; however, S is not equal to EI). A 200 S number is equal to 1 mR of exposure to the plate. The optimal range when using this system is approximately 250 to 300 for the torso and 75 to 125 for the extremities. Carestream (Kodak) uses EI numbers, and the value is directly related to the exposure to the plate and the changes are logarithmic expressions. For example, a change in EI from 1500 to 1800, a difference of 300, is equal to a factor of 2 and represents twice as much exposure to the plate. The optimal range of EI values for grid or Bucky examinations is 1800 to 1900. Agfa uses log mean (lgM) numbers; the value is directly related to exposure to the plate and changes are also logarithmic expressions. For example, a change in lgM from 2 to 2.3, a change of 0.3, is equal to a factor of 2 and represents twice as much exposure to the plate. The optimal range of lgM values is 1.9 to 2.1. These optimum ranges are vendor specified. However, the ultimate determination of optimum ranges will be made by the interpreting radiologists and facility. When using CR systems, the radiographer should monitor the exposure indicator values as a guide for optimum technique. If the exposure indicator value is within the acceptable range, adjustments can be made for contrast and brightness with postprocessing functions and will not degrade the image. If, however, the exposure is outside of the acceptable range, attempting to adjust the image data with postprocessing functions will not correct for improper receptor exposure and may result in suboptimal images that should not be submitted for interpretation. For CR systems, histogram analysis is the basis for determining the exposure indicator value. The radiographer has a role in the selection of the appropriate anatomic part and projection before processing the PSP plate. This step tells the computer which histogram to use. If the radiographer selects a part other than the one imaged, a histogram analysis error may occur.

### CR Exposure Indicators

The radiographer should use exposure indicators of CR systems as indicators of optimal technique and strive to keep selected exposures within the indicated optimal range for that system.

DR systems use **dose-area product (DAP)** as an indicator of exposure. DAP is a measure of exposure in air, followed by computation to estimate absorbed dose to the patient. It is measured by a DAP meter embedded in the collimator. The DAP value depends on the exposure factors and field size and is expressed in centigray-meter squared ($cGY\text{-}m^2$). DAP reflects both the dose to the patient and the total volume of tissue being irradiated.

Standardization of exposure values is making some headway, and the following would apply to all digital radiography systems. In 2008, the International Electrotechnical Commission published an exposure terminology standard. In 2009, the AAPM published its report. At the 2010 summit of the Image Gently consortium, all stakeholders agreed to adopt the International Electrotechnical Commission 62494-1 standard, which presents three terms of value to radiographers: EI, target exposure index ($EI_T$), and deviation index (DI). EI represents the exposure at the detector relevant to the region being imaged and is defined by the signal-to-noise ratio (SNR). EI will respond linearly to changes in mAs when the kVp is held constant. $EI_T$ is the target reference exposure obtained from a properly exposed image receptor. $EI_T$ values will vary with each anatomic area of interest. Finally, DI is a measure of the deviation of the EI from projection-specific $EI_T$ values. It is the DI value that indicates to the radiographer proper exposure for the body part being examined by indicating the deviation (above or below) the ideal value determined for that part.

The **detective quantum efficiency (DQE)** of the detector is an expression of the radiation exposure level that is required to produce an optimal image. DQE is a measurement of the efficiency of an image receptor in converting the x-ray exposure it receives to a quality radiographic image. If an image receptor system can convert x-ray exposure into a quality image with 100% efficiency (meaning no information loss), the DQE would measure 100% or 1.0. However, no imaging system has 100% conversion efficiency. Nevertheless, the higher the DQE of a system, the lower the radiation exposure required to produce a quality image, thereby decreasing patient exposure. DQE "predicts" patient dose. A higher DQE indicates a potentially lower patient dose. However, if the DQE is too high, the patient dose will be very low, but the image will also be very noisy (grainy) because there was an insufficient quantity of radiation to create the image. DQE is evaluated by comparing the image noise of a detector with that of an "ideal" detector with the same signal-response characteristics. DQE is a measure of how well the SNR is preserved in an image. SNR is an expression of how clearly a very faint object appears in an image.

### Detective Quantum Efficiency

DQE is an expression of the exposure level required to produce an image.

Image noise and spatial resolution are additional considerations in digital systems. Image noise is any undesirable fluctuation in the brightness of an image (Fig. 10.10). In addition to the inherent x-ray quantum noise, the electronic components of digital imaging systems also contribute undesirable noise. Spatial resolution is a characteristic of a digital system and by definition is equal to one-half the Nyquist frequency. The Nyquist frequency is the highest spatial frequency (number of line pairs per millimeter) that a digital detector can record and is determined by the sampling frequency of CR systems and the DEL spacing of DR systems (recall that DEL is the smallest resolvable area of a DR system).

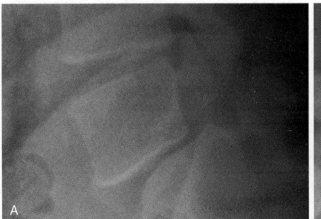
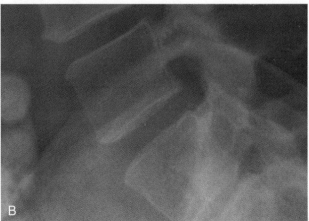

**Fig. 10.10 Image Noise. (A)** Excessive noise caused by an insufficient mAs. **(B)** The same part with a sufficient mAs. An optimal mAs should be selected to provide sufficient quanta to expose the receptor and avoid excessive noise. (Courtesy Andrew Woodward R.T.(R) and The University of North Carolina at Chapel Hill.)

There are two measures of spatial resolution: limiting spatial resolution (LSR) and **modulation transfer function (MTF)**. LSR is the ability of a detector to resolve small structures and is measured using a bar pattern. LSR is limited by the number of pixels and pixel size. Because LSR depends on the contrast of the target and the exposure and display conditions, it is not as accurate as MTF. MTF is a measure of the ability of the system to preserve signal contrast (display the contrast of anatomic objects varying in size) as a function of spatial resolution and describes the fraction of each component that preserves the captured image. It is considered the ideal expression of digital detector image resolution.

The primary factor influencing radiographic contrast with digital systems is the lookup table (LUT). LUTs are histograms of luminance values used as a reference to evaluate the input intensities and assign predetermined grayscale values—VOI, as previously mentioned. Rescaling occurs at this stage. Rescaling is the adjusting of the image by the computer program to present an image of predetermined image brightness (Fig. 10.11). An image receptor that is overexposed is rescaled lighter, and an image receptor that is underexposed is rescaled darker. In this way, the display computer presents a consistent and uniform image over a wide range of exposures.

Digital receptors are more sensitive to low-energy radiation. They capture and record the low-energy scatter photons, and image quality suffers as a result. There are two ways to effectively control scatter radiation's effect on the image: collimation and grid use.

Precise collimation limits the area of exposed tissues and, with it, the effective dose and amount of scatter that can be produced. The use of the postprocessing cropping tool to give the appearance of collimation of the finished radiograph does not serve the same purpose and is unethical. The use of this tool does not reduce patient dose as with actual collimation; furthermore, it removes from display image data that may be important to the diagnostic quality. The use of a grid reduces the amount of scatter reaching the image receptor by taking advantage of the greater divergent angle of scatter (scatter is absorbed by the lead strips of the grid and useful photons pass between). For digital systems, a fairly high-frequency grid is recommended.

**Critical Concept**

**Digital Systems and Low-Energy Radiation**

Digital systems are more sensitive to low-energy radiation and are therefore more sensitive to scatter radiation.

Just because digital systems automatically rescale overexposed images does not mean one should take advantage of this in an effort to avoid repeats. This is flawed logic and violates the radiographers' code of ethics and the As Low as Reasonably Achievable (ALARA) principle.

Finally, troubleshooting with digital imaging involves the recognition of those image processing errors that can degrade image clarity. As has been discussed previously, the image acquisition and display functions in digital systems are separated. With these

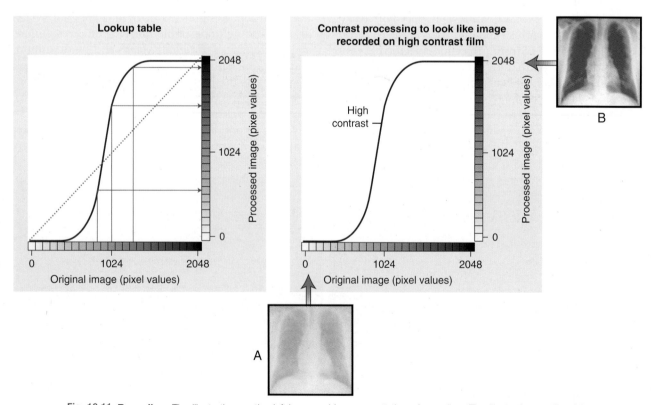

**Fig. 10.11 Rescaling.** The illustration on the *left* is a graphic representation of rescaling. The illustration on the *right* includes radiographs to further illustrate the concept. **(A)** An example of what an image may look like before rescaling. **(B)** An example of what an image may look like after rescaling. (Courtesy Sprawls: *Physical principles of medical imaging online*, ed 2, http://www.sprawls.org/ppmi2/.)

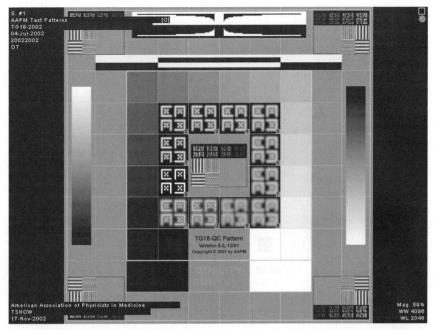

**Fig. 10.12 TG18-QC Test Pattern.** The TG18-QC test pattern is used to evaluate general image quality. It also looks for artifacts and evaluates geometric distortion and resolution. (Courtesy Samei E, et al.: Assessment of display performance for medical imaging systems. Draft report of the American Association of Physicists in Medicine [AAPM] Task Group 18, Version 10.0, August 2004.)

systems, the radiographer must pay attention to the exposure indicator values as an indicator of proper exposure. No amount of postprocessing will correct for poor image-acquisition procedures. Next, the radiographer must review those factors that may result in a histogram analysis error. Exposure field recognition errors, proper collimation, excessive scatter radiation, processing under the correct menu, and proper technical factor selection must be considered. Finally, the radiographer must evaluate proper positioning and tube-part-receptor alignment.

## QUALITY ASSURANCE AND QUALITY CONTROL

Digital imaging quality control focuses on the display monitors and viewing environment. The AAPM published an online report, Report No. OR-03, to provide guidelines for proper performance of display devices intended for medical use. This report presents 26 test patterns that can be used to assess display device performance. The complete report with a list of tests, test procedures, necessary tools, acceptance criteria, and corrective action may be found online at http://www.aapm.org/pubs/reports/OR_03.pdf.

The following tests may be performed by a quality control radiographer. Additional tests are performed annually by a qualified medical physicist (see AAPM Report No. OR-03 for a complete list).

### DAILY

• Overall visual assessment: Uses the TG18-QC test pattern. This test looks at general image quality and for the presence of any artifacts (Fig. 10.12).

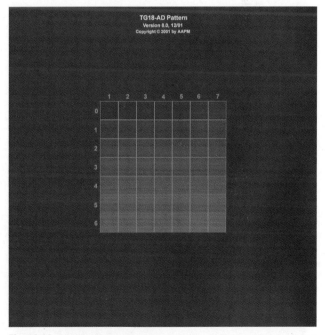

**Fig. 10.13 TG18-AD Test Pattern.** The TG18-AD test pattern is used to evaluate ambient light contribution. (Courtesy Samei E, et al.: Assessment of display performance for medical imaging systems. Draft report of the American Association of Physicists in Medicine [AAPM] Task Group 18, Version 10.0, August 2004.)

### MONTHLY OR QUARTERLY

• Geometric distortion: Uses the TG18-QC test pattern (see Fig. 10.12). This test checks for a variation in the shape of the displayed image from the original image.
• Reflection: Uses a TG18-AD test pattern. This test evaluates the ambient light contribution to the light reflected by the display monitor (Fig. 10.13).

- Luminance response: Uses the TG18-LN01, TG18-LN08, and TG18-LN18 test patterns. This test assesses the displayed luminance values versus the input values from the display system (Fig. 10.14A–C). Luminance may also be evaluated visually using the TG18-CT test pattern (Fig. 10.14D).
- Luminance dependencies: Uses the TG18-UNL10 and TG18-UNL80 test patterns. This test evaluates the image for nonuniformity and effects of viewing at different angles (Fig. 10.15).
- Resolution: Uses the TG18-QC (see Fig. 10.12) and TG18-CX (Fig. 10.16) test patterns. This test assesses

the system's ability to display images of different parts of an image with high fidelity.

The following are a few additional notes of consideration regarding quality assurance and quality control. First, those using CR systems should create a maintenance schedule for the plates. The plates should be cleaned and inspected every 3 months or as needed based on workload and conditions, using approved cleaning products only. The plates should also be erased every 48 hours if unused. Furthermore, for all digital systems within a facility, identical processing codes should be used to ensure the consistency of image appearance.

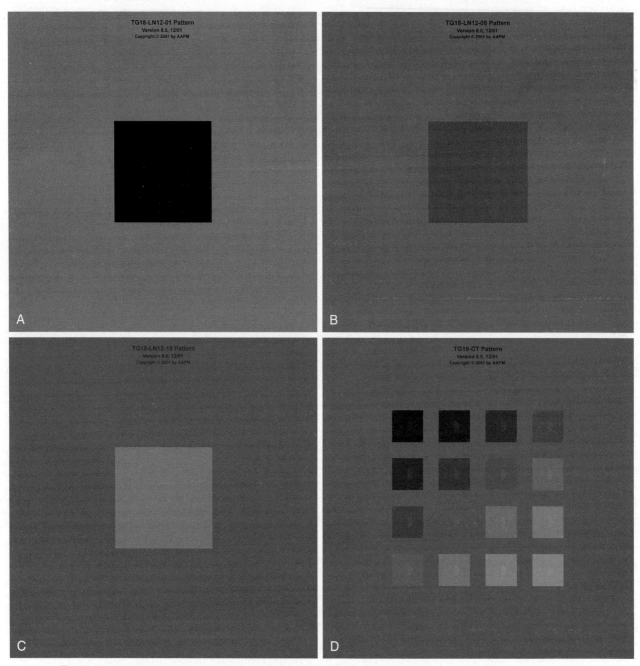

Fig. 10.14 **TG18-LN01, TG18-LN08, TG18-LN18, and TG18-CT Test Patterns.** TG18-LN01 **(A)**, TG18-LN08 **(B)**, and TG18-LN18 **(C)** test patterns are used to evaluate the displayed luminance values versus the input values from the display system. The TG18-CT **(D)** test pattern may also be used to visually evaluate luminance. (Courtesy Samei E, et al.: Assessment of display performance for medical imaging systems. Draft report of the American Association of Physicists in Medicine [AAPM] Task Group 18, Version 10.0, August 2004.)

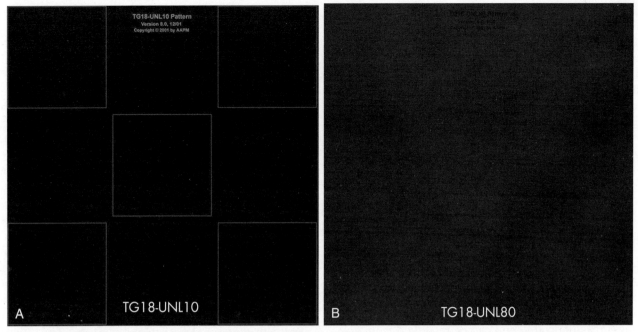

Fig. 10.15 **TG18-UNL10 and TG18-UNL80 Test Patterns.** The TG18-UNL10 **(A)** and TG18-UNL80 **(B)** test patterns are used to evaluate the image for nonuniformity and effects of viewing at different angles. (Courtesy Samei E, et al.: Assessment of display performance for medical imaging systems. Draft report of the American Association of Physicists in Medicine [AAPM] Task Group 18, Version 10.0, August 2004.)

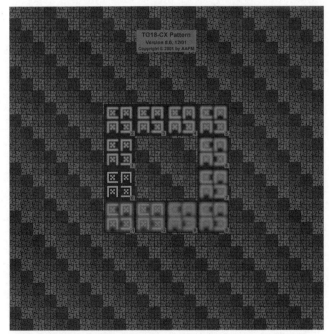

Fig. 10.16 **TG18-CX Test Pattern.** The TG18-CX test pattern (along with the TG18-QC test pattern) is used to assess the system's ability to display images of different parts of an image with high fidelity. (Courtesy Samei E, et al.: Assessment of display performance for medical imaging systems. Draft report of the American Association of Physicists in Medicine [AAPM] Task Group 18, Version 10.0, August 2004.)

## PICTURE ARCHIVING AND COMMUNICATION SYSTEMS

The **Picture Archiving and Communication System (PACS)** is an integral part of the digital radiology imaging department. A PACS can generally be divided into acquisition (imaging modalities), a secure network for transmitting and exchange of patient images and data, display (viewing and workstations), and storage (archive server) systems. Storage, in particular, is an ever-increasing challenge because of the increased use of multislice modalities (computed tomography, magnetic resonance imaging, ultrasound) and the increasing quantity of data generated by all digital modalities. With increasing size and number of examination files comes an increased demand for storage. For example, the average size of a digital radiography study is 38 MB. Each of the major systems of a PACS is discussed here, as are trends and challenges.

PACS is an electronic network for communication between the image acquisition modalities, display stations, and storage. For these different systems to communicate with each other, a common language is necessary. The **Digital Imaging and Communications in Medicine (DICOM)** standard was first formulated in 1983 for this purpose and has been refined over time. This standard allows for the exchange of medical images and information among modalities, display stations, and storage. With the introduction of a common language, equipment has been designed and manufactured to be DICOM-compatible as well.

As previously mentioned, many modalities have been digital for some time. The process of digital acquisition for radiography has already been discussed. The digital format is necessary for radiography to be integrated as a part of the PACS. The role of the PACS is to allow for the display and storage of these medical images. Now that this information is in a digital form and DICOM allows it to be transferred to a display and storage medium, radiography can occur in an environment that is completely digital. The patient's medical information and imaging studies can be viewed and stored as an electronic file. Through **teleradiology**, image files can be accessed from various workstations located throughout the facility or even by clients outside the facility if they are given access to the system. The radiologist, operating room staff, and emergency department staff can access image files at the same time if needed. For example, this system allows an ordering physician to log into the network from their office outside of the facility and view a patient's radiographic images without printing films or burning and sending over a CD. In addition to the images, information management systems such as the Radiology Information System serve to handle textual and other information portions stored on the PACS. All such systems are networked on the PACS so that information and images are integrated and can be retrieved from any number of locations.

## ! Critical Concept

### Picture Archiving and Communication System

PACS is an electronic network for communication between the image acquisition modalities, display stations, and storage, using the common language of DICOM. Its role is to allow for the display and storage of medical images and information.

A display station is simply a desktop computer that allows for the retrieval and viewing of medical images from one of the modalities or storage components of the PACS. The quality and function of one of these stations depend on the user. The quality of the display monitor and the complexity of the software are major variables. A 1-megapixel (Mp) (1280 × 1024 pixel) monitor is sufficient for general viewing by noninterpreting physicians and other health care workers, whereas a 2-Mp (1600 × 1200 pixel) monitor is necessary for general interpretation by a radiologist or viewing for quality control by a radiologic technologist. A 5-Mp (2048 × 2560 pixel) monitor is necessary for interpretation of digital mammograms.

The software loaded to each display station also depends on the user. For general viewing by noninterpreting physicians and other health care workers, a very basic package allowing minimal adjustment may be all that is available. Quality control display stations and reading stations have greater function and capability, such as more advanced image manipulation (windowing and leveling), annotation, patient demographic information, masking, and magnification (zoom). Even among radiologic technologists, each may have access to different functions protected by login and password to limit which aspects of a medical image may be changed (and by whom) to prevent accidentally damaging or negatively altering the record.

As the complexity of medical images and patient data has grown, new approaches to PACS have developed. One particular challenge has been expansion and maintenance of PACS, access to and storage of data over decades, not to mention changes in vendors. One latest solution is the trend toward vendor neutral archives (VNAs). VNAs allow for images and data from different systems and in different formats to be stored using a singular system on a common infrastructure. VNAs may be used as replacements to existing PACS to avoid very expensive transition costs. They may also be used to consolidate a number of systems that exist within a single facility or across a system of facilities. Another growing trend is the creation of health information exchanges for the purpose of sharing patient information across systems and creating networks of service providers. To accomplish this, Cross-Enterprise Document sharing standards have been developed. These Cross-Enterprise Documents are also supported by VNAs.

As previously mentioned, one of the biggest challenges of a PACS is storage. With increasingly complex modalities feeding large image files into the system, the demand for storage is ever increasing. This is further complicated by the Health Insurance Portability and Accountability Act requirement to store images and data for years. There is also the requirement to address disaster recovery processes. This is basically a requirement to duplicate all files in a remote location so that recovery is possible in the event of a disaster and the primary files are lost.

To support this ever-increasing demand for data storage, PACS has taken on new directions. Traditionally, PACS were created and maintained in house. This required the purchase and maintenance of a very large computer servers and storage systems. The forms of storage are discussed next. One recent trend to address storage space and expense is cloud-based storage. This process consists of offsite storage and servers supported by a secure network and third-party vendor. This also shifts the DA requirement to the vendor along with the maintenance and storage equipment purchase. The user basically pays for the service and storage space as needed.

There are also hybrid versions of this configuration whereby the facility maintains current image and patient data in-house and longer-term storage externally or in the cloud. The advantages and disadvantages of these systems are facility dependent and change according to the imaging volume, facility size, and need for access. The speed of access, for example, depends on connectivity speed and file size.

The basic archiving components of PACS comprise the image manager and image storage. The image manager is the component that handles the workflow of the system by moving images back and forth between viewing stations and storage. The storage component is that portion that archives the data on a storage medium, such as optical disk or flash drive.

Storage is usually classified as:

- Online: Data are stored on hard drives with access times in milliseconds and transfer times in the range of tens and hundreds of megabytes per second.
- Nearline: A jukebox uses robotic arms to retrieve the data storage device automatically and inserts it into a drive to read or write data. This type can access data within 60 seconds and is able to transfer data at a few megabytes per second.
- Offline: Removable media are stored on a shelf in a catalog and retrieved manually.

The online storage component is networked to the PACS via direct attached storage, network attached storage, or storage area network. The direct attached storage has hard drives directly on the server. The network attached storage is a free-standing storage attached to the network. Storage area network is a dedicated network for connecting the storage devices to computers (network to the PACS).

Magnetic tape is the oldest storage technology and is a linear storage medium; that is, a ferromagnetic material is bonded to a length of plastic "tape." As the medium is passed by an electromagnet, it is modulated (varied) by an electronic signal and magnetizes the medium accordingly. In read mode, an electric field is induced in the electromagnet by the moving magnetic field of the tape. Because of the density of digital data, this form is very limited in use.

Optical disk is a common storage technology. An optical disk (a compact disc) has a reflective surface layer followed by a photosensitive layer that is "burned" by light from a laser, creating a series of light and dark spots on the disk modulated by the data signal. Recall that the digital signal is a series of ones and zeros. The light spots represent ones and the dark spots represent zeros. The data are recorded in a spiral from the center of the disk outward. In read mode, a laser light is aimed on the disk following the spiral, beginning at any point on it according to where the file is stored. If the laser light hits a light spot, it is reflected to the optical reader and is transmitted as a one; if it hits a dark spot, it is transmitted as a zero. These disks may be arranged as an array and referred to as a *redundant array of independent disks*. The data are stored across the array to create backups and maximize efficiency of retrieval and storage.

As the demand for data storage space increases, research continues to find ways to store more in a smaller space. Optical disk technology has improved, but the spiral can be only so tight. Ways of compressing the data files without loss of data are also being researched, but this is also self-limiting. Recently introduced potential solutions include the use of high-capacity flash drive arrays. The flash drives are available in 73-GB and 146-GB capacities. They are arranged as an array and used in much the same way as an array of optical disks. Another solution recently introduced is the holographic storage device. This technology makes use of a special recording medium and laser technology to record data throughout the depth of the medium. A holographic disk device stores data through its entire depth rather than just the surface. This approach has the potential of storing 1 TB per cubic centimeter.

## On the Spot

- The PSP plate of a CR system contains a phosphor that is ionized when exposed to x-rays. Approximately half of the liberated electrons are trapped in the conduction band. When the plate is scanned in the reader, the energy is released and converted to an electronic signal, becoming a manifest image.
- DR systems use a detector array that converts the remnant beam to a signal for almost immediate viewing. There are two forms of DR systems: indirect and direct capture. The two forms of indirect capture use a scintillator that converts remnant radiation to light and then to an electronic signal, which causes some loss of resolution. The direct-capture method does not use a scintillator, instead using amorphous selenium and TFT array, thereby avoiding the loss of spatial resolution.
- During image acquisition a histogram is created from the exposure received to the detector. This histogram is compared with a stored histogram (*a priori* model) for that anatomic part and VOI identified. From the VOI, the computer determines which section of the histogram will be included in the displayed image.
- In CR systems, the image is stored in the plate as trapped electrons in the conduction bands. This "image" is extracted by exposing the plate to a laser. The released energy is in the form of light and is passed through an ADC, where it is digitized. The digitized signal is converted to a matrix and assigned grayscale values.
- In DR systems, the image-forming radiation is processed as it exposes the detector array and digitized. The digitized signal is then converted to a matrix and assigned grayscale values.
- The digital image has a linear response to x-ray exposure and a wide dynamic range. Digital receptors can respond to low and high exposure levels and display many shades of gray.
- Postprocessing functions are manual manipulative functions of the displayed image available to the radiologic technologist and radiologist. Care should be taken in the use of these functions so as not to negatively alter the digital data set.
- In CR systems, the exposure indicators should be monitored as a guide for optimal technical factor selection. In DR systems, the DAP should be used for the same purpose.
- DQE is a measure of how well the signal-to-noise ratio is preserved. It is related to the radiation exposure level required to produce an optimal image.
- Image noise is any undesirable fluctuation in the brightness of an image and is caused by the inherent x-ray quantum noise and electronic components of the digital system.

- Spatial resolution of digital systems is equal to one-half of the Nyquist frequency and is best measured using MTF.
- Troubleshooting with digital systems involves the recognition of those image-processing errors that can degrade image visibility, and the radiographer should consider exposure field recognition errors, proper collimation, excessive scatter radiation, processing under the correct menu, and proper technical factor selection.
- Digital imaging quality control focuses on the display monitors and viewing environment.
- The PACS is an integral part of the digital radiology imaging department and is generally divided into acquisition, display, and storage systems.
- PACS is an electronic network for communication between the image acquisition modalities, display stations, and storage using the common language, DICOM. Its role is to allow for the display and storage of medical images and information.
- VNAs allow for images and data from different systems and in different formats to be stored using a singular system on a common infrastructure.
- A display station is simply a desktop computer that allows for the retrieval and viewing of medical images from one of the modalities or storage components of the PACS. The quality and function of these stations depend on the user.
- One of the biggest challenges of a PACS is storage. With increasingly complex modalities feeding large image files into the system, the demand for storage is ever-increasing.
- Storage of a PACS is generally classified as *online*, *nearline*, or *offline*.

## CRITICAL THINKING QUESTIONS

1. What are the considerations for use of different digital detectors?
2. What are the image display and ethical problems associated with processing an image under the wrong histogram?

## REVIEW QUESTIONS

1. What represents the latent image in a PSP CR system?
   a. Electrons trapped in conduction band
   b. Ionized silver halide crystals
   c. Scattered photons in the patient
   d. Chemical reaction in the processor
2. Which PACS storage option offers the fastest retrieval of data?
   a. Offline
   b. Nearline
   c. Online
   d. All are equal in retrieval speed.

3. Which of the following controls brightness of a digital system?
   a. mAs
   b. kVp
   c. The display monitor
   d. Room lighting
4. Rescaling a digital image adjusts the histogram to reflect which of the following?
   a. kVp
   b. mAs
   c. LUT
   d. VOI
5. Which of the following is used by both forms of indirect cassette-less systems?
   a. Scintillator
   b. CCD
   c. Optics
   d. TFT
6. Which of the following does not involve the conversion of x-rays to light?
   a. Direct capture DR system
   b. Indirect capture DR system
   c. CR system
   d. Cassette-based system
7. Which component of the CR reader digitizes the signal?
   a. Photodetector
   b. ADC
   c. Optics
   d. Laser
8. What is this test pattern used for?

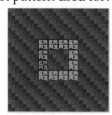

(Courtesy *Mosby's radiography online: radiographic imaging*, ed 2, St Louis, 2009, Mosby.)

   a. Luminance response
   b. Luminance dependence
   c. Reflection
   d. Resolution
9. The emission of light by a phosphor when exposed to a laser is known as _____.
   a. phosphorescence
   b. sensitometry
   c. conversion efficiency
   d. photostimulable luminescence

# Radiographic Exposure Technique

## Outline

## Objectives

- Explain the relationship between milliamperage and exposure time with radiation production and image receptor exposure.
- Calculate changes in milliamperage and exposure time to change or maintain exposure to the image receptor.
- Explain how kVp affects radiation production and image receptor exposure.
- Calculate changes in kVp to change or maintain exposure to the image receptor.
- Recognize the factors that affect spatial resolution and distortion.
- Calculate changes in mAs for changes in source-to-image receptor distance.

- Calculate the magnification factor and object percent magnification and determine image and object size.
- Describe the use of grids and beam restriction and their effect on image receptor exposure and image quality.
- Calculate changes in mAs when adding or removing a grid.
- Recognize patient factors that may affect image receptor exposure.
- State exposure technique modifications for patient factors, such as body habitus and part thickness.
- Identify the exposure factors that can affect patient radiation exposure.

## Key Terms

15% rule
body habitus
direct square law
exposure maintenance formula

inverse square law
magnification factor (MF)
object-to-image receptor
   distance (OID)

source-to-image receptor
   distance (SID)
source-to-object distance (SOD)

## INTRODUCTION

In Chapter 6, variables that affect both the quantity and quality of the x-ray beam were presented. Milliamperage and time affect the quantity of radiation produced and kilovoltage affects both the quantity and quality. Chapter 9 emphasized that a diagnostic-quality radiographic image accurately represents the anatomic area of interest. The characteristics evaluated for image quality are brightness, radiographic contrast, spatial resolution, distortion, and quantum noise. This chapter focuses on radiographic exposure techniques and the use of accessory devices and their effect on the radiation reaching the image receptor (IR) and the image produced. Radiographers have the responsibility of selecting the combination of exposure factors to produce a quality image. Knowledge of how these factors affect the image individually and in combination helps radiographers produce a radiographic image with the amount of information desired for diagnostic interpretation. In addition, the patient should be exposed to the least amount of radiation necessary to produce a diagnostic-quality radiographic image.

This chapter discusses all the primary and secondary factors and their effects on the radiation reaching the IR and image quality.

## PRIMARY FACTORS

The primary exposure technique factors the radiographer selects on the control panel are milliamperage (mA), time of exposure (s), and kilovoltage peak (kVp). Depending on the type of control panel, milliamperage and exposure time may be selected separately or combined as one factor, milliamperage/second (mAs). Regardless, it is important to understand how changing each separately or in combination affects the radiation reaching the IR and the radiographic image.

### MILLIAMPERAGE AND EXPOSURE TIME

The quantity of radiation exiting the x-ray tube and reaching the patient affects the amount of remnant radiation reaching the IR. The product of milliamperage and exposure time has a directly proportional relationship with the quantity of x-rays produced.

 **Make the Physics Connection**

**Chapter 6**

Because the milliamperage/second (mAs) controls the number of electrons boiled off the filament and available to produce x-rays, it is considered the primary factor controlling quantity. All other factors remaining constant, an increase in milliamperage increases the amplitude of both the continuous and discrete portions of the x-ray emission spectrum (Fig. 11.1).

Once the anatomic part is adequately penetrated, as the quantity of x-rays is increased, the exposure to the IR proportionally increases (Fig. 11.2). Conversely, when the quantity of x-rays is decreased, the exposure to the IR decreases. Therefore exposure to the IR can

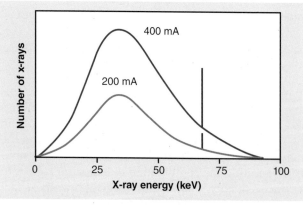

**Fig. 11.1 Change in Milliamperage.** Two emission spectra illustrating the result of an increase in mA *(purple curve)*. Increases in mA increase the quantity of radiation. *keV,* Kilovoltage volt; *mA,* milliamperage.

be increased or decreased by adjusting the amount of radiation (mAs).

 **Critical Concept**

**mAs and Quantity of Radiation**

As the mAs is increased, the quantity of radiation reaching the IR is increased proportionally. As the mAs is decreased, the amount of radiation reaching the IR is decreased proportionally.

Because the mAs is the product of milliamperage and exposure time, increasing milliamperage or time has the same effect on radiation exposure.

 **Math Application**

**Adjusting Milliamperage or Exposure Time**

$$100\,mA \times 0.1\,s = 10\,mAs$$

To increase the mAs to 20, you could use:

$$100\,mA \times 0.2\,s = 20\,mAs$$
$$200\,mA \times 0.1\,s = 20\,mAs$$

As demonstrated in the Math Application, mAs can be doubled by doubling the milliamperage or doubling the exposure time. A change in either milliamperage or exposure time proportionally changes the mAs. To maintain the same mAs, the radiographer must increase the milliamperage and proportionally decrease the exposure time.

 **Critical Concept**

**Milliamperage and Exposure Time**

Milliamperage and exposure time have an inverse proportional relationship when maintaining the same mAs.

 **Math Application**

**Adjusting Milliamperage and Exposure Time to Maintain mAs**

$$100\,mA \times 100\,ms\,(0.1s) = 10\,mAs$$

To maintain the mAs, use:

$$50\,mA \times 200\,ms\,(0.2\,s) = 10\,mAs$$
$$200\,mA \times 50\,ms\,(0.05\,s) = 10\,mAs$$

It is important for the radiographer to determine the amount of mAs needed to produce a diagnostic image. This is not an easy task because there are so many variables that can affect the amount of mAs required. For example, thin parts (such as the hand) require less radiation than thicker parts (such as the pelvis).

A patient's age, condition, and the presence of a pathologic condition also affect the amount of mAs

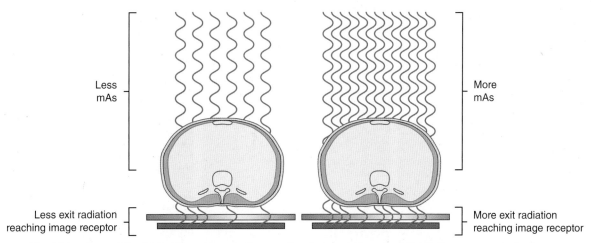

Fig. 11.2 **mAs and Radiation Exposure.** As the quantity of x-rays is increased (mAs), the exposure to the image receptor proportionally increases.

required for the procedure. Additionally, for a given mAs, IRs respond differently. For example, mAs does not control the amount of brightness displayed within a digital image. Digital IRs can detect a wider range of radiation intensities (wider dynamic range) exiting the patient and therefore are not dependent on the mAs. However, exposure errors can adversely affect the quality of the digital image. If the mAs is too low (low exposure to the digital IR), image brightness is adjusted during computer processing to achieve the desired level. Although the level of brightness has been adjusted, there may be increased quantum noise visible within the image (Fig. 11.3). If the mAs selected is too high (high exposure to the digital IR), the brightness

can also be adjusted, but the patient has received more radiation than necessary (Fig. 11.4).

> ### ! Critical Concept
>
> **mAs and Image Brightness**
>
> The mAs does not control image brightness when using digital IRs. During computer processing, image brightness is maintained when the mAs is too low or too high. A lower-than-required mAs produces an image with increased quantum noise and a higher-than-needed mAs exposes the patient to unnecessary radiation.

In general, for repeat radiographic images necessitated by exposure errors, the mAs is adjusted by a

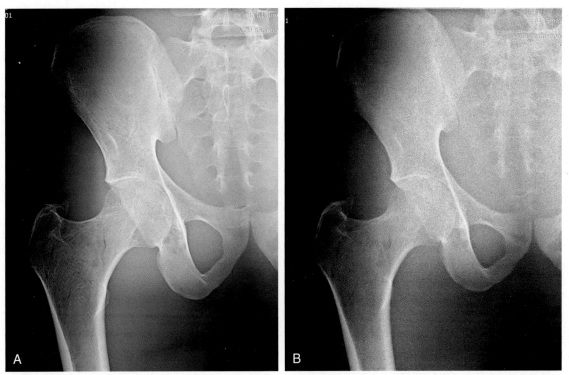

Fig. 11.3 **Quantum Noise. (A)** Quality image created using sufficient mAs. **(B)** Image created using insufficient mAs and results in increased quantum noise visible within the image.

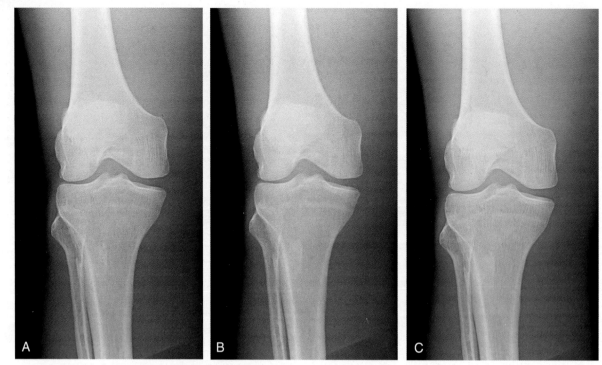

**Fig. 11.4 Exposure Errors and Image Brightness.** Exposure errors can be computer adjusted to maintain image brightness. **(A)** Image created with sufficient mAs. **(B)** Image created with insufficient mAs and results in increased quantum noise visible. **(C)** Image created with excessive mAs and results in decreased quantum noise visible.

factor of 2; therefore, a minimum change involves doubling or halving the mAs.

If a radiographic image must be repeated because of another error, such as positioning, the radiographer may also use the opportunity to make an adjustment in the exposure to the IR to produce an image of diagnostic quality. A radiographic image repeated because of insufficient or excessive exposure generally requires a change in mAs by a factor of at least 2.

To best visualize the anatomic area of interest, the mAs selected must produce a sufficient amount of radiation reaching the IR. Excessive or insufficient mAs adversely affects image quality and affects patient radiation exposure. The radiographer should be diligent in monitoring exposure indicator values to ensure that quality images are obtained with the lowest possible radiation dose to the patient (Box 11.1).

## KILOVOLTAGE

The kVp affects the exposure to the IR because it alters the intensity and penetrating ability of the x-ray beam (Fig. 11.5).

| Box 11.1 | Radiation Protection: Excessive Radiation Exposure and Digital Imaging |
|---|---|

Although the computer can adjust image brightness for technique exposure errors, routinely using more radiation than required for the procedure in digital radiography unnecessarily increases patient exposure. Even though the digital system can adjust for overexposures, it is an unethical practice to knowingly overexpose a patient.

**Make the Physics Connection**

## Chapter 6

When the kVp is increased at the control panel, a larger potential difference occurs in the x-ray tube, giving more electrons the kinetic energy to produce x-rays and increasing the kinetic energy overall. The result is more photons (quantity) and higher-energy photons (quality) (Fig. 11.6).

The area of interest must be adequately penetrated before the mAs can be adjusted to produce a diagnostic-quality radiographic image. When adequate penetration is achieved, further increasing the kVp results in more radiation reaching the IR. Unlike mAs, the kVp also affects the subject contrast produced within the image.

**Critical Concept**

## kVp and the Subject Contrast

Increasing or decreasing the kVp changes the amount of radiation exposure to the IR and the subject contrast produced within the image.

Assuming the anatomic part is adequately penetrated, changing the kVp does not affect the brightness of the digital image. Because kVp affects the amount of radiation reaching the IR, its effect on the digital image is similar to the effect of mAs. Too much radiation reaching the IR (within reason) produces a digital

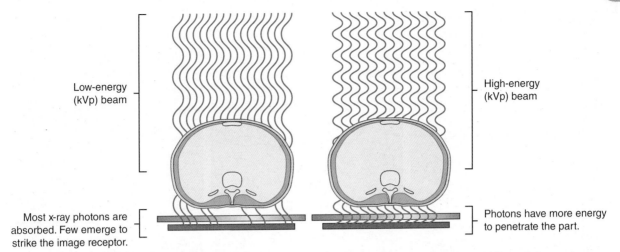

**Fig. 11.5 kVp and Radiation Exposure.** Increasing the kVp increases the penetrating power of the radiation and increases the exposure to the image receptor.

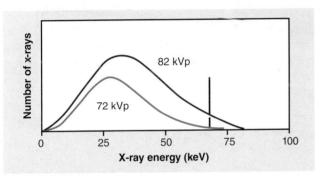

**Fig. 11.6 Change in Kilovoltage Peak.** Two emission spectra illustrating the result of an increase in kVp (*purple curve*). Increases in kVp increase the quantity and quality of radiation. *keV,* Kiloelectron volt; *kVp,* kilovoltage peak.

image with the appropriate level of brightness because of computer adjustment during image processing; however, the patient has been overexposed. Similarly, too little radiation reaching the IR (within reason) produces a digital image with the appropriate level of brightness, but the increased noise may decrease image quality.

A diagnostic quality image (Fig. 11.7A) was produced using 70 kVp at 2 mAs. Fig. 11.7B was produced using 50 kVp at 2 mAs, and Fig. 11.7C was produced using 93 kVp at 2 mAs. Although the brightness was adjusted by the computer, the exposure indicator for each of the images varied greatly and reflected the exposure to the IR. When a kVp that is too low is selected, the brightness is adjusted, but quantum noise may be visible. Additionally, when a kVp that is too high is selected, the image brightness is adjusted, but patient exposure may be increased. Although brightness can be computer adjusted when using a kVp that is too high, increased scatter radiation reaches the IR and may adversely affect image quality.

> ### ❗ Critical Concept
> #### Kilovoltage and Digital Image Quality
> Assuming the anatomic part is adequately penetrated, changing the kVp does not affect the brightness of the digital image. Image brightness is primarily controlled during computer processing.

Kilovoltage is not a factor typically manipulated to vary the amount of exposure to the IR because the kVp also affects subject contrast. However, it is sometimes necessary to manipulate the kVp to maintain the required exposure to the IR. For example, using portable or mobile x-ray equipment may limit choices of mAs settings; therefore, the radiographer must adjust the kVp to maintain sufficient exposure to the IR.

Maintaining or adjusting exposure to the IR can be accomplished with kVp by using the **15% rule**. The 15% rule states that changing the kVp by 15% has the same effect as doubling the mAs or reducing the mAs by 50%; for example, increasing the kVp from 82 to 94 (15%) produces the same exposure to the IR as increasing the mAs from 10 to 20.

> ### ❗ Critical Concept
> #### kVp and the 15% Rule
> A 15% increase in kVp has the same effect as doubling the mAs. A 15% decrease in kVp has the same effect as decreasing the mAs by half.

Increasing the kVp by 15% increases the exposure to the IR, unless the mAs is decreased. Also, decreasing the kVp by 15% decreases the exposure to the IR, unless the mAs is increased.

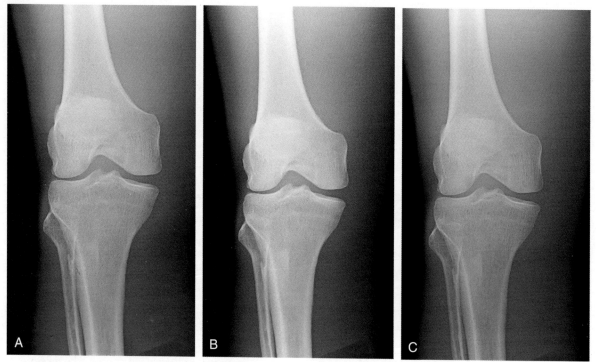

Fig. 11.7 **Changes in kVp and Image Quality. (A)** Image produced using 70 kVp at 2 mAs. **(B)** Image produced using 50 kVp at 2 mAs results in higher subject contrast and computer adjusted to maintain brightness; however, increased quantum noise is visible. **(C)** Image produced using 93 kVp at 2 mAs results in lower subject contrast and computer adjustment to maintain brightness; however, patient exposure is increased.

### 123 Math Application

#### Using the 15% Rule

To increase exposure to the IR, multiply the kVp by 1.15 (original kVp + 15%).

$$80 \text{ kVp} \times 1.15 = 92 \text{ kVp}$$

To decrease exposure to the IR, multiply the kVp by 0.85 (original kVp − 15%).

$$80 \text{ kVp} \times 0.85 = 68 \text{ kVp}$$

To maintain exposure to the IR, when increasing the kVp by 15% (kVp × 1.15), divide the original mAs by 2.

$$80 \text{ kVp} \times 1.15 = 92 \text{ kVp and mAs/2}$$

When decreasing the kVp by 15% (kVp × 0.85), multiply the mAs by 2.

$$80 \text{ kVp} \times 0.85 = 68 \text{ kVp and mAs} \times 2$$

result, images with lower subject contrast are produced (Fig. 11.8). When a low kVp is used, the x-ray beam penetration is decreased, resulting in more absorption and less transmission, which results in greater variation in the x-ray intensities exiting the patient. This produces an image with higher subject contrast (Fig. 11.9).

### ⚠ Critical Concept

#### kVp and Subject Contrast

A high kVp results in less absorption and more transmission in the anatomic tissues, which results in less variation in the x-ray intensities exiting the patient (remnant), producing lower subject contrast. A low kVp results in more absorption and less transmission in the anatomic tissues, but with more variation in the x-ray intensities exiting the patient, resulting in higher subject contrast.

Altering the penetrating power of the x-ray beam affects its absorption and transmission through the anatomic tissue being radiographed. Higher kVp increases the penetrating power of the x-ray beam and results in less absorption and more transmission in the anatomic tissues, which results in less variation in the x-ray intensities exiting the patient. As a

Changing the kVp affects its absorption and transmission as it interacts with anatomic tissue; however, using a higher kVp reduces the total number of interactions and increases the number of x-rays transmitted. In these interactions, more Compton scattering than x-ray absorption occurs (photoelectric effect) and more scatter exits the patient.

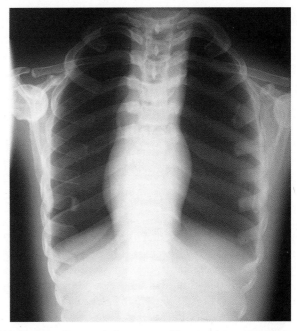

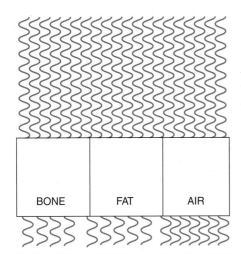

Fig. 11.8 **kVp and Exit-Beam Intensities.** Higher kVp increases the penetrating power of the x-ray beam and results in less absorption and more transmission in the anatomic tissues, which results in less variation in the x-ray intensities exiting the patient. As a result, images with lower subject contrast are produced. (Courtesy Fauber TL: *Radiographic imaging and exposure*, ed 3, St Louis, 2009, Mosby.)

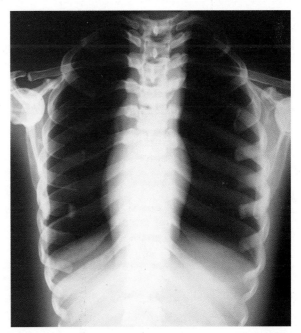

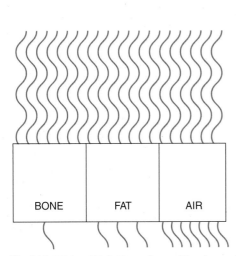

Fig. 11.9 **kVp and Exit-Beam Intensities.** Lower kVp decreases the x-ray beam penetration, resulting in more absorption and less transmission, which results in greater variation in the x-ray intensities exiting the patient. As a result, images with higher subject contrast are produced. (Courtesy Fauber TL: *Radiographic imaging and exposure*, ed 3, St Louis, 2009, Mosby.)

 **Make the Physics Connection**

**Chapter 7**

The probability of Compton scattering is related to the energy of the photon. As x-ray photon energy increases, the probability of that photon penetrating a given tissue without interaction increases. However, with this increase in photon energy, the likelihood of Compton interactions relative to photoelectric interactions also increases. Scatter radiation remains a concern at higher kVp, provides no useful information, and always decreases radiographic contrast.

 **Critical Concept**

**Kilovoltage, Scatter Radiation, and Radiographic Contrast**

At higher kVp, a greater proportion of Compton scattering occurs compared with x-ray absorption (photoelectric effect), which decreases radiographic contrast. Decreasing the kVp decreases the proportion of Compton scattering and increases radiographic contrast.

The level of subject contrast desired, and therefore the kVp selected, depends on the type and composition of the

Box 11.2 **Radiation Protection: kVp and mAs**

Whenever possible, a higher kVp and lower mAs should be used to reduce patient exposure. Increasing kVp requires less mAs to maintain the correct exposure to the IR and decreases the radiation dose to the patient. For example, changing from 70 to 81 when radiographing a pelvis is a 15% increase in kVp and requires half the mAs needed at 70 kVp. Higher kVp increases the beam penetration, and therefore lower quantity of radiation is needed to achieve the required amount of radiation reaching the IR and produce a diagnostic-quality image.

anatomic tissue, the structures that must be visualized, and to some extent the diagnostician's preference. For most anatomic regions, an accepted range of kVp provides an appropriate level of subject contrast. As long as the kVp selected is sufficient to penetrate the anatomic part, the radiographic contrast can be adjusted by the computer to display the desired contrast for the anatomic region.

Radiographic images generally are not repeated because of radiographic contrast errors. If a repeat radiograph is necessary and kVp is to be adjusted to either increase or decrease the level of subject contrast, the 15% rule provides an acceptable method of adjustment. In addition, whenever a 15% change is made in the kVp, the radiographer must adjust the mAs by a factor of 2 to maintain the exposure to the IR. The selection of kVp alters its absorption and transmission through the anatomic part regardless of the type of IR used and therefore must be selected wisely. Exposure techniques using higher kVp with lower mAs exposure techniques are recommended in digital imaging because radiographic contrast is primarily controlled during computer processing (Box 11.2).

## SECONDARY FACTORS

Many secondary factors affect the radiation reaching the IR and image quality. It is important for the radiographer to understand their effects individually and in combination.

### FOCAL SPOT SIZE

On the control panel, the radiographer can select whether to use a small or large focal spot size. The physical dimensions of the focal spot on the anode target in x-ray tubes used in standard radiographic applications usually range from 0.5 to 1.2 mm. Small focal spot sizes are usually 0.5 or 0.6 mm and large focal spot sizes are usually 1 or 1.2 mm. Focal spot size is determined by the filament size. When the radiographer selects a particular focal spot size, they are actually selecting a filament size that is energized during x-ray production. Focal spot size is an important consideration for the radiographer because the focal spot size affects sharpness but not IR exposure. Lower mA settings are associated with the small filament, whereas higher mA settings energize the large filament.

 **Make the Physics Connection**

**Chapter 5**

The actual focal spot is the area bombarded by the filament electrons. The size of the electron stream depends on the size of the filament. The smaller this stream, the greater the heat generated in a small area; therefore, it is desirable to have a larger actual focal spot area for heat dissipation. The effective focal spot is the origin of the x-ray beam and is the area as seen from the patient's perspective. The smaller this area of origin, the sharper the image. It is desirable to keep this as small as practical to improve image quality (Fig. 11.10).

 **Critical Concept**

**Focal Spot Size and Spatial Resolution**

As focal spot size increases, unsharpness increases and spatial resolution decreases; as focal spot size decreases, unsharpness decreases and spatial resolution increases.

In general, the smallest focal spot size available should be used for every exposure. Unfortunately, exposure is limited with a small focal spot size. When a small focal spot is used, the heat created during the x-ray exposure is concentrated in a smaller area and could cause tube damage. The radiographer must weigh the importance of improved spatial resolution for a particular examination or anatomic part against the amount of radiation exposure used. For example, a radiographer should ensure the small focal spot is not selected for a lumbar spine examination. Modern radiographic x-ray generators are equipped with safety circuits that prevent an exposure from being made if that exposure exceeds the

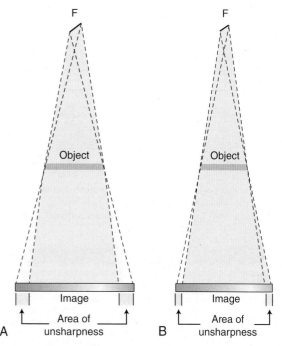

**Fig. 11.10 Focal Spot Size and Spatial Resolution.** Focal spot size influences the amount of unsharpness recorded in the image. As focal spot size changes, so does the amount of unsharpness. **(A)** Larger focal spot. **(B)** Smaller focal spot.

tube-loading capacity for the focal spot size selected. Repeated exposures made just under the limit over a long period can still jeopardize the life of the x-ray tube.

## SOURCE-TO-IMAGE RECEPTOR DISTANCE

The distance between the source of the radiation and the IR, **source-to-image receptor distance (SID)**, affects the amount of radiation reaching the patient. Because of the divergence of the x-ray beam, the intensity of the radiation varies at different distances.

 **Make the Physics Connection**

### Chapter 6

X-ray photons diverge as they travel away from the source. If the distance is shorter, they do not have the opportunity to diverge as much and are concentrated in a smaller area.

This relationship between distance and x-ray beam intensity is best described by the **inverse square law**. The inverse square law states that the intensity of the x-ray beam is inversely proportional to the square of the distance from the source. Because beam intensity varies as a function of the square of the distance, SID affects the quantity of radiation reaching the IR. As SID is increased, the x-ray intensity is spread over a larger area. This decreases the overall intensity of the x-ray beam reaching the IR (Fig. 11.11).

 **Critical Concept**

### SID and X-Ray Beam Intensity

As SID increases, the x-ray beam intensity is spread over a larger area. This decreases the overall intensity of the x-ray beam reaching the IR.

 **Math Application**

### Inverse Square Law Formula

$$\frac{I_1}{I_2} = \frac{(D_2)^2}{(D_1)^2}$$

The intensity of radiation at an SID of 40 inches (100 cm) is equal to 500 mR. What is the intensity of radiation when the distance is increased to 56 inches (140 cm)?

$$\frac{500\ mR}{X} = \frac{(56)^2}{(40)^2}$$

$$500\ mR \times 1600 = 3136X;$$

$$\frac{800,000}{3136} = X; 255.1\ mR = X$$

Because increasing the SID decreases x-ray beam intensity, the mAs must be increased accordingly to maintain the proper exposure to the IR. When the SID is decreased, the beam intensity increases; therefore, the mAs must be decreased accordingly to maintain proper exposure to the IR.

 **Critical Concept**

### SID and mAs

Increasing the SID requires that the mAs be increased to maintain exposure to the IR and decreasing the SID requires a decrease in the mAs to maintain exposure to the IR.

Maintaining consistent radiation exposure to the IR when the SID is altered requires that the mAs be adjusted to compensate. The **direct square law** or **exposure maintenance formula** provides a mathematical calculation for adjusting the mAs when changing the SID.

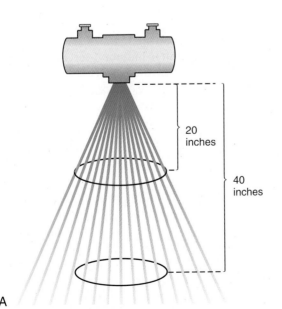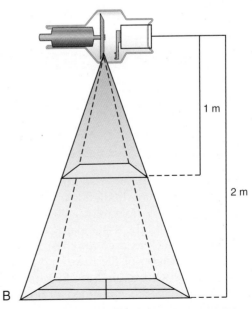

Fig. 11.11 **SID and Radiation Intensity.** Beam intensity varies as a function of the square of the distance. **(A)** This decreases the overall intensity of the x-ray beam reaching the image receptor, and **(B)** as SID is increased, the x-ray intensity is spread over a larger area.

## Math Application

### Direct Square Law or Exposure Maintenance Formula

$$\frac{mAs_1}{mAs_2} = \frac{(SID_1)^2}{(SID_2)^2}$$

Proper exposure to the IR is achieved at an SID of 40 inches using 25 mAs. The SID must be increased to 56 inches. What adjustment in mAs is needed to maintain exposure to the IR?

$$\frac{25}{mAs_2} = \frac{(40)^2}{(56)^2};$$

$$1600X = 78,400 \frac{78,400}{1600};$$

$$mAs_2 = 49$$

Standard distances are used in radiography to provide more consistency in radiographic quality. Most diagnostic radiography is performed at an SID of 40, 48, or 72 inches. Certain circumstances, such as trauma or mobile radiography, do not allow for standard distances to be used often. In these circumstances, the radiographer must determine the change needed in the mAs to obtain a diagnostic-quality radiograph. When a 72-inch (180-cm) SID cannot be used, adjusting the SID to 56 inches (140 cm) requires half the mAs. When a 40-inch (100-cm) SID cannot be used, adjusting the SID to 56 inches (140 cm) requires twice the mAs. This quick method of calculating mAs changes should produce sufficient exposure to the IR.

In addition to altering the intensity of radiation, SID also affects size distortion (magnification) and spatial resolution. As the distance between the source and IR increases, the diverging x-rays become more perpendicular to the object radiographed and influence the amount of size distortion produced on a radiographic image (Fig. 11.12).

## Critical Concept

### SID, Size Distortion, and Spatial Resolution

As SID increases, size distortion (magnification) decreases and spatial resolution increases; as SID decreases, size distortion (magnification) increases and spatial resolution decreases.

Standard distances for SID are used in radiography to accommodate equipment limitations. Except for chest and cervical spine radiography, a 40-inch (100-cm) or 48-inch (120-cm) SID is standard. A greater 72-inch (180-cm) SID, such as used for chest imaging, decreases the magnification of the heart and records its size more accurately. Increasing the SID from the standard distances may be recommended for positions that result in increased OID. For example, using an SID between 60 inches (150 cm) and 72 inches (180 cm) for the lateral and oblique positions of the cervical spine is recommended to compensate for the unavoidable

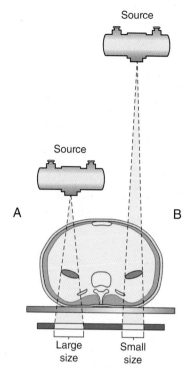

Fig. 11.12 **SID and Size Distortion.** A long SID creates less magnification than a short SID. The image in **(A)** is larger than that in **(B)** because the object is closer to the source.

increase in OID. In these situations, increasing the SID will increase spatial resolution.

## OBJECT-TO-IMAGE RECEPTOR DISTANCE

When distance is created between the object radiographed and the IR, known as **object-to-image receptor distance (OID)**, decreased beam intensity may result. As the exit radiation continues to diverge, less overall intensity of the x-ray beam reaches the IR.

When sufficient distance between the object and IR exists, an air gap is created, preventing some scatter radiation from striking the IR (Fig. 11.13). Whenever the amount of scatter radiation reaching the IR is reduced, radiographic contrast is increased. The amount of OID required to increase radiographic contrast depends in part on the percentage of scatter radiation exiting the patient. For anatomic areas that produce a high percentage of scatter radiation, less OID is needed to increase radiographic contrast than for anatomic areas that produce less scatter.

In addition to affecting the intensity of radiation reaching the IR, the OID also affects the amount of size distortion (magnification) and spatial resolution. Optimal spatial resolution is achieved when the OID is zero. Unfortunately, this cannot realistically be achieved in radiographic imaging because there is always some distance created between the area of interest and the IR. As the exit beam leaves the patient, it continues to diverge. When distance is created between the area of interest and the IR, the diverging exit beam records the anatomic part with increased size distortion (magnification) (Fig. 11.14).

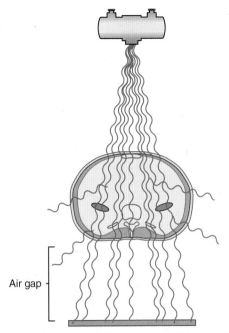

**Fig. 11.13 OID and Air Gap.** Distance created between the object and the image receptor reduces the amount of scatter radiation reaching the image receptor.

---

### ! Critical Concept

**OID, Size Distortion, and Spatial Resolution**

Increasing the OID increases magnification and decreases spatial resolution, whereas decreasing the amount of OID decreases magnification and increases spatial resolution.

---

OID is the factor that affects the intensity of radiation reaching the IR, image contrast, magnification, and spatial resolution. The distance between the area of interest and the IR has the greatest effect on the amount of size distortion. The radiographer must position the area of interest as close to the IR as possible to minimize the amount of distortion. Although the amount of OID necessary to adversely affect image quality has not been standardized, the radiographer should minimize the amount of OID whenever possible. In some situations, it is difficult to minimize OID because of factors or conditions beyond the radiographer's control. In these instances, size distortion can still be reduced by increasing SID. However, this would also necessitate a corresponding increase in mAs to ensure appropriate IR exposure.

## CALCULATING MAGNIFICATION

To observe the effect of distance (SID and OID) on size distortion, it is necessary to consider the magnification factor. The **magnification factor (MF)** indicates how much size distortion or magnification is demonstrated on a radiographic image. The MF can be expressed mathematically by the following formula:

$$MF = SID \div SOD$$

**Source-to-object distance (SOD)** refers to the distance from the x-ray source (focal spot) to the object being imaged. SOD can be expressed mathematically as follows:

$$SOD = SID - OID$$

SOD is demonstrated in Fig. 11.15.

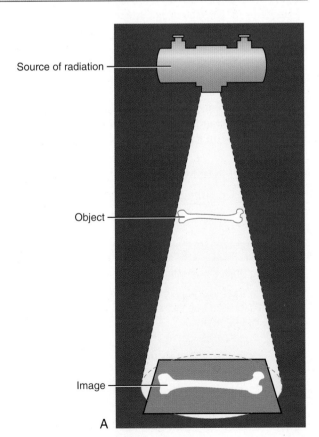

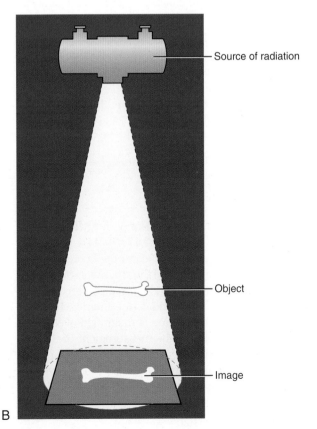

**Fig. 11.14 OID and Size Distortion.** A long OID creates more magnification than a short OID. The image in **(A)** is larger than that in **(B)** because the object is farther from the image receptor.

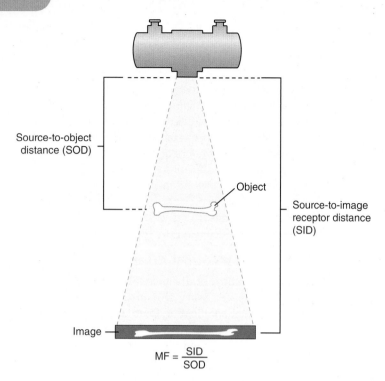

$$MF = \frac{SID}{SOD}$$

**Fig. 11.15 Source-to-Object Distance (SOD).** The SOD is the distance between the source of the x-ray and the object radiographed.

An MF of 1 indicates no magnification, which means that the size of the radiographic image matches the true object size. True object size on an image is impossible to achieve because some magnification exists on every image because of the internal location of anatomic structures. An MF greater than 1 can be expressed as a percentage of magnification. For example, an MF of 1.2 indicates the image size is 20% (0.2 × 100) larger than the object size.

**Math Application**

**The Magnification Factor**

A posteroanterior (PA) projection of the chest is produced with an SID of 72 inches and an OID of 3 inches (SOD is equal to 69 inches). What is the MF?

$$SOD = SID - OID \quad MF = \frac{72 \text{ inches}}{69 \text{ inches}}$$

$$69 = 72 - 3 \qquad MF = 1.044$$

In the case of the Math Application for MF, an MF of 1.044 means that the image is 4.4% (0.044 × 100) larger than the true object size. The MF computed here is a minimum. A 3-inch OID implies that the anterior surface of the patient's chest was 3 inches away from the IR for a PA projection. Anatomy that is posterior to the anterior chest wall is farther away from the IR and is magnified even more. It may be helpful to know the measurement of the true object size in comparison with its size on a radiographic image. Once the MF is known, the object size can then be determined. This requires the use of another formula:

$$\text{Object size} = \frac{\text{Image size}}{MF}$$

**Math Application**

**Determining Object Size**

On a PA chest image taken with an SID of 72 inches and an OID of 3 inches (SOD is equal to 69 inches), the size of a round lesion in the right lung measures 1.5 inches in diameter on the radiographic image. The MF has been determined to be 1.044. What is the object size of this lesion?

$$\text{Object size} = \frac{1.5 \text{ inches}}{1.044}$$

The object size is 1.44 inches.

If both the object size and image size are known, then the percentage of magnification of the object can be calculated with the formula:

$$\text{Object \% of Magnification}$$
$$= \frac{\text{Image size} - \text{Object size}}{\text{Object size}} \times 100$$

**Math Application**

**Determining Object % of Magnification**

A lesion on the radiographic image measures 1.68 cm, and the lesion's (object) true size measures 1.56 cm. What is the object % of magnification?

$$\text{Object \% of Magnification}$$
$$= \frac{1.68 - 1.56}{1.56 \text{ cm}} \times 100$$

$$0.12 / 1.56 \times 100 = 0.0769 \times 100$$
$$= 7.69\% \text{ object magnification}$$

Perhaps the most practical use of these formulas is to observe how changing the SID and OID affects the image size. Size distortion (magnification) can be increased by decreasing the SID or by increasing the OID. This increase in magnification can be demonstrated mathematically by using the MF, then calculating the change in the size of the object on the radiographic image. It is important to note that any time magnification is increased, spatial resolution decreases.

## CENTRAL RAY ALIGNMENT

Shape distortion of the anatomic area of interest can occur from inaccurate central ray (CR) alignment to the part being radiographed and/or the IR. Any misalignment of the CR among these three factors alters the shape of the part on the radiographic image.

For example, Fig. 11.16 demonstrates shape distortion when the anatomic part and IR are misaligned.

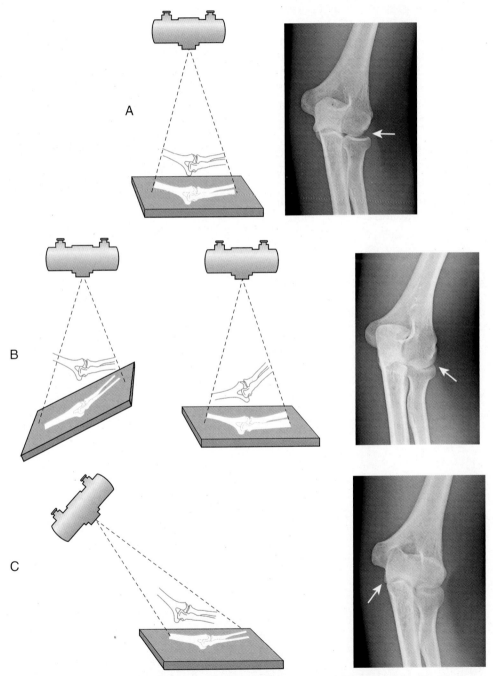

Fig. 11.16 **Misalignment and Shape Distortion. (A)** Proper alignment among the x-ray tube, part, and image receptor. Image **(A)** is a quality image with minimal distortion. Note the proper alignment of the radial head with capitulum in the image. **(B)** Improper alignment among the x-ray tube, part, and image receptor. The illustration on the left shows the image receptor misaligned to the part and the one on the right shows the part not parallel to image receptor. Image **(B)** has shape distortion resulting from misalignment of the part and image receptor. Note the improper alignment of the radial head with capitulum in the image. **(C)** Improper alignment among the x-ray tube, part, and image receptor. Image **(C)** has shape distortion from the central ray not being perpendicular to the part. Note the elongation of the olecranon process.

In addition, shape distortion can occur if the CR of the primary beam is not directed to enter or exit the anatomy as required for the particular projection or position (off centering). This happens because the path of individual photons in the primary beam becomes more divergent as the distance increases from the CR. The radiographer must properly control alignment of the tube, part, and IR, and properly direct the CR to minimize shape distortion. The ideal method to minimize shape distortion is for the radiographer to align the CR perpendicular to the part and IR and align the long axis of the part parallel to the IR.

In addition to creating shape distortion, CR angulation and misalignment of the tube, part, and IR could affect the exposure to the IR. For example, when the CR is angled, the distance between the source of the radiation and the IR is increased. As a general rule, when the CR is angled, the SID is decreased accordingly (1 inch for every 5 degrees of angulation) to maintain exposure to the IR. If misalignment occurs among the tube, part, or IR, the distance between the source of radiation and the IR or the part and the IR could be increased or decreased. This could affect the amount of exposure to the IR, and therefore the mAs may need adjustment.

## GRIDS

A radiographic grid is a device that is placed between the anatomic area of interest and the IR to absorb scatter radiation exiting the patient. Limiting the amount of scatter radiation that reaches the IR improves the quality of the image. Much of the scatter radiation exiting the patient will not reach the IR when absorbed by a grid (Fig. 11.17). The effect of less scatter, or unwanted

exposure, on the image is increased radiographic contrast. Grids are typically used only when the anatomic part is 10 cm (4 inches) or greater in thickness, and more than 60 kVp is needed for the examination.

 **Critical Concept**

### Grids, Scatter, and Contrast

Placing a grid between the anatomic area of interest and the IR absorbs scatter radiation exiting the patient and increases radiographic contrast.

The more efficient a grid is in absorbing scatter, the greater its effect on radiographic contrast. Unfortunately, grids also absorb some of the transmitted radiation exiting the patient; therefore, the amount of radiation reaching the IR is reduced.

 **Critical Concept**

### Grids and Image Receptor Exposure

Adding, removing, or changing a grid requires an adjustment in mAs to maintain radiation exposure to the IR.

When grids are used, the mAs must be adjusted to maintain exposure to the IR. In addition, the more efficient a grid is at absorbing scatter, the greater increase in mAs is required. The grid conversion formula is a mathematical formula for adjusting the mAs for changes in grid ratio (Table 11.1).

When a grid is added, the radiographer must use the correct grid conversion factor to multiply by the mAs to compensate for the decrease in exposure. When a grid is removed, the correct conversion grid

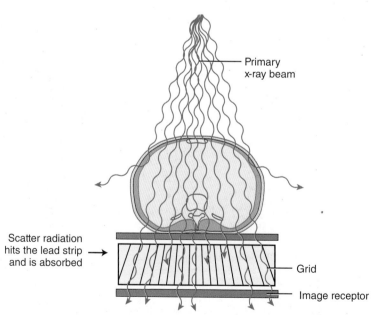

Fig. 11.17 **Grids and Scatter Absorption.** Much of the scatter radiation toward the image receptor is absorbed when a grid is used.

## Table 11.1   Grid Conversion Chart

| GRID RATIOS | GRID CONVERSION FACTOR (GCF) |
|---|---|
| No grid | 1 |
| 5:1 | 2 |
| 6:1 | 3 |
| 8:1 | 4 |
| 12:1 | 5 |
| 16:1 | 6 |

## Box 11.3   Radiation Protection: Grid Selection

Decisions regarding the use of a grid and grid ratio should be made by balancing image quality and patient protection. To keep patient exposure as low as possible, grids should be used only when appropriate, and the grid ratio should be the lowest that will provide sufficient radiographic contrast improvement.

factor must be divided into the mAs to compensate for the increase in exposure (Box 11.3). When the grid ratio is changed, the following formula should be used to adjust the exposure:

$$\frac{mAs_1}{mAs_2} = \frac{\text{Grid conversion factor}_1}{\text{Grid conversion factor}_2}$$

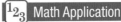

## Math Application

### Adjusting mAs for Changes in Grid

A quality image is obtained using 2 mAs at 70 kVp without using a grid. What new mAs is needed when adding a 12:1 grid to maintain the same exposure to the IR?

$$\frac{2\,mAs}{X} = \frac{1}{5}$$
$$2\,mAs \times 5 = 1\,X; 10\,mAs = X$$

The new mAs produces an exposure comparable to the IR.

It is important to note that brightness can be computer adjusted when the mAs is not properly adjusted for adding or changing a grid (Fig. 11.18). However, without proper mAs adjustment when adding or changing a grid, increased quantum noise or unnecessary patient exposure could be the result. Currently published grid conversion factors were designed for use with past film-screen technology. Research indicates a need to revisit these factors. Radiologic technologists and imaging departments should reevaluate traditional grid conversion factors to ensure digital image receptors receive appropriate exposure and patients receive the lowest amounts of radiation exposure.

Grid construction and efficiency are discussed in greater detail in Chapter 12.

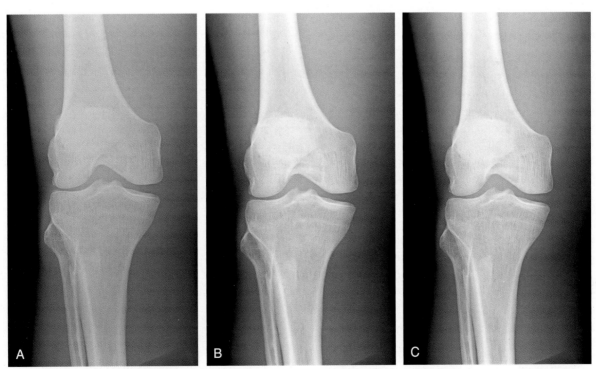

**Fig. 11.18 Grid Use and Image Quality. (A)** Quality image created without a grid. **(B)** Image created with a grid but no adjustment in mAs. Image has higher contrast but increased quantum noise visible. **(C)** Image created with a grid and appropriate mAs adjustment. Image has higher contrast than image **(A)** and less quantum noise visible compared with image **(B)**.

## BEAM RESTRICTION

Any change in the size of the x-ray field alters the amount of tissue irradiated (Box 11.4). A larger field size (decreasing collimation) increases the amount of tissue irradiated, causing more scatter radiation to be produced, and increases the amount of radiation reaching the IR. The increased amount of scatter reaching the IR results in lower radiographic contrast. Conversely, a smaller field size (increasing collimation) reduces the amount of tissue irradiated, reduces the amount of scatter radiation produced, and reduces the amount of radiation reaching the IR. The decreased amount of scatter radiation reaching the IR results in higher radiographic contrast but requires an increase in the mAs. The effect of collimation is greater when imaging large anatomic areas, performing examinations without a grid, and using a high kVp.

 **Critical Concept**

### Beam Restriction and Image Receptor Exposure

Changes in beam restriction alter the amount of tissue irradiated and therefore affect the amount of exposure to the IR. The effect of collimation is greater when imaging large anatomic areas, performing examinations without a grid, and using a high kVp.

## GENERATOR OUTPUT

Exposure techniques and the amount of radiation output depend on the type of x-ray generator used. Generators with more efficient output, such as three-phase or high-frequency units, require lower exposure technique settings to produce an image comparable to those of single-phase units. The radiographer must be aware of the generator output when using different types of equipment, especially when performing examinations in different departments. For example, imaging a knee using a single-phase generator requires more mAs than imaging a knee using a three-phase generator. In addition, x-ray generators must be calibrated periodically to ensure they are producing consistent radiation output.

 **Make the Physics Connection**

### Chapter 6

High-frequency units produce x-rays much more efficiently than single-phase units. A high-frequency unit produces more x-rays using the same amount of electricity (Fig. 11.19).

## TUBE FILTRATION

According to the National Council on Radiation Protection and Measurement, x-ray tubes operated above

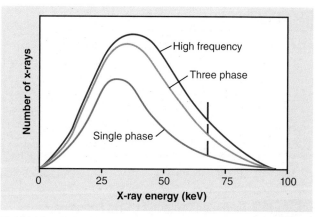

Fig. 11.19 **Change in Generator Type.** Three emission spectra illustrating the result of a change in generator type. Note as the efficiency of the generator type increases, so does x-ray quantity given the same amount of electricity used. *keV*, Kiloelectron volt.

70 kVp are required to have a minimum of 2.5 mm of aluminum filtration. Small variations in the amount of tube filtration should not have any effect on radiographic quality.

 **Make the Physics Connection**

### Chapter 6

The use of filtration decreases x-ray quantity to the extent that it depends on the thickness and type of filtration material. Filtration absorbs low-energy photons that do not contribute to the image. Added filtration placed at the collimator serves to reduce patient dose by removing such photons (Fig. 11.20).

Variability of the x-ray tube filtration should be checked as a part of routine quality control evaluation of the radiographic equipment. X-ray tubes with excessive or insufficient filtration may begin to affect image quality. Increasing the amount of tube filtration increases the percentage of higher-penetrating x-rays to lower-penetrating x-rays. As a result, the x-ray beam has increased energy and can increase the amount of scatter radiation reaching the IR. The increased x-ray energy (kVp) and scatter production decrease

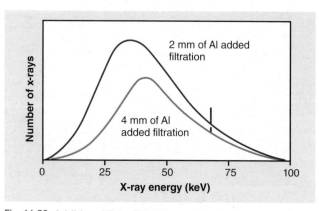

Fig. 11.20 **Additional Tube Filtration.** Two emission spectra illustrating the result of added filtration (*green curve*). Increases in filtration decreases the quantity and increases quality of radiation. *Al*, aluminum; *keV*, kiloelectron volt.

radiographic contrast. The amount of tube filtration should not vary greatly; therefore, small changes do not have a visible effect on radiographic contrast.

## COMPENSATING FILTERS

When imaging an anatomic area that varies greatly in tissue thickness, a compensating filter can be placed in the primary beam to produce a more uniform exposure to the IR. The use of compensating filters requires an increase in mAs to maintain the overall exposure to the IR. The amount of increase in the mAs depends on the thickness and type of compensating filter. Additionally, a compensating filter increases the exposure to the patient and is not typically used in routine radiography.

## PATIENT FACTORS

### BODY HABITUS

**Body habitus** refers to the general form or build of the body, including size. It is important for the radiographer to consider body habitus when establishing exposure techniques. There are four types of body habitus: sthenic, hyposthenic, hypersthenic, and asthenic (Fig. 11.21).

The sthenic body habitus accounts for approximately 50% of the adult population and is commonly called a *normal* or *average* build. Hyposthenic accounts for approximately 35% of adults and refers to a similar type of body habitus as sthenic but with a tendency toward a more slender and taller build. Together, the sthenic and hyposthenic types of body habitus are, in terms of establishing radiographic techniques, classified as *normal* or *average* of the adult population. These two types of body habitus combined account for approximately 85% of adults.

Hypersthenic and asthenic body habitus types are more extreme and are more rare. The hypersthenic body habitus—a large, stocky build—accounts for only 5% of adults. These individuals have thicker part sizes compared with sthenic or hyposthenic individuals, so exposure factors for their radiographic examinations are higher.

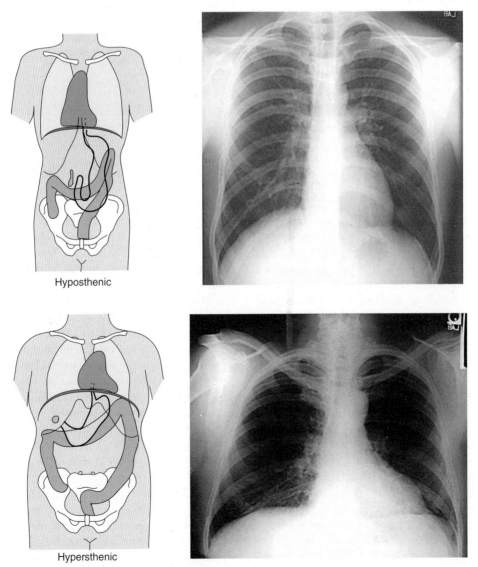

Hyposthenic

Hypersthenic

Fig. 11.21 **Four Types of Body Habitus.** (Courtesy Long BW, Rollins JH, Smith BJ: *Merrill's atlas of radiographic positioning and procedures,* vol 1, ed 13, St Louis, 2016, Mosby.)

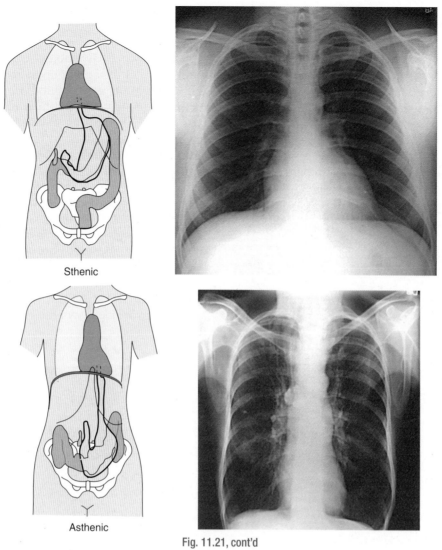

Sthenic

Asthenic

Fig. 11.21, cont'd

## PART THICKNESS AND SUBJECT CONTRAST

*Asthenic* refers to a very slender body habitus and accounts for only 10% of adults. Exposure factors for asthenic individuals are at the low end of exposure technique charts because their respective part sizes are thinner than those of sthenic and hyposthenic individuals.

The thickness of the anatomic part being imaged affects the amount of x-ray beam attenuation that occurs. A thick part absorbs more radiation, whereas a thin part transmits more radiation.

Maintaining the exposure to the IR when imaging a thicker part requires the mAs to be increased accordingly (Fig. 11.22). In addition, when a thinner anatomic part is radiographed, the mAs must be decreased accordingly. Brightness can be computer adjusted when the mAs is not properly altered for changes in part thickness; however, increased quantum noise or unnecessary patient exposure could result.

Because x-rays are attenuated exponentially, a general guideline is that for every change in part thickness of 4 to 5 cm, the radiographer should adjust the mAs by a factor of 2 (Fig. 11.23). For example, an optimal image was obtained using 20 mAs on an anatomic part that measured 18 cm. The same anatomic part is imaged in another patient, and it measures 22 cm. What new mAs is needed to expose the IR? Because the part thickness was increased by 4 cm, the original mAs is multiplied by 2, yielding 40 mAs. If another patient for the same part measures 26 cm, what new mAs is needed? Because the part thickness increased by another 4 cm, the mAs is multiplied by 2, yielding 80 mAs. This mAs is four times greater than for the original patient who measured 8 cm less.

As the thickness of a given type of anatomic tissue increases, the amount of scatter radiation also increases and radiographic contrast decreases. Using a higher kVp for a thicker part only adds to the increase in scatter radiation. Increased scatter radiation will continue to degrade the quality of the image because it creates fog, which decreases the radiographic contrast. The amount of radiographic contrast achieved is also influenced by the anatomic part to be radiographed.

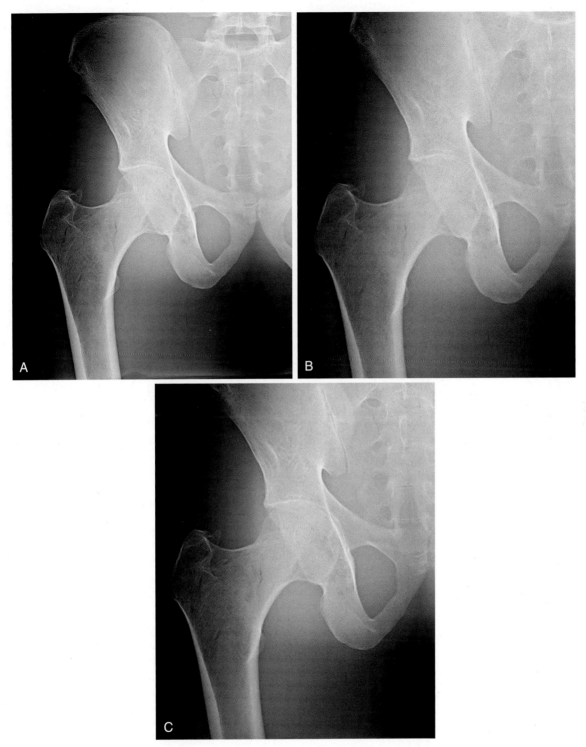

Fig. 11.22 **Patient Thickness and Image Quality. (A)** Quality Image. **(B)** Image created with added thickness and no mAs adjustment, which results in increased quantum noise visible. **(C)** Image created with added patient thickness and appropriate mAs adjustment, which results in decreased quantum noise visible.

As mentioned in Chapter 9, subject contrast is one of the categories of radiographic contrast. The atomic number and thickness of the tissue and cell compactness affect its absorption characteristics. The absorption characteristics of the anatomic tissue create the range of brightness levels produced on a radiograph. Tissues that have a higher atomic number absorb more radiation than those with a lower atomic number.

Anatomic structures that have a wide range of tissue composition demonstrate high subject contrast (Fig. 11.24). Alternately, anatomic structures that consist of similar type tissue demonstrate low subject contrast (Fig. 11.25). The radiographer cannot control the composition of the anatomic part to be radiographed; however, changing the kVp alters its absorption and transmission within anatomic tissues and affects

100 x-rays incident

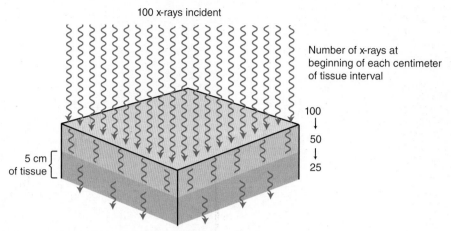

Number of x-rays at
beginning of each centimeter
of tissue interval

100
↓
50
↓
25

5 cm
of tissue

Fig. 11.23 **Tissue Beam Attenuation.** X-rays are attenuated exponentially and generally reduced by approximately 50% for each 4 to 5 cm of tissue thickness.

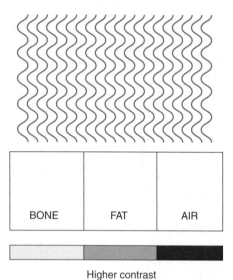

BONE    FAT    AIR

Higher contrast

Fig. 11.24 **High Subject Contrast Tissues.** Higher contrast resulting from great differences in the radiation absorption for tissues that have greater variation in composition.

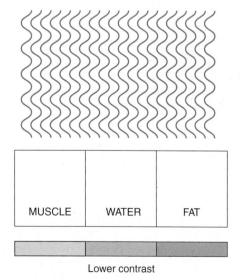

MUSCLE    WATER    FAT

Lower contrast

Fig. 11.25 **Low Subject Contrast Tissues.** Lower contrast resulting from fewer differences in the radiation absorption for tissues that are more similarly composed.

subject contrast. Knowledge about the absorption characteristics of anatomic tissues and the effect of kVp helps the radiographer produce a desired level of radiographic contrast.

The quality of the radiographic image depends on a multitude of variables. Knowledge of these variables and their effects assist the radiographer in producing quality radiographic images. Table 11.2 provides a chart demonstrating how the variables discussed in this chapter affect the primary and remnant x-ray beam, and Table 11.3 provides a chart demonstrating how the variables discussed in this chapter affect the IR exposure and image quality.

## RADIATION PROTECTION REVIEW

### KILOVOLTAGE PEAK AND MAS

Whenever possible, a higher kVp and lower mAs should be used to reduce patient exposure. Increasing kVp requires less mAs to maintain sufficient exposure to the IR and decreases the radiation dose to the patient. For example, changing from 70 to 81 when radiographing a pelvis is a 15% increase in kVp peak and requires half the mAs needed at 70 kVp. Higher kVp increases the beam penetration, and therefore less quantity of radiation is needed to achieve the required amount of radiation reaching the IR and produce a quality image. The actual settings may vary by department and reflect the preference of the radiologists.

### BEAM RESTRICTION

In performing a radiographic examination, the radiographer should be aware of the anatomic area of interest and limit the x-ray field size to just beyond this area. Collimating to the appropriate anatomic area is a basic method for protecting the patient from unnecessary exposure.

### GRID SELECTION

Decisions regarding the use of a grid and grid ratio should be made by balancing image quality and

**Table 11.2** Exposure Factors and Their Effect on the Primary and Exit X-Ray Beam

| | PRIMARY BEAM REACHING THE PATIENT | EXIT BEAM REACHING THE IMAGE RECEPTOR |
|---|---|---|
| **mAs** | | |
| Increasing mAs | ↑ Quantity | ↑ Quantity |
| Decreasing mAs | ↓ Quantity | ↓ Quantity |
| **kVp** | | |
| Increasing kVp | ↑ Quantity and quality | ↑ Quantity and quality |
| Decreasing kVp | ↓ Quantity and quality | ↓ Quantity and quality |
| **Focal Spot Size** | | |
| Smaller focal spot size | No effect | No effect |
| Larger focal spot size | No effect | No effect |
| **SID** | | |
| Increasing SID | ↓ Quantity | ↓ Quantity |
| Decreasing SID | ↑ Quantity | ↑ Quantity |
| **OID** | | |
| Increasing OID | No effect | ↓ Quantity and scatter |
| Decreasing OID | No effect | ↑ Quantity and scatter |
| **Central Ray Angle** | | |
| Increase | ↓ Quantity | ↓ Quantity |
| **Grid** | | |
| Increasing grid ratio | No effect | ↓ Quantity and scatter |
| Decreasing grid ratio | No effect | ↑ Quantity and scatter |
| **Beam Restriction** | | |
| Increasing collimation | ↓ Quantity | ↓ Quantity and scatter |
| Decreasing collimation | ↑ Quantity | ↑ Quantity and scatter |
| **Generator Output** | | |
| Single-phase generator | ↓ Quantity and quality | ↓ Quantity and quality |
| High frequency generator | ↑ Quantity and quality | ↑ Quantity and quality |
| **Compensating Filter** | | |
| Adding a compensating filter | ↓ Quantity | ↓ Quantity |

**Table 11.3** Exposure Technique Factors and Image Quality: Individual Factor Change Without Exposure Technique Compensation

| EXPOSURE FACTOR | IR EXPOSURE | BRIGHTNESS[a] | CONTRAST[a,b] | SPATIAL RESOLUTION | DISTORTION |
|---|---|---|---|---|---|
| **mAs** | | | | | |
| Increase | Increase | No effect | No effect | No effect | No effect |
| Decrease | Decrease | | | | |
| **kVp[c]** | | | | | |
| Increase | Increase | No effect | Decrease | No effect | No effect |
| Decrease | Decrease | | Increase | | |
| **Focal Spot Size** | | | | | |
| Increase | No effect | No effect | No effect | Decrease | No effect |
| Decrease | | | | Increase | |
| **SID** | | | | | |
| Increase | Decrease | No effect | No effect | Increase | – Magnification |
| Decrease | Increase | | | Decrease | + Magnification |
| **OID** | | | | | |
| Increase | Decrease | No effect | Increase[d] | Decrease | + Magnification |
| **Central Ray Angle** | | | | | |
| Increase | Decrease | No effect | No effect | Decrease | + Shape distortion |

*Continued*

| Table 11.3 | Exposure Technique Factors and Image Quality: Individual Factor Change Without Exposure Technique Compensation—cont'd | | | | |
| --- | --- | --- | --- | --- | --- |
| EXPOSURE FACTOR | IR EXPOSURE | BRIGHTNESS[a] | CONTRAST[a,b] | SPATIAL RESOLUTION | DISTORTION |
| **Grid Use** | | | | | |
| Add grid | Decrease | No effect | Increase | No effect | No effect |
| Remove grid | Increase | | Decrease | | |
| **Collimation** | | | | | |
| Increase | Decrease | No effect | Increase | No effect | No effect |
| Decrease | Increase | | Decrease | | |
| **Tube Filtration** | | | | | |
| Excessive | Decrease | No effect | Decrease | No effect | No effect |
| Insufficient | Increase | | Increase | | |
| **Patient Thickness** | | | | | |
| Increase | Decrease | No effect | Decrease | Decrease | + Magnification |
| Decrease | Increase | | Increase | Increase | – Magnification |
| **Patient Motion** | | | | | |
| | No effect | No effect | No effect | Decrease | No effect |

[a]Brightness and radiographic contrast can be adjusted by the computer.
[b]Increase is higher radiographic contrast and decrease is lower radiographic contrast.
[c]kVp affects subject contrast
[d]Increase (higher) radiographic contrast because of less scatter reaching IR; this effect is dependent on anatomic region, thickness, and amount of OID.

patient protection. To keep patient exposure as low as possible, grids should be used only when appropriate, and the grid ratio should be the lowest that will provide sufficient radiographic contrast improvement.

## EXCESSIVE RADIATION EXPOSURE AND DIGITAL IMAGING

Although the computer can adjust image brightness for technique exposure errors, routinely using more radiation than required for the procedure in digital radiography unnecessarily increases patient exposure. Even though the digital system can adjust for overexposures, it is an unethical practice to knowingly overexpose a patient.

### On the Spot

- The product of milliamperage and exposure time (mAs) has a directly proportional relationship with the quantity of x-rays produced and exposure to the IR.
- Milliamperage and exposure time have an inverse relationship to maintain exposure to the IR.
- The kVp changes the penetrating power of the x-ray beam and has a direct effect on exposure to the IR.
- Changing the kVp by 15% has the same effect on the x-ray beam as changing the mAs by a factor of 2.
- kVp has an inverse relationship with subject contrast: A high kVp creates an image with low subject contrast, and a low kVp creates an image with high subject contrast.
- Focal spot size affects only spatial resolution. A smaller focal spot size increases spatial resolution.
- SID has an inverse squared relationship with the intensity of radiation reaching the patient and the IR.
- Increasing OID decreases exposure to the IR.

- Decreasing SID and increasing OID increases size distortion (magnification) and decreases spatial resolution.
- Grids absorb scatter exiting the patient and increase radiographic contrast.
- Beam restriction affects the amount of tissue irradiated, scatter produced, and the exposure to the IR.
- Changes in SID, grids, and patient thickness require a change in mAs to maintain the exposure to the IR.
- X-ray generators with more efficient output, such as three-phase or high frequency, require lower exposure techniques to produce the same exposure to the IR as a single-phase generator.
- Exposure factors may need to be modified for body habitus and part thickness.

## CRITICAL THINKING QUESTIONS

1. Given a diagnostic image, describe how the exposure technique would be adjusted for individual changes in mA or exposure time, kVp, grid ratio, beam collimation, SID, and patient thickness.
2. Given patient and exposure factor variability, how do radiographers select exposure techniques to produce diagnostic-quality radiographic images?
3. What considerations can be made when selecting exposure techniques to minimize patient exposure?

## REVIEW QUESTIONS

1. What type of relationship does mAs have with the exposure reaching the image receptor?
   a. Direct
   b. Inverse
   c. Directly proportional
   d. Inversely proportional

2. Which of the following describes the relationship between mA and time to maintain exposure to the image receptor?
   a. Direct
   b. Inverse
   c. Directly proportional
   d. Inversely proportional

3. Increasing the mAs (within reason) has _____ effect on brightness displayed in digital imaging.
   a. direct
   b. proportional
   c. inverse
   d. no

4. Given the anatomic part is adequately penetrated, changing the kVp will affect:
   a. brightness.
   b. Compton scattering.
   c. subject contrast.
   d. b and c.

5. Which of the following factors do not affect spatial resolution?
   a. Focal spot size
   b. SID
   c. OID
   d. Grid

6. The amount of remnant radiation will *decrease* when *increasing*:
   a. focal spot size.
   b. tissue thickness.
   c. mAs.
   d. kVp.

7. A diagnostic image was produced using 70 kVp, 15 mAs at 40-inch SID. Which of the following exposure techniques would maintain the exposure to the image receptor when decreasing the SID to 30 inches?
   a. 80 kVp at 15 mAs
   b. 70 kVp at 8.4 mAs
   c. 70 KVp at 11.3 mAs
   d. 60 kVp at 27 mAs

8. What factor affects the amount of radiation intensity and scatter reaching the image receptor, magnification, and spatial resolution?
   a. OID
   b. SID
   c. Grid ratio
   d. Beam restriction

9. A diagnostic image is created using 80 kVp, 10 mAs, and a grid ratio of 12:1. Which of the following exposure techniques would maintain exposure to the image receptor when the grid is removed?
   a. 68 kVp at 10 mAs
   b. 80 kVp at 2 mAs
   c. 92 kVp at 5 mAs
   d. 80 kVp at 50 mAs

10. What is the magnification factor when using a 72-inch SID and 1.5-inch OID?
    a. 0.979
    b. 1.021
    c. 1.5
    d. 2.0

11. How is the primary beam affected when increasing the tube filtration?
    a. Increase in the number of x-ray photons
    b. Increase in the proportion of lower-energy x-rays
    c. Increase in the proportion of higher-energy x-rays
    d. Increase in the speed of the x-ray photons

**WORD PROBLEMS**

12. A digital image of the T-spine was created using 75 kVp at 10 mAs, 12:1 grid, 40 inch SID, and small focal spot size. The exposure indicator value denotes insufficient exposure to the image receptor, and the image displays excessive noise. What adjustments to the exposure technique would improve the quality of the image if repeated?

13. A good-quality anteroposterior (AP) projection of the hip was created in the radiology department using 80 kVp at 15 mAs, a 40-inch SID, and a 12:1 grid ratio. A request to image a similar-sized patient's hip with the mobile x-ray unit requires the SID to be increased to 48 inches and the use of an 8:1 grid ratio. What adjustments in the exposure technique would provide a similar quality image?

14. A good-quality anteroposterior (AP) projection of the abdomen was created on a patient measuring 10 cm using 70 kVp at 30 mAs, 40-inch SID, 12:1 grid, and large focal spot size. What adjustment in exposure technique would be done if the next patient requiring a KUB measured 15 cm?

# 12

# Scatter Control

## Outline

## Objectives

- State the purpose of beam-restricting devices.
- Describe each of the types of beam-restricting devices.
- State the purpose of automatic collimators or positive beam-limiting devices.
- Describe the purpose of a radiographic grid.
- Describe the construction of grids, including the different types of grid pattern and grid focus.
- Calculate grid ratio.
- List the various types of stationary grids and describe the function and purpose of a moving grid.
- Demonstrate use of the grid conversion formula.
- Describe different types of grid cutoff that can occur and their radiographic appearance.
- Identify the factors to be considered in using a grid.
- Recognize how beam restriction and use of grids affect patient radiation exposure.
- Describe a virtual grid and its effect on patient radiation exposure
- Explain the air gap technique and describe its use.
- Describe the use of shielding accessories to absorb scatter radiation.

## Key Terms

air gap technique
aperture diaphragm
automatic collimator
beam-restricting device
beam restriction
Bucky
Bucky factor
collimation
collimator
cone
convergent line
convergent point

cross-hatched grid
crossed grid
cylinder
focal distance
focal range
focused grid
grid
grid cap
grid cassette
grid conversion factor (GCF)
grid cutoff
grid focus

grid frequency
grid pattern
grid ratio
interspace material
lead mask
linear grid
Moiré effect
nonfocused grid
parallel grid
positive beam-limiting (PBL) device
virtual grid
wafer grid

## INTRODUCTION

Chapters 7 and 8 discuss the interactions of x-rays with matter. Scatter radiation is primarily the result of the Compton interaction, in which the incoming x-ray photon loses energy and changes direction.

Two major factors affect the amount of scatter radiation produced and exiting the patient: the volume of tissue irradiated and the kilovoltage peak (kVp). The volume of tissue depends on the thickness of the part and the x-ray beam field size. Increasing the volume of tissue irradiated results in increased scatter production. In addition, using a higher kVp increases x-ray transmission and reduces its overall absorption (photoelectric interactions); however, a higher kVp

150

increases the energy of scatter radiation exiting the patient.

## Make the Physics Connection
### Chapter 7

Compton scattering is one of the most prevalent interactions between x-ray photons and the human body in general diagnostic imaging and is responsible for most of the scatter that fogs the image. The probability of Compton scattering does not depend on the atomic number of atoms involved. Compton scattering may occur in both soft tissue and bone. The probability of Compton scattering is related to the energy of the photon. As x-ray photon energy increases, the probability of that photon penetrating a given tissue without interaction increases. However, with this increase in photon energy, the likelihood of Compton interactions relative to photoelectric interactions also increases.

Chapter 9 introduces the characteristics of a quality image and explains that scatter radiation provides no useful information about the anatomic area of interest. Controlling the amount of scatter radiation produced in the patient and ultimately reaching the image receptor (IR) is essential in creating a diagnostic-quality image. Scatter radiation is detrimental to radiographic quality because it adds unwanted exposure (fog) to the image without adding any patient information. Digital IRs are more sensitive to lower-energy levels of radiation, such as scatter, which results in increased fog in the image. Additionally, scatter radiation decreases radiographic contrast; however, radiographic contrast can be computer manipulated by changing the window width. Increased scatter radiation either produced within the patient or higher-energy scatter exiting the patient affects the exposure to the patient and anyone within close proximity. Therefore, the radiographer must act to minimize the amount of scatter radiation produced and reaching the IR.

## Critical Concept
### Factors Affecting the Amount of Scatter Radiation

The greater the volume of tissue irradiated because of part thickness or x-ray beam field size, the greater the amount of scatter radiation produced. The higher the kVp used, the greater the energy of scattered x-rays exiting the patient.

Beam-restricting devices and radiographic grids are tools the radiographer can use to limit the amount of scatter radiation that affects the radiographic image and exposure to the patient or personnel. Beam-restricting devices decrease the x-ray beam field size and the amount of tissue irradiated, thereby reducing the amount of scatter radiation produced. Radiographic grids are used to improve radiographic image quality by absorbing scatter radiation that exits

the patient, reducing the amount of scatter reaching the IR. Grids do nothing to prevent scatter *production;* they merely reduce the amount of scatter reaching the IR.

## BEAM RESTRICTION

It is up to each radiographer to limit the x-ray beam field size to the anatomic area of interest. Beam restriction serves two purposes: limiting patient exposure and reducing the amount of scatter radiation produced within the patient.

The unrestricted primary beam is cone shaped and projects a round field on the patient and IR (Fig. 12.1). If not restricted in some way, the primary beam goes beyond the boundaries of the anatomic area of interest and IR size, resulting in unnecessary patient exposure. Any time the x-ray field extends beyond the anatomic area of interest, the patient receives unnecessary exposure. Limiting the x-ray beam field size is accomplished with a beam-restricting device. Located just below the x-ray tube housing, the **beam-restricting device** changes the shape and size of the primary beam. The terms **beam restriction** and **collimation** are used interchangeably; they refer to a decrease in the size of the projected radiation field. The term *collimation* is used more often than *beam restriction* because collimators are the most popular type of beam-restricting device. *Increasing* collimation means *decreasing* field size and *decreasing* collimation means *increasing* field size.

## Critical Concept
### Beam Restriction and Patient Dose

Collimating to the appropriate field size is a basic method for protecting the patient from unnecessary exposure. As beam restriction or collimation increases, field size decreases and patient dose decreases. As beam restriction or collimation decreases, field size increases and patient dose increases.

### BEAM RESTRICTION AND SCATTER RADIATION

In addition to decreasing patient dose, beam-restricting devices also reduce the amount of scatter radiation produced within the patient, reducing the amount of scatter the IR is exposed to and thereby increasing the radiographic contrast.

The relationship between collimation (field size) and quantity of scatter radiation is illustrated in Fig. 12.2. As stated previously, collimation means decreasing the size of the projected field, so increasing collimation means decreasing field size and decreasing collimation means increasing field size.

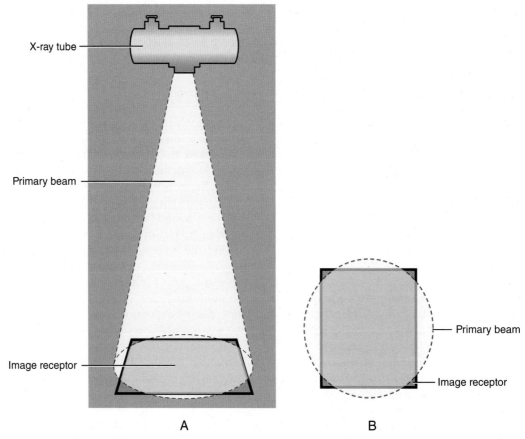

**Fig. 12.1 The Unrestricted Primary Beam.** The unrestricted primary beam is cone shaped, projecting a circular field. **(A)** Side view. **(B)** View from above.

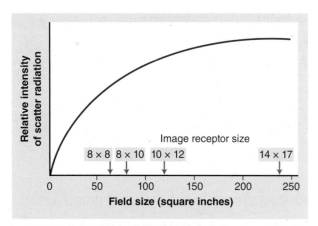

**Fig. 12.2 X-ray Field Size and Scatter Radiation.** As the field size increases, the relative quantity of scatter radiation increases.

## COLLIMATION AND CONTRAST

Because collimation decreases the x-ray beam field size, less scatter radiation is produced within the patient. Therefore less scatter radiation reaches the IR. As described in Chapter 9, this affects the radiographic contrast.

> **Critical Concept**
>
> **Collimation and Radiographic Contrast**
>
> As collimation increases, the quantity of scatter radiation decreases and radiographic contrast increases; as collimation decreases, the quantity of scatter radiation increases and radiographic contrast decreases.

## COMPENSATING FOR COLLIMATION

An increase in collimation also affects the number of x-ray photons reaching the IR to produce the latent image. Increasing collimation decreases the number of photons that strike the patient and decreases the amount of scatter radiation produced. Therefore, exposure factors should be increased when increasing collimation. For example, when collimating significantly (changing from an 11 × 14-inch field size to a small,

> **Critical Concept**
>
> **Collimation and Scatter Radiation**
>
> As collimation increases, the field size decreases and the quantity of scatter radiation decreases; as collimation decreases, the field size increases and the quantity of scatter radiation increases.

## Table 12.1 Restricting the Primary Beam

| INCREASED FACTOR | RESULT |
| --- | --- |
| Collimation | Patient dose **decreases.** |
| | Scatter radiation **decreases.** |
| | Radiographic contrast **increases.** |
| | Quantum noise **increases without appropriate increase in mAs.** |
| X-ray field size | Patient dose **increases.** |
| | Scatter radiation **increases.** |
| | Radiographic contrast **decreases.** |
| | Quantum noise **decreases.** |

4-inch-diameter cone), the radiographer must increase exposure to compensate for the decrease in the number of x-ray photons that otherwise occurs. The kVp is typically not increased because it increases the proportion of scatter produced in the patient and results in decreased image contrast. To maintain exposure to the IR, the mAs (milliamperes/second) should be altered.

Important relationships regarding the restriction of the primary beam are summarized in Table 12.1.

### TYPES OF BEAM-RESTRICTING DEVICES

Several types of beam-restricting devices are available; they differ in sophistication and utility. All beam-restricting devices are made of a metal or a combination of metals that readily absorb x-rays.

### Aperture Diaphragms

The simplest type of beam-restricting device is the aperture diaphragm. An **aperture diaphragm** is a flat piece of lead (diaphragm) that has a hole (aperture) in it. Commercially made aperture diaphragms are available (Fig. 12.3), as are those that are "homemade"

(hospital-made) for purposes specific to a radiographic unit. Aperture diaphragms are easy to use. They are placed directly below the x-ray tube window. An aperture diaphragm can be made by cutting rubberized lead to the size needed to create the diaphragm and cutting the center to create the shape and size of the aperture.

Although the aperture's size and shape can be changed, the aperture cannot be adjusted from the designed size; therefore, the projected field size is not adjustable. In addition, because of the aperture's proximity to the radiation source (focal spot), a large area of unsharpness surrounds the radiographic image (Fig. 12.4). Although aperture diaphragms are still used in some applications, their use is not as widespread as that of other types of beam-restricting devices.

### Cones and Cylinders

Cones and cylinders are shaped differently (Fig. 12.5), but they have many of the same attributes. A **cone** or **cylinder** is essentially an aperture diaphragm that has an extended flange attached to it. The flange can vary in length and can be shaped as either a cone or a cylinder. The flange can also be made to telescope, thereby increasing its total length (Fig. 12.6). Like aperture diaphragms, cones and cylinders are easy to use. They slide onto the tube directly below the window. Cones and cylinders limit unsharpness surrounding the radiographic image more than aperture diaphragms do, with cylinders accomplishing this task slightly better than cones (Fig. 12.7). However, they are limited in terms of the sizes that are available, and they are not necessarily interchangeable among tube housings. Cones have a disadvantage compared with cylinders. If the angle of the flange of the cone is greater than the angle of divergence of the primary beam, the base

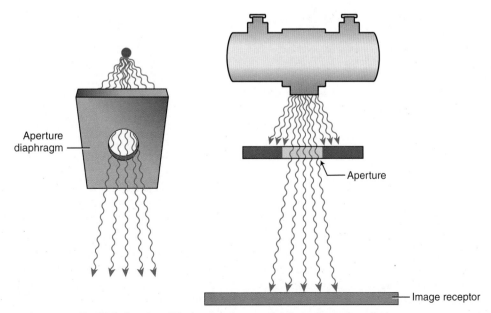

Fig. 12.3 **Aperture Diaphragm.** A commercially made aperture diaphragm.

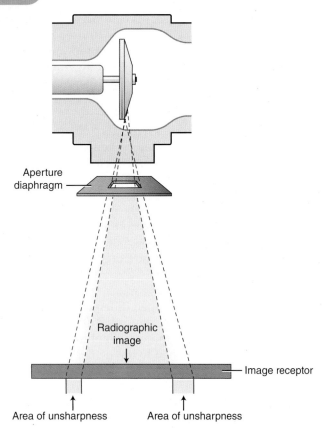

Fig. 12.4 **Image Unsharpness and Aperture Diaphragm.** Radiographic image unsharpness using an aperture diaphragm.

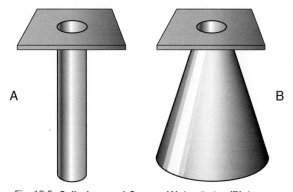

Fig. 12.5 **Cylinders and Cones. (A)** A cylinder. **(B)** A cone.

plate or aperture diaphragm of the cone is the only metal restricting the primary beam; therefore, cylinders generally are more useful than cones. Cones and cylinders are almost always made to produce a circular projected field, and they can be used to advantage for some radiographic procedures (Fig. 12.8).

## Collimators

The most sophisticated, useful, and accepted beam-restricting device is the collimator. Collimators are considered the best beam-restricting device available for radiography. Beam restriction accomplished with the use of a collimator is referred to as *collimation*. Again, the terms *collimation* and *beam restriction* are used interchangeably.

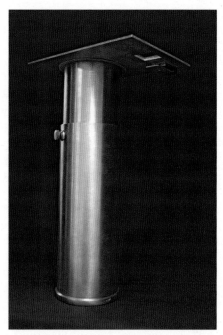

Fig. 12.6 **Telescoping Cylinder.** A telescoping cylinder.

A **collimator** has two or three sets of lead shutters (Fig. 12.9). Located immediately below the tube window, the entrance shutters limit the x-ray beam much as the aperture diaphragm does. One or more sets of adjustable lead shutters are located 3 to 7 inches (8-18 cm) below the tube. These shutters consist of longitudinal and lateral leaves or blades, each with its own control. This makes the collimator adjustable in that it can produce projected fields of varying sizes. The field shape produced by a collimator is always rectangular or square unless using a lead mask, cone, or cylinder placed below the collimator. A **lead mask** is similar to an aperture diaphragm in that it will change the shape and size of the projected x-ray field. Collimators are equipped with a white light source and a mirror to project a light field onto the patient. This light is intended to accurately indicate where the primary x-ray beam will be projected during exposure. In case of failure of this light, an x-ray field measurement guide (Fig. 12.10) is present on the front of the collimator. The guide indicates the projected field size based on the adjusted size of the collimator opening at source-to-image receptor distances (SIDs). This helps ensure that the radiographer does not open the collimator to produce a field that is larger than the IR. Another problem that may occur is the lack of accuracy of the light field. The mirror that reflects the light down toward the patient or the light bulb itself could be slightly out of position, projecting a light field that inaccurately indicates where the primary beam will be projected. There is a means of testing the accuracy of this light field and the location of the center of projected beam (Box 12.1).

A plastic template with crosshairs is affixed to the bottom of the collimator to indicate where the center of the primary beam—the central ray (CR)—will be

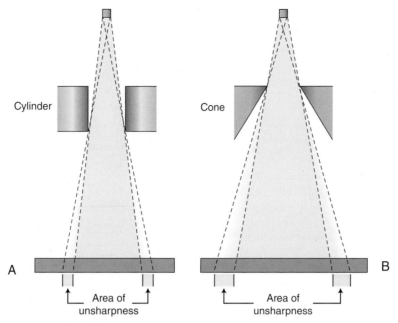

**Fig. 12.7 Cylinder/Cone and Unsharpness.** A cylinder **(A)** is better than a cone **(B)** at limiting the area of unsharpness.

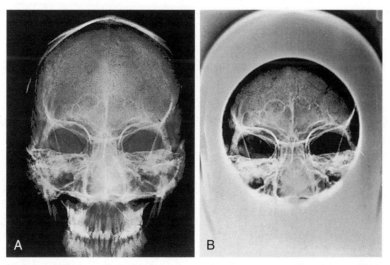

**Fig. 12.8 Images With and Without a Cylinder.** Radiograph of the frontal and maxillary sinuses. **(A)** Not using a cylinder. **(B)** Using a cylinder. (Courtesy *Mosby's radiographic instructional series: radiographic imaging*, St Louis, 1998, Mosby.)

directed. This is of great assistance to the radiographer in accurately centering the x-ray field to the patient.

## Automatic Collimators

An **automatic collimator**, also called a **positive beam-limiting (PBL) device**, automatically limits the size and shape of the primary beam to the size and shape of the IR. For a few years, automatic collimators were required by U.S. federal law on all new radiographic installations. This law has since been rescinded, and automatic collimators are no longer a requirement on any radiographic equipment. However, they are still widely used. Automatic collimators mechanically adjust the primary beam size and shape to that of the IR when the IR is placed in the Bucky tray, just below

the tabletop. Automatic collimation makes it difficult for the radiographer to increase the size of the primary beam to a field larger than the IR, which would result in increasing the patient's radiation exposure. PBL devices were a way of protecting patients from overexposure to radiation. However, automatic collimators have an override mechanism that allows the radiographer to disengage this feature and decrease the size of the exposure field appropriate to the part.

Whether automatic collimation is used, the radiographer should always be sure that the size of the x-ray field is the same as or less than the size of the IR, except for digital flat-panel detectors. When using a flat-panel detector, the x-ray field size should be restricted to the anatomic area of interest. These digital IRs are typically

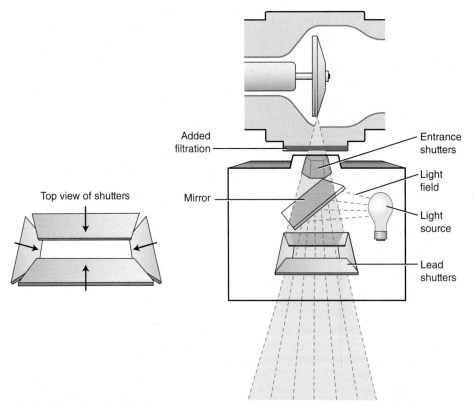

**Fig. 12.9 Collimators.** Collimators have two sets of lead shutters that are used to change the size and shape of the primary beam.

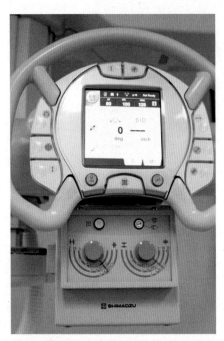

**Fig. 12.10 X-ray Field Measurement Guide.** The x-ray field measurement guide on the front of a collimator.

| Box 12.1 | Quality-Control Check: Collimator and Beam Alignment |
| --- | --- |

- Lack of congruence of the x-ray field and the exposure field, and misalignment of the light and Bucky tray, may affect the quality of the radiographic image. In addition, if the x-ray central ray is not perpendicular to the table and Bucky tray, radiographic quality may be compromised. A collimator and beam alignment test tool template and cylinder can easily be imaged and evaluated for proper alignment.
- Collimator misalignment should be less than 2% of the SID used, and the perpendicularity of the x-ray central ray must be less than or equal to 1 degree misaligned.

*SID*, Source-to-image receptor distance.

## RADIOGRAPHIC GRIDS

The radiographic grid was invented in 1913 by Gustave Bucky and continues to be the most effective means for limiting the amount of scatter radiation that reaches the IR. Approximately $^{1}/_{4}$-inch thick and ranging from 8 × 10 inches (20 × 25 cm) to 17 × 17 inches (43 × 43 cm), a **grid** is a device that has very thin lead strips with radiolucent interspaces; it is intended to absorb scatter radiation emitted from the patient. Placed between the patient and the IR, grids are invaluable in the practice of radiography. They work well to improve radiographic contrast but are not without drawbacks. As is discussed later in this chapter, using

14 × 17 or 17 × 17 and, in many instances, are larger than the anatomic area of interest. It is therefore even more crucial for the radiographer to collimate appropriately for the imaging procedure so the patient is not exposed to radiation unnecessarily.

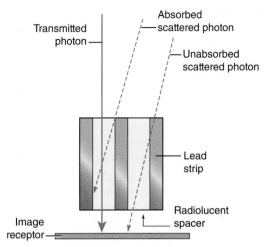

Fig. 12.11 **Grid Absorption of Scatter.** Ideally, grids would absorb all scattered radiation and allow all transmitted photons to reach the image receptor. In reality, however, some scattered photons pass through to the image receptor and some transmitted photons are absorbed.

a grid requires additional mAs, resulting in a higher patient dose. Therefore, grids are typically used only when the anatomic part is 10 cm (4 inches) or greater in thickness and for imaging procedures requiring more than 60 kVp. Radiographers should follow the department protocol for adding a grid because of the significant increase in patient radiation exposure.

As scatter radiation leaves the patient, a significant amount is directed at the IR. As stated previously, scatter radiation is detrimental to radiographic quality because it adds unwanted exposure (fog) to the image without adding any patient information. Scatter radiation decreases radiographic contrast. Ideally, grids would absorb, or clean up, all scattered photons directed toward the IR and would allow all transmitted photons emitted from the patient to pass from the patient to the IR. Unfortunately, this does not happen (Fig. 12.11). When used properly, however, grids can greatly increase the contrast of the radiographic image.

### ! Critical Concept

**Scatter Radiation and Image Quality**

Scatter radiation adds unwanted exposure (fog) to the radiographic image and decreases image quality.

## GRID CONSTRUCTION

Grids contain thin lead strips or lines that have a precise height, thickness, and space between them. Radiolucent **interspace material** separates the lead lines. Interspace material is typically made of aluminum. An aluminum front and back panel cover the lead lines and interspace material of the grid.

Grid construction can be described by grid frequency and grid ratio. **Grid frequency** expresses the number of lead lines per unit length in inches, centimeters, or both. Grid frequencies can range in value from 25 to 45 lines/cm (60–110 lines/inch). A typical value for grid frequency might be 40 lines/cm or 103 lines/inch. Another way of describing grid construction is by its grid ratio. **Grid ratio** is defined as the ratio of the height of the lead strips to the distance between them (Fig. 12.12).

Grid ratio can also be expressed mathematically as follows:

$$\text{Grid ratio} = h/D$$

in which $h$ is the height of the lead strips and $D$ is the distance between them.

### $^1_{2_3}$ Math Application

**Calculating Grid Ratio**

What is the grid ratio when the lead strips are 3.2 mm high and separated by 0.2 mm?

$$\text{Grid ratio} = h/D$$
$$\text{Grid ratio} = 3.2/0.2$$
$$= 16 \text{ or } 16:1$$

Grid ratios range from 4:1 to 16:1. High-ratio grids remove, or clean up, more scatter radiation than lower-ratio grids and thus further increase radiographic contrast.

### ! Critical Concept

**Grid Ratio and Radiographic Contrast**

As grid ratio increases, for the same grid frequency, scatter cleanup improves and radiographic contrast increases; as grid ratio decreases, for the same grid frequency, scatter cleanup is less effective and radiographic contrast decreases.

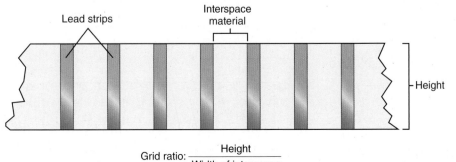

Fig. 12.12 **Grid Ratio.** Grid ratio is the ratio of the height of the lead strips to the distance between them.

There is a relationship among grid ratio, grid frequency, and the amount of lead content (measured in mass per unit area). Increasing the grid ratio for the same grid frequency will increase the amount of lead content and therefore increase scatter absorption. If the grid frequency is increased for the same grid ratio, there is overall less lead content, because the width of the interspace and/or the thickness of the lead strips have been decreased. Decreasing the overall lead content will result in decreased scatter absorption.

Information about a grid's construction is contained on a label placed on the tube side of the grid. This label usually states the type of interspace material used, grid frequency, grid ratio, grid size, and information about the range of SIDs that can be used with the grid. The radiographer should read this information before using the grid because these factors influence grid performance, exposure factor selection, grid alignment, and image quality.

### Grid Pattern

**Grid pattern** refers to the linear pattern of the lead lines of a grid. Two types of grid pattern exist: linear and crossed or cross-hatched. A **linear grid** has lead lines that run in only one direction (Fig. 12.13). Linear grids are the most popular in terms of grid pattern because they allow angulation of the x-ray tube along the length of the lead lines. A **crossed grid** or **cross-hatched grid** has lead lines that run at right angles to one another (Fig. 12.14). Crossed grids remove more scattered photons than linear grids because they contain more lead strips that are oriented in two directions. However, applications are limited with a crossed

grid because the x-ray tube cannot be angled in any direction without producing grid cutoff (i.e., absorption of the transmitted x-rays). Grid cutoff, which is undesirable, is discussed later in this chapter.

### Grid Focus

**Grid focus** refers to the orientation of the lead lines to one another. Two types of grid focus exist: parallel (nonfocused) and focused. A **parallel grid** or **nonfocused grid** has lead lines that run parallel to one another (Fig. 12.15). Parallel grids are used primarily in fluoroscopy and mobile imaging. A **focused grid** has lead lines that are angled, or canted, to approximately match the angle of divergence of the primary beam (Fig. 12.16). The advantage of focused grids compared with parallel grids is that focused grids allow more transmitted photons to reach the IR. As seen in Fig. 12.17, transmitted photons are more likely to pass through a focused grid to reach the IR than they are to pass through a parallel grid.

**Critical Concept**

**Focused Versus Parallel Grids**

Focused grids have lead lines that are angled to approximately match the divergence of the primary beam. Thus focused grids allow more transmitted photons to reach the IR than parallel grids.

As seen in Fig. 12.18, if imaginary lines were drawn from each of the lead lines in a linear focused grid, these lines would meet to form an imaginary point, called the **convergent point**. If points were connected along the length of the grid, they would form an imaginary line, called the **convergent line**. Both the convergent line and convergent point are important because they determine the focal distance of a focused grid. The focal distance (sometimes referred to as *grid radius*) is the distance between the grid and the convergent line or point. The **focal distance** is important because it is used to determine the **focal range** of a focused grid. The focal range is the recommended range of SIDs that

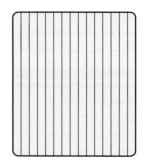
Fig. 12.13 **Linear Grid Pattern.**

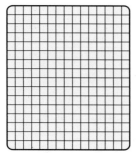
Fig. 12.14 **Crossed Grid Pattern.** Crossed or cross-hatched grid pattern.

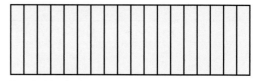
Fig. 12.15 **Parallel Grid.** Parallel or nonfocused grid.

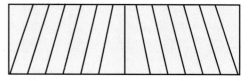
Fig. 12.16 **Focused Grid.** Focused grid.

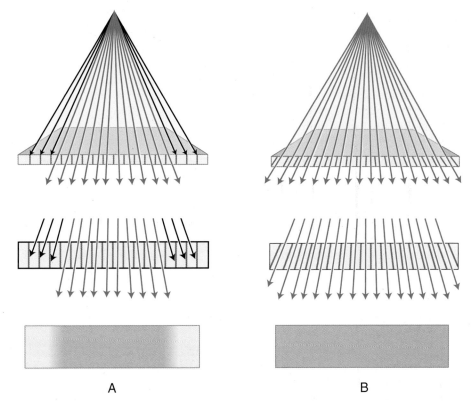

**Fig. 12.17 Comparison of Parallel and Focused Grids.** Comparison of transmitted photons passing through a parallel grid **(A)** and a focused grid **(B)**.

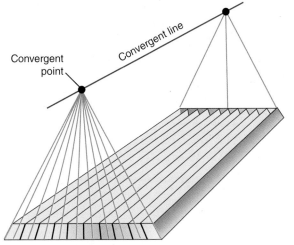

**Fig. 12.18 Convergent Line.** Imaginary lines drawn above a linear-focused grid from each lead strip meet to form a convergent point. The points form a convergent line along the length of the grid.

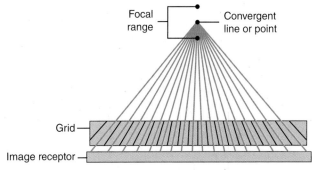

**Fig. 12.19 Convergent Point.** The convergent line or point of a focused grid falls within a focal range.

can be used with a focused grid. The convergent line or point always falls within the focal range (Fig. 12.19). For example, a common focal range is 36 to 42 inches (90–105 cm), with a focal distance of 40 inches (100 cm). Another common focal range is 66 to 74 inches (165–185 cm), with a focal distance of 72 inches (180 cm). Some equipment manufacturers have designed grids with a focal range of 40 to 72 inches. Radiographers can use these grids for almost all projections performed in the clinical environment. These grids feature very little angulation of the lead strips and increased width between the strips.

Because the lead lines in a parallel grid are not angled, they have a focal range extending from a minimum SID to infinity.

## TYPES OF GRIDS

Grids are available for use by the radiographer in several forms and can be stationary or moving. Stationary, nonmoving grids include the wafer or slip-on grid, grid cassette, and grid cap. A **wafer grid** matches the size of the cassette and is used by placing it on top of the IR. Wafer grids typically are taped to the IR to prevent them from sliding during the radiographic procedure. A **grid cassette** is an IR that has a grid permanently mounted to its front surface. A **grid cap** contains a permanently mounted grid and allows the IR to slide in behind it. This is useful because the grid is secure, and many IRs can be interchanged behind the grid before processing the image.

## Stationary and Reciprocating Grids

When grids are stationary, it is possible to closely examine and see the grid lines on the radiographic image. Slightly moving the grid during the x-ray exposure blurs the grid lines.

Moving or reciprocating grids are part of the **Bucky**, more accurately called the *Potter-Bucky diaphragm*. The grid is located directly below the radiographic tabletop and just above the tray that holds the IR. Grid motion is controlled electrically by the x-ray exposure switch. The grid moves slightly back and forth in a lateral direction over the IR during the entire exposure. These grids typically have dimensions of 17 × 17 inches (43 × 43 cm), so that a 14 × 17-inch (35 × 43-cm) IR can be positioned under the grid either lengthwise or crosswise, depending on the examination requirements.

## Long- Versus Short-Dimension Grids

Linear grids can be either constructed as long dimension or short dimension. A long-dimension linear grid has lead strips running parallel to the long axis of the grid. A short-dimension linear grid has lead strips running perpendicular to the long axis of the grid (Fig. 12.20). For example, a 14 × 17-inch-long (35 × 43-cm) dimension grid has lead strips 17 inches (43 cm) long, whereas a short-dimension grid has lead strips 14 inches (35 cm) long. A short-dimension grid may be useful for examinations in which it is difficult to center the CR correctly for the long-dimension grid.

## GRID PERFORMANCE

The purpose of using grids in radiography is to increase radiographic contrast. In addition to improving contrast by cleaning up scatter, grids reduce the total amount of x-rays reaching the IR. The better the grid is at absorbing scattered photons, such as with

a higher-ratio grid, the fewer the photons reaching the IR. To compensate for this reduction, additional mAs must be used to produce diagnostic images. The **grid conversion factor (GCF)**, or **Bucky factor**, can be used to determine the adjustment in mAs needed when changing from using a grid to nongrid (or vice versa) or for changing to grids with different grid ratios.

 **Critical Concept**

### Grid Ratio and Exposure to the IR

As grid ratio increases, radiation exposure to the IR decreases; as grid ratio decreases, radiation exposure to the IR increases.

The GCF can be expressed mathematically as:

$$GCF = \frac{\text{mAs with the grid}}{\text{mAs without the grid}}$$

Table 12.2 presents specific grid ratios and grid conversion factors. When a grid is added to the IR, mAs must be increased by the factor indicated to maintain the same number of x-ray photons reaching the IR. This requires multiplication by the GCF for the grid ratio.

 **Math Application**

### Adding a Grid

If a radiographer produces a knee image with a nongrid exposure using 2 mAs and next wants to use an 8:1 ratio grid, what mAs should be used to produce a comparable-quality image?

Nongrid exposure = 2 mAs

GCF (for 8:1 grid) = 4 (from Table 12.2)

$$GCF = \frac{\text{mAs with the grid}}{\text{mAs without the grid}}$$

$$4 = \frac{\text{mAs with the grid}}{2}$$

$$8 = \text{mAs with the grid}$$

When adding an 8:1 ratio grid, the mAs must be increased by a factor of 4, in this case to 8 mAs.

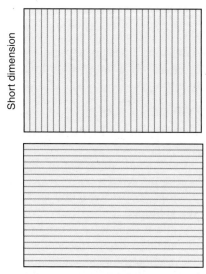

**Fig. 12.20 Long- Versus Short-Dimension Grid.** Orientation of lead strips for a long- and short-dimension grid.

| Table **12.2** | The Grid Conversion (Bucky) Factor | |
| --- | --- |
| **GRID FACTOR** | **GCF** |
| No grid | 1 |
| 5:1 | 2 |
| 6:1 | 3 |
| 8:1 | 4 |
| 12:1 | 5 |
| 16:1 | 6 |

*GCF,* Grid conversion factor.

Likewise, if a radiographer chooses to not use a grid during a procedure but only knows the appropriate mAs when a grid is used, the mAs must be decreased by the GCF. This requires division by the GCF for the grid ratio.

 **Math Application**

### Removing a Grid

If a radiographer produces a knee image using a 16:1 ratio grid and 18 mAs, and on the next exposure wants to use a nongrid exposure, what mAs should be used to produce an image with comparable quality?

Grid exposure = 18 mAs

GCF (for 16:1) = 6 (from Table 12.2)

$$GCF = \frac{mAs \text{ with the grid}}{mAs \text{ without the grid}}$$

$$6 = \frac{18}{mAs \text{ without the grid}}$$

$$3 = mAs \text{ without the grid}$$

When removing a 16:1 ratio grid, the mAs must be decreased by a factor of 6, in this case to 3 mAs.

The GCF is also useful when changing between grids with different grid ratios.

When changing from one grid ratio to another, the following formula should be used to adjust the mAs:

$$\frac{mAs_1}{mAs_2} = \frac{GCF_1}{GCF_2}$$

 **Math Application**

### Increasing the Grid Ratio

If a radiographer performs a routine portable abdomen examination using 30 mAs with a 6:1 ratio grid, what mAs should be used if a 12:1 ratio grid is substituted?
Exposure 1: 30 mAs, 6:1 grid, GCF = 3
Exposure 2: __mAs, 12:1 grid, GCF = 5

$$\frac{mAs_1}{mAs_2} = \frac{GCF_1}{GCF_2}$$

$$\frac{30}{mAs_2} = \frac{3}{5}$$

$$mAs_2 = 50$$

Increasing the grid ratio requires additional mAs.

The increase in the mAs required to maintain the same exposure to the IR results in an increase in patient dose. This increase in patient dose is significant, as the numbers for the GCF indicate.

 **Math Application**

### Decreasing the Grid Ratio

If a radiographer uses 40 mAs with an 8:1 ratio grid, what mAs should be used with a 5:1 ratio grid to maintain the same exposure to the IR?
Exposure 1: 40 mAs, 8:1 grid, GCF = 4
Exposure 2: __mAs, 5:1 grid, GCF = 2

$$\frac{mAs_1}{mAs_2} = \frac{GCF_1}{GCF_2}$$

$$\frac{40}{mAs_2} = \frac{4}{2}$$

$$mAs_2 = 20$$

Decreasing the grid ratio requires a lower mAs.

 **Critical Concept**

### Grid Ratio and Patient Dose

As grid ratio increases, patient dose increases; as grid ratio decreases, patient dose decreases.

It is important to remember that patient dose is increased because of the following:
1. Using a grid compared with not using a grid
2. Using a higher-ratio grid

Decisions regarding the use of a grid and grid ratio should be made by balancing image quality and patient protection. To keep patient exposure as low as possible, grids should be used only when appropriate, and the grid ratio should be the lowest that will provide sufficient contrast improvement. Currently published grid conversion factors were designed for use with past film-screen technology. Research indicates a need to revisit these factors. Radiologic technologists and imaging departments should reevaluate traditional grid conversion factors and adjust them to ensure digital image receptors receive appropriate exposure and patients receive the lowest amounts of radiation exposure.

### GRID CUTOFF

In addition to the disadvantage of increased patient dose associated with grid use, another disadvantage is the possibility of grid cutoff. **Grid cutoff** is defined as a decrease in the number of transmitted photons that reach the IR because of some misalignment of the grid. The primary radiographic effect of grid cutoff is a further reduction in the number of photons reaching the IR, resulting in an increase in noise caused by a decrease in x-ray photons reaching the digital IR. Grid cutoff may require that the radiographer repeat the image, thereby increasing patient dose yet again. Grid ratio has a significant effect on grid cutoff, with higher grid ratios resulting in more potential cutoff.

Grid cutoff can occur because of four types of errors in grid use. To reduce or eliminate grid cutoff, the radiographer must have a thorough understanding of

**Fig. 12.21 Image of Upside-Down Focused Grid.** Radiograph produced with an upside-down focused grid. (Courtesy Fauber TL: *Radiographic imaging and exposure*, ed 3, St Louis, 2009, Mosby.)

the importance of proper grid alignment in relation to the IR and x-ray tube.

### Upside-Down Focused

Upside-down focused grid cutoff occurs when a focused grid is placed upside down on the IR, resulting in the grid lines going opposite to the angle of divergence of the x-ray beam. This appears radiographically as a significant loss of exposure along the edges of the image (Fig. 12.21). Photons easily pass through the center of the grid because the lead lines are perpendicular to the IR surface. Lead lines that are more peripheral to the center are angled more and thus absorb the transmitted photons. Upside-down focused

grid error is easily avoided because every focused grid should have a label indicating "tube side." This side of the grid should always face the tube, away from the IR.

### Off-Level

Off-level grid cutoff results when the x-ray beam is angled across the lead strips. It is the most common type of cutoff and can occur from either the tube or grid being angled (Fig. 12.22 and Fig. 12.23). Off-level grid cutoff can often be seen with mobile radiographic studies or horizontal beam examinations and appears as a loss of exposure across the entire IR. This type of grid cutoff is the only type that occurs with both focused and parallel grids.

### Off-Center

Also called *lateral decentering,* off-center grid cutoff occurs when the CR of the x-ray beam is not aligned from side to side with the center of a focused grid. Because of the arrangement of the lead lines of the focused grid, the divergence of the primary beam does not match the angle of these lead strips when not centered (Fig. 12.24). Off-center grid cutoff appears radiographically as an overall loss of exposure to the IR (Fig. 12.25).

### Off-Focus

Off-focus grid cutoff occurs when using an SID outside of the recommended focal range. Grid cutoff occurs if the SID is less than or greater than the focal range. Radiographically, both appear the same—that is, as a loss of exposure at the periphery of the image.

A radiographic image that is underexposed can be the result of many factors, one of which is grid cutoff. Before assuming that an underexposed image is due to insufficient mAs and then reexposing the patient with the mAs increased, the radiographer should evaluate grid alignment. If misalignment is the cause of the underexposure, the patient can be protected from repeating the image with increased mAs. Table 12.3

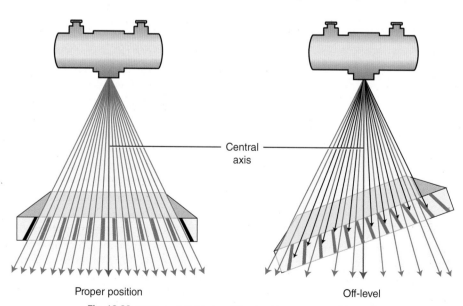

Proper position                                    Off-level

**Fig. 12.22 Off-Level Grid.** An off-level grid can cause grid cutoff.

Central axis

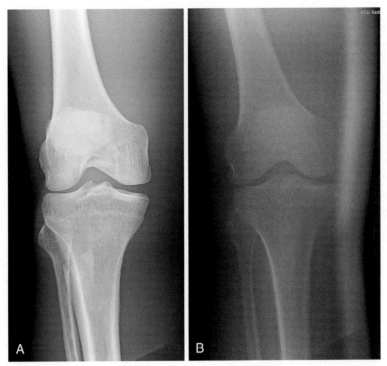

**Fig. 12.23 Grid Cutoff. (A)** Image created with proper alignment of CR and no grid cutoff. **(B)** Image created with off-level grid cutoff. The overall brightness was adjusted but image quality is poor.

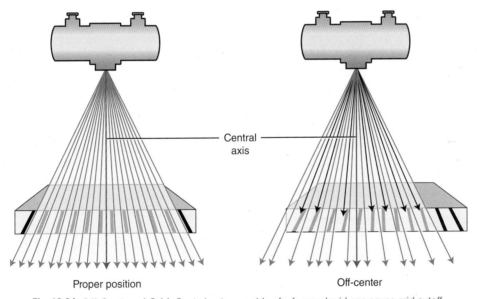

Proper position                                    Off-center

**Fig. 12.24 Off-Centered Grid.** Centering to one side of a focused grid can cause grid cutoff.

summarizes grid cutoff errors and their radiographic effect. Table 12.4 summarizes important relationships regarding the use of radiographic grids.

It is important to note that the brightness of a digital image will be computer adjusted for reduction in exposure to the IR because of grid errors. However, increased quantum noise may be visible and image quality reduced.

## MOIRÉ EFFECT

The **Moiré effect**, or zebra pattern, is an artifact that can occur when a stationary grid is used during CR imaging.

If the grid frequency is similar to the laser scanning frequency during CR image processing, then a zebra pattern can result on the digital image. Use of a higher grid frequency or a moving grid with CR digital imaging eliminates this type of grid error. In addition, if a grid cassette is placed in a Bucky, imaging the double grids creates a zebra pattern on the radiograph (Fig. 12.26).

## GRID USAGE

The radiographer must consider several factors when deciding which type of grid, if any, to use for an examination. Although quite efficient at preventing scatter

**Fig. 12.25 Off-Center Grid Cutoff.** Radiograph demonstrating grid cutoff caused by off-centering. (Courtesy Fauber TL: *Radiographic imaging and exposure*, ed 3, St Louis, 2009, Mosby.)

| Table 12.3 | Grid Cutoff Errors and Their Radiographic Effects |
|---|---|
| **GRID ERROR** | **RADIOGRAPHIC EFFECT** |
| Upside-down focused grid: Placing a focused grid upside down on the IR | Significant underexposure to the lateral edges of the IR |
| Off-level error: Angling the x-ray tube across the grid lines or angling the grid itself during exposure | Decrease in radiation exposure to the IR |
| Off-center error: The center of the x-ray beam is not aligned from side to side with the center of a focused grid | Decrease in radiation exposure to the IR |
| Off-focus error: Using an SID outside of the focal range | A loss of exposure at the periphery of the IR |

*IR*, Image receptor; *SID*, source-to-image receptor distance.

| Table 12.4 | Radiographic Grid Ratio |
|---|---|
| **INCREASED FACTOR** | **RESULT** |
| Grid ratio[a] | Contrast **increases**. |
| | Patient dose **increases**. |
| | The likelihood of grid cutoff **increases**. |

[a]Milliamperage/second adjusted to maintain exposure to image receptor.

radiation from reaching the IR, grids are not appropriate for all examinations. When appropriate, selection of a grid involves consideration of contrast improvement, patient dose, and the likelihood of grid cutoff. Radiographers typically choose between parallel and focused grids, high- and low-ratio grids, grids with different focal ranges, and whether to use a grid at all.

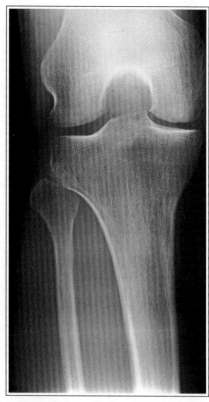

**Fig. 12.26 Moiré Effect.** Radiograph demonstrating the zebra pattern as a result of the Moiré effect. Rights were not granted to include this content in electronic media. Please refer to the printed book. (Courtesy Cesar LI, et al.: Artifacts found in computed radiography, *Br J Radiol* 74:195–202, 2001. Used with permission from the British Institute of Radiology. Permission conveyed through Copyright Clearance Center, Inc.)

As indicated earlier, the choice of whether to use a grid is based on the kVp necessary for the examination and the thickness of the part. Parts 10 cm (4 inches) or larger, together with a kVp higher than 60, produce enough scatter to necessitate the use of a grid. The next decision is which grid to use. There is no single best grid for all situations. A 16:1 focused grid provides excellent contrast improvement, but the patient's dose will be high and the radiographer must ensure that the grid and x-ray tube are perfectly aligned to prevent grid cutoff. The 5:1 parallel grid will do a mediocre job of scatter cleanup, especially at 80 kVp or more. However, the patient dose will be significantly lower, and the radiographer need not be concerned with cutoff caused by being off-center, SID used, or having the grid upside down. Selection between grids with different focal ranges depends on the radiographic examination. Supine abdomen studies should use a grid that includes 40 inches (100 cm) in the focal range; upright chest studies should have grids that include 72 inches (180 cm). In general, most radiographic rooms are equipped with a 10:1 or 12:1 focused grid, which provides a compromise between contrast improvement and patient dose. Stationary grids for mobile examinations may be lower ratio, parallel, or both to allow the radiographer greater positioning latitude.

## Box 12.2 The Typical Grid

- Is long-dimension linear instead of crossed.
- Is focused instead of parallel.
- Is of mid-ratio (8:1-12:1).
- Has a focal range that includes an SID of 40 or 72 inches (100 or 180 cm).

*SID*, Source-to-image receptor distance.

## Box 12.3 Quality-Control Check: Grid Uniformity and Alignment

- Nonuniformity of a grid (lack of uniform lead strips) may create artifacts on the image. Grid uniformity can be easily evaluated by imaging a grid with a homogeneous phantom. The displayed image can be visually assessed for any image artifacts and the pixel brightness levels measured throughout areas of the image. Pixel brightness levels throughout the displayed image should measure within 20% for proper uniformity.
- Misalignment of a focused grid (off center) can reduce the exposure to the IR because of grid cutoff. A grid alignment tool made of radiopaque material with cutout holes in a line can be imaged to evaluate correct alignment of the grid with the x-ray field.

*IR*, Image receptor.

Grids differ from one another in performance, especially in the areas of grid ratio and focal distance. Before using a grid, the radiographer must determine the grid ratio so that the appropriate exposure factors can be selected. Also, the radiographer must be aware of the focal range of focused grids so that the appropriate SID is selected. Box 12.2 lists attributes of the grid typically used in radiography.

Box 12.3 provides information on quality-control checks for grid uniformity and alignment.

## RADIATION PROTECTION

Limiting the size of the x-ray field to the anatomic area of interest will decrease scatter production and reduce patient exposure. Although the mAs may be increased to compensate for decreasing the size of the x-ray field, the tissues located closest to the lateral edge or outside of the collimated x-ray beam will receive the least amount of radiation exposure. Those tissues that lie inside the collimated edge of the x-ray beam will receive the greatest amount of radiation exposure. Collimating to the anatomic area of interest is an important radiation safety practice that should be routinely performed.

The use of grids requires an increase in mAs to maintain exposure to the image receptor. As a result, patient radiation exposure is increased when using grids. The higher the grid ratio, the greater the mAs needed to maintain exposure to the image receptor, increasing patient radiation exposure. Limiting the use of grids or using a grid with a lower grid ratio will decrease the radiation exposure to the patient.

## VIRTUAL GRIDS

Some equipment manufacturers have created virtual grids with computer software that reduces the appearance of grid lines. The use of physical grids is not required. The effectiveness of virtual grids at minimizing the appearance of grid lines is similar to the effectiveness of physical grids. Often, radiographers can select from a variety of grid ratios when applying a virtual grid. Virtual grids provide radiographers the opportunity to significantly decrease patient exposure dose. Because physical grids are not required, grid cutoff is not possible, which reduces the possibility of a repeat image. In addition, radiographers can lower mAs because virtual grids do not absorb primary radiation like physical grids do.

## THE AIR GAP TECHNIQUE

The radiographer may use the grid most often to prevent scatter from reaching the IR, but the grid is not the only available tool. Although limited in its usefulness, the air gap technique provides another method for limiting the scatter reaching the IR. The **air gap technique** is based on the simple concept that, because scatter radiation travels in every direction, much of the scatter will miss the IR if there is increased distance between the patient and IR (increased object-to-image receptor distance [OID]) (Fig. 12.27). The greater the gap, the greater the reduction in scatter reaching the IR. Similar to a grid, image contrast is increased, the number of photons reaching the IR is reduced because less scatter reaches the IR, and the mAs must be increased to compensate. The most common application of the air gap technique is the lateral projection of the cervical spine. Due to the patient's shoulder, the radiographer is limited in how close they can position the patient's cervical spine to the IR.

The air gap technique is limited in its usefulness because the necessary OID results in decreased sharpness. To overcome this decrease in sharpness, an increase in SID is required, which may not always be feasible. The air gap technique results in patient dose that is the same as, or slightly less than, using a comparable grid. Exposure may be slightly less because a grid absorbs some of the transmitted photons (grid cutoff) whereas the air gap technique does not.

### Critical Concept

**Air Gap Technique and Scatter Control**

The air gap technique is an alternative to using a grid to control scatter reaching the IR. By moving the IR away from the patient, more of the scatter radiation misses the IR. The greater the gap, the less scatter reaches the IR.

Using an increased OID is necessary for the air gap technique. However, this decreases image quality. To decrease unsharpness and increase spatial resolution, the radiographer must increase SID, which would also necessitate an increase in mAs to maintain receptor exposure.

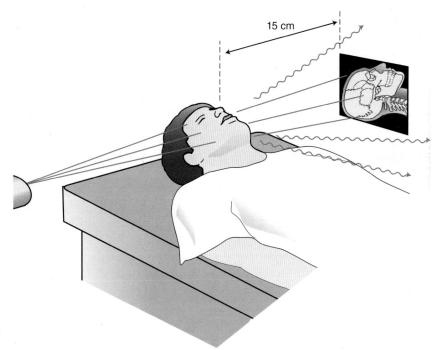

15 cm

Fig. 12.27 **Air Gap Technique.** The air gap technique showing scatter radiation missing the image receptor.

## SHIELDING ACCESSORIES

Efforts to control the amount of scatter radiation produced within the patient and reaching the IR are important considerations during radiography. Restricting the size of the x-ray beam to the anatomic area of interest reduces the radiation exposure to the patient and improves image quality. There are situations in which it is beneficial to use shielding devices to absorb scatter radiation exiting the patient. Placing a lead shield on the x-ray table close to the collimated edge of the area of interest absorbs scatter exiting the patient that could degrade image quality. The lateral lumbar spine projection and the lateral spot are projections in which a significant amount of scatter exits the patient. Placing a lead shield behind the patient's lower back absorbs the scatter and reduces the amount striking the IR (Fig. 12.28). Accurate

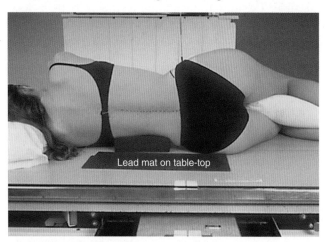

Lead mat on table-top

Fig. 12.28 **Shielding Accessory.** Lead shield placed to absorb scatter radiation from patient. (Courtesy Bontrager KL, Lampignano JP: *Textbook of radiographic positioning and related anatomy*, ed 7, St Louis, 2010, Mosby.)

placement of the lead shield is important so it does not affect the processing of the digital image. Placing a lead shield on the table to limit the scatter radiation reaching the IR does not reduce the exposure to the patient.

Because the patient is the greatest source of scatter radiation, any individual remaining in the radiographic room during an exposure must wear a lead apron. Wearing a lead apron and standing as far from the patient as possible decreases the amount of occupational exposure to scatter radiation.

It is the radiographer's responsibility to reduce the amount of scatter radiation produced and reaching the IR. Reducing the amount of scatter produced through beam restriction, reducing the amount of scatter reaching the IR by using a grid, avoiding grid cutoff errors, and making appropriate exposure adjustments as needed all help produce diagnostic quality radiographic images.

### On the Spot

- Scatter radiation, the result of Compton interactions, is detrimental to radiographic image quality. Excessive scatter results in additional unwanted x-ray exposure (fog) to the IR and reduced contrast.
- The effect of scatter radiation can be reduced by limiting the amount produced and by absorbing the scatter before it reaches the IR.
- The amount of scatter exiting the patient increases as the volume of irradiated tissue increases.
- A higher kVp increases the energy of scatter radiation exiting the patient.
- Beam restriction limits the area exposed to radiation, the patient dose, and the amount of scatter produced in the patient. Aperture diaphragms, cones and cylinders, and collimators are types of beam restrictors.

- Increasing collimation reduces the volume of anatomic tissue irradiated, reduces scatter production, and reduces patient exposure.
- Radiographic grids are devices placed between the patient and IR to absorb scatter radiation. Consisting of a series of lead strips and radiolucent interspaces, grids allow transmitted radiation to pass through while scatter radiation is absorbed.
- Grid designs include linear parallel, focused parallel, crossed, and long and short dimension, each with advantages and disadvantages.
- The use of a grid in a radiographic examination results in fewer x-ray photons reaching the IR. The grid conversion or Bucky factor is used to calculate the increase in exposure needed when grids are used.
- Grid errors that produce grid cutoff include using a focused grid upside down and errors caused by off-level, off-center, and off-focus misalignment.
- The type of grid used depends on the thickness of the part, the kVp, patient dose, contrast improvement, and the likelihood of grid errors.
- Adding a grid will require an increase in mAs to maintain exposure to the image receptor and, therefore, increase the radiation exposure to the patient.
- The air gap technique is another method, although seldom used, for reducing the amount of scatter reaching the IR.
- Scatter control is of the same, or greater, importance in digital imaging because of the IR's increased sensitivity to low-energy radiation.

## CRITICAL THINKING QUESTIONS

1. What are the advantages and disadvantages of beam restriction?
2. How can patient exposure be reduced when restricting the x-ray beam if exposure factors are increased to maintain image quality?
3. What are the advantages and disadvantages of using a grid?

## REVIEW QUESTIONS

1. Which of the following will decrease the amount of scatter radiation produced?
   a. Increasing the x-ray field size
   b. Decreasing the x-ray field size
   c. Increasing the grid ratio
   d. Decreasing the grid ratio
2. Which of the following is not a type of beam restrictor?
   a. Aperture diaphragm
   b. Positive beam-limiting device
   c. Cylinder
   d. Lead shield

3. As collimation decreases, the quantity of scatter radiation decreases.
   a. True
   b. False
4. What type of beam-restricting device provides the most flexibility in adjusting the x-ray field size?
   a. Cylinder
   b. Aperture diaphragm
   c. Collimator
   d. Cone
5. What describes the number of lead lines per unit length?
   a. Grid frequency
   b. Grid pattern
   c. Grid convergent point
   d. Grid ratio
6. A radiographic image was created using a 12:1 grid and 70 kVp at 10 mAs. What exposure technique change would maintain a similar exposure to the image receptor when converting to a 6:1 ratio grid?
   a. 81 kVp at 5 mAs
   b. 70 kVp at 16.7 mAs
   c. 70 kVp at 6 mAs
   d. 60 kVp at 20 mAs
7. What type of grid has lead strips running parallel to the long axis of the grid?
   a. Focused
   b. Short dimension
   c. Cross hatched
   d. Long dimension
8. Angling the x-ray tube along the long axis of a crossed grid would result in:
   a. increased scatter absorption.
   b. grid cutoff.
   c. Moiré effect.
   d. lateral decentering.
9. For the air gap technique to be effective in reducing scatter radiation reaching the image receptor, what must be increased?
   a. SID
   b. Focal spot size
   c. kVp
   d. OID
10. With exposure technique compensation, _____ the grid ratio will _____ patient radiation exposure.
    a. decreasing, increase
    b. increasing, decrease
    c. increasing, increase
    d. decreasing, will not affect

## Outline

## Objectives

- State the purpose of automatic exposure control (AEC) in radiography.
- Differentiate among the types of radiation detectors used in AEC systems.
- Recognize how the detector size and configuration affect the response of the AEC device.
- Explain how alignment and positioning affect the response of the AEC device.
- Discuss patient and exposure technique factors and their effect on the response of the AEC device.
- Analyze poor-quality images produced using AEC and identify possible causes.
- Recognize the effect of the type of image receptor on AEC calibration, its use, and image quality.

- Describe patient radiation protection issues associated with AEC.
- State the importance of calibration of the AEC system to the type of image receptor used.
- List the quality-control tests used to evaluate AEC.
- Define anatomically programmed radiography.
- Differentiate between the types of exposure technique charts.
- State exposure technique modifications for the following considerations: pediatric, geriatric, and bariatric patients; projections and positions; soft tissue; casts and splints; contrast media; and pathologic conditions.

## Key Terms

anatomically programmed radiography (APR)
automatic exposure control (AEC)
backup time
calipers
comparative anatomy
contrast medium

density controls
detectors
exposure adjustment
exposure technique chart
fixed kVp–variable mAs technique chart
ionization or ion chamber

mAs readout
minimum response time
optimal kVp
photomultiplier (PM) tube
phototimer
variable kVp–fixed mAs technique chart

## INTRODUCTION

The radiographer is tasked with selecting exposure factor techniques to produce quality radiographic images for a wide variety of equipment and patients. There are many thousands of possible combinations of kilovoltage peak (kVp), milliamperage (mA), source-to-image receptor distance (SID), exposure time, image receptors, and grid ratios. When combined with patients of various sizes and with various pathologic conditions, the selection of proper exposure factors becomes a formidable task. An **automatic exposure control (AEC)** system is a tool available on most modern radiographic units to assist the radiographer.

AEC is a system used to consistently control the amount of radiation reaching the image receptor by terminating the length of exposure. AEC systems also are called *automatic exposure devices*, and sometimes they are erroneously referred to as *phototiming*. Technique charts make setting technical factors much more manageable, but there are always patient factors that require the radiographer's assessment and judgment. When using AEC systems, the radiographer must still use individual discretion to select an appropriate kVp, mA, image receptor, and grid. However, the AEC device determines the exposure time (and therefore total exposure).

 **Critical Concept**

**Principle of Automatic Exposure Control Operation**

Once a predetermined amount of radiation is transmitted through a patient, the x-ray exposure is terminated. This determines the exposure time and therefore the total amount of radiation exposure to the image receptor.

AEC systems are excellent at producing consistent levels of exposure when used properly, but the radiographer should also be aware of the technical limitations of using an AEC system.

## AEC RADIATION DETECTORS

All AEC devices work by the same principle: Radiation is transmitted through the patient and the activated AEC chambers, where it is converted into an electrical signal, terminating the exposure time. This occurs when a predetermined amount of radiation has been detected, as indicated by the level of electrical signal that has been produced. Service personnel calibrate the predetermined level of radiation to meet the departmental standards of image quality.

The difference in AEC systems lies in the type of device used to convert radiation into electricity. Two types of AEC systems have been used: phototimers and ionization chambers. Phototimers represent the first generation of AEC systems used in radiography, and it is from this type of system that the term *phototiming* has evolved. *Phototiming* specifically refers to the use of an AEC device that uses photomultiplier tubes or photodiodes; these systems are not common today. Therefore, the use of the term *phototiming* is usually in error. The more common type of AEC system uses ionization chambers. Regardless of the specific type of AEC system used, almost all systems use a set of three radiation-measuring detectors arranged in some specific manner (Fig. 13.1). The radiographer selects the configuration of these devices, determining which of the three (individually or in combination) measures radiation exposure reaching the image receptor. These devices are variously referred to as *sensors*, *chambers*, *cells*, or *detectors*. These radiation-measuring devices are referred to here for the remainder of the discussion as **detectors**. In this chapter, AEC detectors are differentiated from flat panel detector type receptors.

 **Critical Concept**

**Radiation-Measuring Devices**

Detectors are the AEC devices that measure the amount of radiation transmitted. The radiographer selects the combination of detectors.

## PHOTOTIMERS

**Phototimers** used a fluorescent (light-producing) screen and a device that converted the light to electricity. A **photomultiplier (PM) tube** is an electronic device that converts visible light energy into electrical energy. A photodiode is a solid-state device that performs the same function. Phototimer AEC devices were considered exit-type devices because the detectors are positioned behind the image receptor (Fig. 13.2) so that radiation must exit the image receptor before it is measured by the detectors. Light paddles, coated with a fluorescent material, served as the detectors, and the radiation interacted with the paddles, producing visible light. This light was then transmitted to remote PM tubes or photodiodes that convert this light into electricity. The timer was tripped and the radiographic exposure was terminated when a sufficiently large

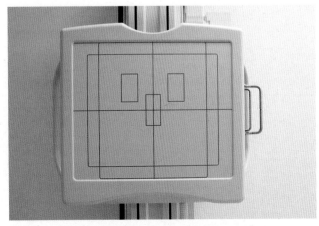

**Fig. 13.1 Automatic Exposure Control Detectors.** Arrangement of three automatic exposure control detectors on an upright Bucky unit.

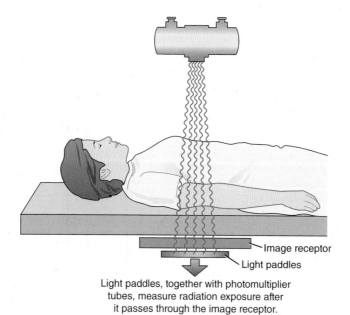

Light paddles, together with photomultiplier
tubes, measure radiation exposure after
it passes through the image receptor.

**Fig. 13.2 Phototimer Automatic Exposure Control.** In the phototimer automatic exposure control system, the detectors are located directly below the image receptor. This is an exit-type device in that the x-rays must exit the image receptor before they are measured by the detectors.

charge had been received. This electrical charge was in proportion to the radiation to which the light paddles have been exposed. Phototimers have largely been replaced with ionization chamber systems.

## IONIZATION CHAMBER SYSTEMS

An **ionization** or **ion chamber** is a hollow cell that contains air and is connected to the timer circuit via an electrical wire. Ionization-chamber AEC devices are considered entrance-type devices, because the detectors are positioned in front of the image receptor (Fig. 13.3) so that radiation interacts with the

detectors just before interacting with the image receptor. When the ionization chamber is exposed to radiation from a radiographic exposure, the air inside the chamber becomes ionized, creating an electrical charge. This charge travels along the wire to the timer circuit. The timer is tripped and the radiographic exposure is terminated when the predetermined amount of electric charge has been received. This electrical charge is in proportion to the radiation to which the ionization chamber has been exposed. Compared with phototimers, ion chambers are less sophisticated and less accurate, but they are

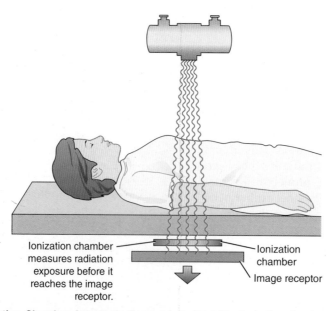

Ionization chamber
measures radiation
exposure before it
reaches the image
receptor.

Ionization
chamber

Image receptor

**Fig. 13.3 Ionization Chamber Automatic Exposure Control.** The ionization chamber automatic exposure control system has detectors located directly in front of the image receptor. This is an entrance-type device because the x-ray exposure is measured just before entering the image receptor.

less prone to failure. Most of today's AEC systems use ionization chambers.

 **Make the Physics Connection**

**Chapter 4**

The AEC serves the same role as the exposure timer in the primary circuit. The AEC is programmed to terminate exposure when a predetermined level of electric charge is received from the detector.

 **Critical Concept**

**Function of the Ionization Chamber**

The ionization chamber interacts with exit radiation before it reaches the image receptor. Air in the chamber is ionized; an electric charge is created that is proportional to the amount of radiation received. This electric charge travels to the timer circuit where the exposure is terminated.

## MILLIAMPERAGE/SECOND READOUT

When a radiographic study is performed using an AEC device, the total amount of radiation (milliamperage/second [mAs]) required to produce the appropriate exposure to the image receptor is determined by the system. Many radiographic units include a **mAs readout** display, on which the actual amount of mAs used for that image is displayed immediately after the exposure (sometimes for only a few seconds). It is critical for the radiographer to take note of this information when it is available. Knowledge of the mAs readout has a number of advantages. It allows the radiographer to become more familiar with manual exposure technique factors. If the image is unacceptable, knowing the mAs readout provides a basis from which the radiographer can make exposure adjustments by switching to the manual technique. There may be procedures with different positions in which AEC and manual techniques are combined because of difficulty with accurate centering. For example, knowing the mAs readout for the anteroposterior lumbar spine gives the radiographer an option to switch to manual technique for the oblique exposures, making technique adjustments based on reliable mAs information.

 **Critical Concept**

**Automatic Exposure Control and Milliamperage/Second Readout**

If the radiographic unit has a mAs readout display, the radiographer should observe the reading after the exposure is made. This information can be invaluable.

## KILOVOLTAGE PEAK AND MILLIAMPERAGE/SECOND SELECTION

AEC controls only the quantity of radiation reaching the image receptor and therefore has no effect on

other image characteristics such as radiographic contrast. The kVp for a particular examination should be selected without regard to whether an AEC device is used. The radiographer must select the kVp level that provides an appropriate subject contrast and is at least the minimum kVp to penetrate the part. Although radiographic contrast can be computer manipulated in digital imaging, the kVp should still be selected to best visualize the area of interest. High kVp is used for chest imaging with a grid to best visualize the anatomy because these tissues have widely varying thicknesses (Fig. 13.4). In addition, the higher the kVp value used, the shorter the exposure time needed by the AEC device. Because high kVp radiation is more

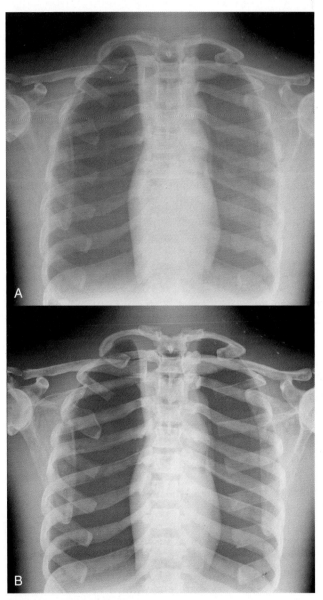

**Fig. 13.4 Kilovoltage. (A)** Radiographic image created using a high kVp (109) and the outer two AEC detectors. The image demonstrates low subject contrast typical for chest imaging. **(B)** Radiographic image created using a low kVp (60) and the outer two AEC detectors. The image demonstrates high subject contrast not typical for chest imaging. The mAs readout indicated significantly more radiation than image (A) as a result of using a low kVp.

penetrating (reducing the total amount of x-ray exposure to the patient because more x-ray photons exit the patient) and the detectors are measuring quantity of radiation, the preset amount of radiation exposure is reached sooner with high kVp. Using higher kVp with AEC decreases the exposure time and overall mAs needed to produce a diagnostic image, significantly reducing the patient's exposure.

### Critical Concept

**Kilovoltage Peak and Automatic Exposure Control Response**

The radiographer must be sure to set the kVp value as needed to ensure adequate penetration and to produce the appropriate subject contrast. The kVp selected determines the length of exposure time when using AEC. A low kVp requires more exposure time to reach the predetermined amount of exposure. A high kVp decreases the exposure time to reach the predetermined amount of exposure and reduces the overall radiation exposure to the patient.

When the radiographer uses a control panel that allows the mA and time to be set independently, they should select the mA without regard to whether an AEC device is used. The mA selected has a direct effect on the exposure time needed by the AEC device. Therefore, if the radiographer wants to decrease exposure time for a particular examination, they may easily do so by increasing the mA. For a given procedure, increasing the mA on the control panel shortens the exposure time and decreasing the mA increases the exposure time.

### Critical Concept

**Milliamperage and Automatic Exposure Control Response**

If the radiographer can set the mA when using AEC, it affects the time of exposure for a given procedure. Increasing the mA decreases the exposure time to reach the predetermined amount of exposure. Decreasing the mA increases exposure time to reach the predetermined amount of exposure.

## MINIMUM RESPONSE TIME

The term **minimum response time** refers to the shortest exposure time that the system can produce. Minimum response time (1 ms with modern AEC systems) usually is longer with AEC systems than with other types of radiographic timers (i.e., other types of radiographic timers usually can produce shorter exposure times than AEC devices). This can be a problem with some segments of the patient population, such as pediatric and uncooperative patients. Typically, the radiographer increases the mA so the time of exposure terminates more quickly. If the minimum response time is longer than the amount of time needed to terminate the preset exposure, an increased amount of radiation reaches the image receptor. With pediatric patients and others who cannot or will not cooperate

with the radiographer by holding still or holding their breath during the exposure, AEC devices may not be the method of choice.

## BACKUP TIME

**Backup time** refers to the maximum length of time the x-ray exposure continues when using an AEC system. The backup time may be set by the radiographer or may be controlled automatically by the radiographic unit. It may be set as backup exposure time or as backup mAs (the product of mA and exposure time). The role of the backup time is to act as a safety mechanism when an AEC system fails or the equipment is not used properly. In either case, the backup time protects the patient from receiving unnecessary exposure and protects the x-ray tube from reaching or exceeding its heat-loading capacity. If the backup time is controlled automatically, it should terminate at a maximum of 600 mAs when equipment is operated at or above 50 kVp.

### Critical Concept

**Function of Backup Time**

Backup time, the maximum exposure time allowed during an AEC examination, serves as a safety mechanism when the AEC is not used properly or is malfunctioning.

The backup time might be reached as the result of operator oversight when an AEC examination, such as a chest x-ray, is performed at the upright Bucky and the radiographer has set the control panel for table Bucky. The table detectors are forced to wait an excessively long time to measure enough radiation to terminate the exposure. The backup time is reached, and the exposure terminated, limiting the patient's exposure and preventing the tube from overloading. However, newer x-ray units with AEC include a sensor in the Bucky tray for the image receptor and will not allow an exposure to activate if the table Bucky detectors are selected, but the x-ray tube is centered to the upright Bucky. When controlled by the radiographer, the backup time should be set high enough to be greater than the exposure needed but low enough to protect the patient from excessive exposure in case of a problem. Setting the backup time at 150% to 200% of the expected exposure time is appropriate. If the backup timer periodically or routinely terminates the exposure, higher mA values should be used to shorten the exposure time.

### Critical Concept

**Setting Backup Time**

Backup time should be set at 150% to 200% of the expected exposure time. This allows the properly used AEC system to appropriately terminate the exposure but protects the patient and tube from excessive exposure if a problem occurs.

To minimize patient exposure, the backup time should be neither too long nor too short. A backup time that is too short results in the exposure ending prematurely, and the image may need to be repeated because of poor quality. A backup time that is too long results in the patient receiving unnecessary radiation if a problem occurs, and the exposure does not end until the backup time is reached. In addition, the image may have to be repeated because of poor quality.

## EXPOSURE ADJUSTMENT

AEC devices are equipped with a mechanism (**exposure adjustment**) that allows the radiographer to adjust the amount of preset radiation detection values (also known as **density controls**). These generally are in the form of buttons on the control panel that are numbered −2, −1, +1, +2, and +3. The actual numbers presented on the exposure adjustment vary, but each button changes exposure time by a predetermined amount or increment expressed as a percentage. A common increment is 25%, meaning that the predetermined exposure level needed to terminate the timer can be either increased or decreased from normal in one increment (+25% or −25%) or two increments (+50% or −50%).

A diagnostic-quality image (Fig. 13.5A) was produced using 81 kVp and the center AEC detector with 0 exposure adjustment. Fig. 13.5B was produced using 81 kVp and the center detector with +3 exposure adjustment, and Fig. 13.5C was produced using

81 kVp and the center detector with −3 exposure adjustment. Although the brightness was adjusted by the computer, the actual mAs applied and exposure indicator for each of the images varied greatly and reflected the exposure to the image receptor (IR). Manufacturers usually provide information on how these exposure adjustments should be used. Common sense and practical experience should also serve as guidelines for the radiographer. Routinely using plus or minus exposure adjustments to produce an acceptable image indicates that a problem exists, possibly with the AEC calibration.

## ALIGNMENT AND POSITIONING CONSIDERATIONS

### DETECTOR SELECTION

Selection of the detector or detectors to be used for a specific examination is critical when using an AEC system. AEC systems with multiple detectors typically allow the radiographer to select any combination of one, two, or three detectors. Radiographic equipment can also be purchased with five AEC detectors (Fig. 13.6), which provide greater flexibility in imaging a wide variety of patients. The selected detectors actively measure radiation during exposure, and the electrical signals are averaged. Typically, the detector that receives the greatest amount of exposure has a greater effect on the total exposure.

Measuring radiation that passes through the anatomic area of interest is important. The general guideline is to select the detectors that will be

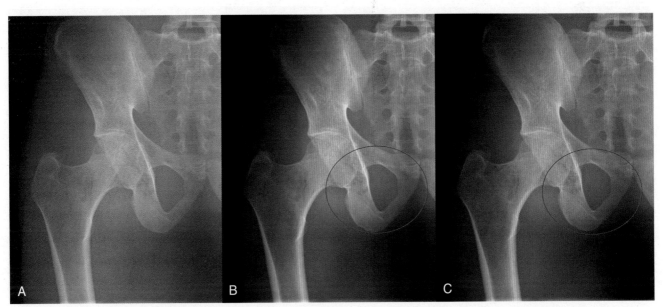

**Fig. 13.5 Exposure Adjustment. (A)** Radiographic image of the hip using 81 kVp, the center AEC detector, and 0 exposure adjustment. **(B)** Radiographic image of the hip using 81 kVp, the center AEC detector, and 13 exposure adjustment. The image demonstrates less quantum noise than image **(A)**. **(C)** Radiographic image of the hip using 81 kVp, the center AEC detector, and 23 exposure adjustment. The image demonstrates more quantum noise than image **(B)**. The mAs readout for images **(B)** and **(C)** reflect the exposure adjustment accordingly.

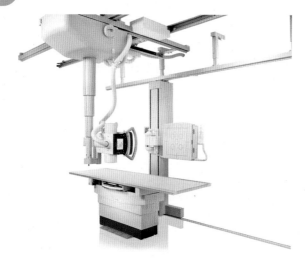

Fig. 13.6 **Multiple Detectors.** Radiographic equipment manufactured with five detector automatic exposure control (AEC). (Courtesy Koninklijke Philips N.V.)

superimposed by the anatomic structures of greatest interest that need to be visualized on the radiographic image. Failure to use the proper detectors could result in either underexposure or overexposure to the image receptor. In the case of a posteroanterior (PA) chest radiograph, the area of radiographic interest includes the lungs and heart; therefore, the outside detectors should be selected to place the detectors directly beneath the critical anatomic area. If the center detector is mistakenly selected, the anatomy superimposing this detector includes the thoracic spine. If the exposure is made,

the resultant image will demonstrate sufficient exposure in the spine, with the lungs overexposed (Fig. 13.7). Although brightness was adjusted by the computer, the mAs readout and exposure indicator reflect overexposure of the image. It is important for radiographers to evaluate image quality, the mAs readout, and the exposure indicator when using the AEC device. AEC device manufacturers provide recommendations for which detectors to use for specific examinations. Recommendations for detector combination can also be found in many radiographic procedures textbooks.

Many radiographic units have AEC devices in both the table Bucky and an upright Bucky. If more than one Bucky per radiographic unit uses AEC, the radiographer must be certain to select the correct Bucky before making an exposure. Failure to do so may result in excessive radiation exposure to the patient and image receptor. The backup time is reached, the exposure terminated, and a repeat radiographic study must be performed, thereby increasing the patient's dose.

A similar problem can occur when not using a Bucky, such as with cross-table, tabletop, stretcher, or wheelchair studies. If the AEC system is activated with these types of examinations, an unusually long exposure results, because the detectors are not exposed to radiation. Again, the backup time will probably be reached, and the patient's dose will be excessive. Some radiographic units are designed so that an exposure does not occur if the AEC device has been selected and there is no image receptor detected in the Bucky.

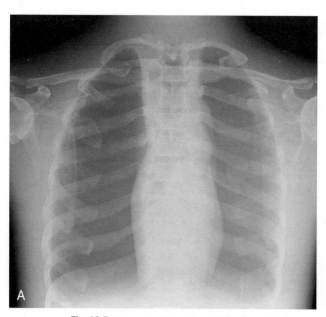
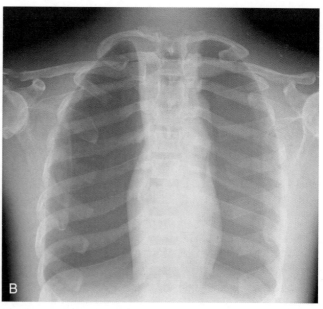

Fig. 13.7 **Detector Selection.** **(A)** Radiographic image created using the outer two AEC detectors appropriate for chest imaging. **(B)** Radiographic image created when the center detector was inappropriately selected for a chest image, placing the thoracic spine directly over the detector. The resulting chest image has increased radiation exposure in the area of the spine and therefore the lungs are overexposed. Although the brightness in the area of interest was computer adjusted, the mAs readout reflected the overexposure of the IR for a chest image.

⚠ **Critical Concept**

**Detector Selection**

> The combination of detectors affects the amount of exposure reaching the image receptor. If the area of radiographic interest is not directly over the selected detectors, that area probably will be over- or underexposed. When performing any radiographic study in which the image receptor is located outside of the Bucky, the AEC system should be deactivated, and a manual technique used.

## PATIENT CENTERING

Proper centering of the part of interest is crucial when using an AEC system. The anatomic area of interest must be centered properly over the detectors that the radiographer has selected. Improper centering of the part over the selected detectors may either underexpose or overexpose the image receptor. For example, when an AEC device is used for a thoracic spine image, if the central ray is positioned over the right lung and the center detector is selected (as appropriate), the soft tissue and ribs will superimpose the detector rather than the spine. In this case, the soft tissue and ribs will demonstrate sufficient exposure, but the spine itself will be underexposed (Fig. 13.8). When the anatomy of interest is not centered directly over the detector, the image will be underexposed or overexposed, possibly requiring the image to be repeated and the patient to receive more radiation than necessary.

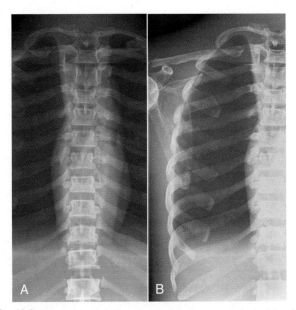

**Fig. 13.8 Centering. (A)** The center detector was selected for this thoracic spine and the central ray (CR) midpoint to the thoracic spine. **(B)** The central ray was centered over the right lung field. The resulting radiograph demonstrates appropriate brightness levels in the right lung and ribs, but the thoracic vertebral bodies are underexposed.

⚠ **Critical Concept**

**Patient Centering**

> Accurate centering of the area of interest over the detectors is critical to ensure proper exposure to the image receptor. If the area of interest is not properly centered to the image receptor, over- or underexposure may occur.

If a digital image receptor is underexposed or overexposed, the brightness is computer adjusted for the exposure error, but the image quality and/or patient exposure are compromised. Underexposure may result in the visibility of quantum noise and overexposure increases patient exposure and may decrease radiographic contrast. It is important for radiographers to evaluate image quality, the mAs readout, and the exposure indicator when using the AEC device. Errors in selecting the appropriate combination of AEC detectors or centering errors may not be visually apparent because of computer adjustment.

## DETECTOR SIZE

The size of the detectors manufactured within an AEC system is fixed and cannot be adjusted. Therefore, it is important for the radiographer to determine whether AEC should be used during the radiographic procedure. The radiographer must first determine whether the patient's anatomic area of interest can adequately cover the detector combination. For example, if the patient for a procedure is very small, such as a toddler, their chest may not adequately cover the outer two detectors. In this case, the patient's chest is smaller than the dimensions of the selected detectors. If a portion of the detector is exposed directly to the primary beam, the radiation exposure level necessary to terminate the exposure is reached prematurely, resulting in underexposure of the area of interest.

It is therefore critical that the radiographer determine whether the anatomic area of interest can adequately superimpose the dimensions of the detector combination. If the detector combination is larger than the area of interest, a manual exposure technique should be used.

## COMPENSATING ISSUES

### PATIENT CONSIDERATIONS

The AEC system is designed to compensate for changes in patient thickness. If the area of interest is thicker because of the patient's size, the exposure time will lengthen to reach the preset exposure to the detectors. AEC systems that do not adequately compensate for changes in patient thickness may need to be adjusted.

Some patients may require greater technical consideration when AEC is used for their radiographic procedures. For example, abdominal examinations using

AEC can be compromised if a patient has an excessive amount of bowel gas. If a detector is superimposed by an area of the abdomen with excessive gas, the timer will terminate the exposure prematurely, resulting in an underexposed image. Likewise, destructive pathologic conditions can cause underexposure of the area of radiographic interest. The presence of positive contrast media, an additive pathologic condition, or a prosthetic device (for example, hip replacement hardware) that superimposes the detector can cause excessive exposure.

### Critical Concept

**Patient Consideration**

Patient factors affect the time the exposure takes to reach the image receptor and ultimately affect image quality. Variations in patient thickness result in changes in the time of exposure accordingly if the AEC system is functioning properly. Pathologic conditions, contrast media, foreign objects, or pockets of gas are patient variations that may affect the proper exposure to the image receptor and ultimately image quality.

If the anatomic area directly over the detector does not represent the anatomic area of interest, inappropriate exposure to the image receptor may result. This can happen when the anatomic area over the detector contains a foreign object, a pocket of air, or contrast media. The radiographer must consider these circumstances individually and determine how best to image the part. Using the exposure adjustment buttons may work in some cases, whereas in others it may be necessary to recenter the patient or part. Sometimes the best solution is a manual technique determined through use of a technique chart. AEC is not a replacement for a knowledgeable radiographer using critical thinking skills.

### COLLIMATION

The size of the x-ray field is a factor when AEC systems are used because the additional scatter radiation produced by failure to accurately restrict the beam may cause the detector to terminate the exposure prematurely. The detector is unable to distinguish transmitted radiation from scattered radiation and, as always, ends the exposure when a preset amount of exposure has been reached. Because the detector is measuring both types of radiation exiting the patient, the exposure timer is turned off too soon when scatter is excessive, which results in underexposure of the area of interest.

Additionally, if the x-ray field size is collimated too closely, the detector does not receive sufficient exposure initially and may prolong the exposure time, which could result in overexposure. The radiographer should open the collimator to the extent that the part is imaged appropriately, but not so much as to cause the AEC device to terminate the exposure before the area is properly exposed.

### Critical Concept

**Collimation and Automatic Exposure Control Response**

Excessive or insufficient collimation may affect the amount of exposure reaching the image receptor. Insufficient collimation may result in excessive scatter reaching the detectors, resulting in the exposure time terminating too quickly. Excessive collimation may result in an exposure time that is too long.

### IMAGE RECEPTOR VARIATIONS

Different types of image receptors cannot be interchanged easily once an AEC device is calibrated to terminate exposures at a preset level. When calibration is performed, it is for a specific type of digital image receptor.

### Critical Concept

**Type of Image Receptor and Automatic Exposure Control Response**

The AEC system is calibrated to the type of image receptor used. If an image receptor of a different type is used, the detectors will not sense the difference, the exposure time will terminate at the preset value, and image quality may be jeopardized.

The AEC device cannot sense when the radiographer uses a different type of image receptor and instead produces an exposure based on the system for which it was calibrated, resulting in either too much or too little exposure for that image receptor.

If a different type of digital image receptor is used, the computer adjusts for the exposure error, but image quality and patient exposure are compromised. Underexposure may result in the visibility of quantum noise, and overexposure increases patient exposure and may decrease radiographic contrast.

### ANATOMICALLY PROGRAMMED RADIOGRAPHY

*Anatomic programming*, or **anatomically programmed radiography**, refers to a radiographic system that allows the radiographer to select a particular button on the control panel that represents an anatomic area for which a preprogrammed set of exposure factors are displayed and can be selected. The appearance of these controls varies depending on the unit (Fig. 13.9), but the operation of all anatomically programmed systems is based on the same principle. Anatomically programmed exposure techniques are controlled by an integrated circuit or computer chip that has been programmed with exposure factors for the projections and positions of different anatomic parts. Once an anatomic part and projection or position has been selected, the radiographer can adjust the exposure factors that are displayed.

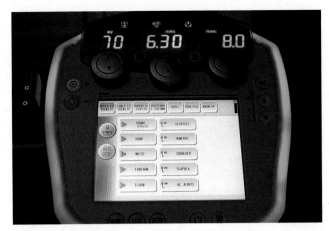

Fig. 13.9 **Anatomically Programmed Radiography.** Anatomically programmed exposure technique selections are displayed on the control panel. Each selection displays the preprogrammed exposure factors that the radiographer can decide to use or adjust.

Anatomically programmed radiography systems and AEC are not related in their functions, other than as systems for making exposures. However, these two different systems are commonly combined on radiographic units because of their similar dependence on integrated computer circuitry and often are used in conjunction with one another. A radiographer can use the anatomically programmed system to select a projection or position for a specific anatomic part and view the kVp, mA, and exposure time for manual technique. When anatomically programmed exposure techniques are used in conjunction with AEC, the system selects and displays not only manual exposure factors but also the AEC detectors to be used for a specific radiographic examination. For example, pressing the "Lungs PA" button results in selection of 120 kVp, the upright Bucky, and the two outside AEC detectors. As with AEC, anatomically programmed radiography is a system that automates some of the work of radiography. However, the individual judgment and discretion of the radiographer is still required to use the anatomically programmed radiography system correctly to produce diagnostic-quality images (Box 13.1).

## QUALITY CONTROL

As with any radiographic unit, it is imperative that systematic equipment testing be performed to ensure proper system performance. Calibration and quality-control testing are essential procedures to maintain the proper functioning of the AEC system.

### CALIBRATION

For an AEC device to function properly, the radiographic unit, the image receptor, and the AEC device must be calibrated to meet departmental standards. When a radiographic unit with AEC is first installed, the AEC device is calibrated, and it is recalibrated at intervals thereafter. The purpose of calibration is to ensure that consistent and appropriate exposures to the image receptor are produced.

Failure to maintain regular calibration of the unit results in the lack of consistent and reproducible exposures to the detectors and could affect image quality. This ultimately leads to overexposure of the patient, poor efficiency of the imaging department, and the possibility of improper interpretation of radiographic images.

| Box **13.1** | Manual Techniques Versus Automatic Exposure Control |

- Manual exposure techniques require the radiographer to select the kVp and mAs necessary for the radiographic procedure. This requires the radiographer to consider the procedure, primary and secondary exposure variables, and patient considerations. Different from manual exposure techniques, the use of AEC systems will terminate the radiation exposure exiting the patient based on the preset calibration of the radiation detectors; therefore, the actual mAs is not set by the radiographer. The decision to select manual exposure techniques or use the AEC device requires the radiographer to consider many variables.

- As previously discussed, the detector(s) selected must be adequately covered by the patient's anatomic area of interest. In the case of a pediatric patient or distal extremities, the area of interest may be too small to adequately cover the detector(s), and therefore the use of a manual exposure technique would be more appropriate.

- Patient factors such as pathology, contrast media, or a foreign object may cause the AEC device to terminate prematurely or result in excessive exposure. The radiographer must consider these patient variations individually and determine whether the use of a manual exposure technique would be best.

- There are a few anatomic regions that may be more challenging for the radiographer when using the AEC device. For example, centering for the axial clavicle to ensure the proper radiation exposure may be more difficult than selecting a manual exposure technique. In addition, any slight movement of the patient before the activation of the radiation exposure could result in the area of interest not being adequately centered to the central ray, such as a lateral cervical spine. In these situations, the radiographer could evaluate the mAs readout for an AP projection and then change to a manual exposure technique for the axial, lateral, or oblique positions.

- For those radiographic procedures best suited, routine use of AEC is recommended. Proper use and calibration of the AEC system will lessen the potential for overexposure. This is especially important during digital imaging, because computer processing will rescale image brightness, and excessive radiation exposure would not be easily apparent to the radiographer.

## QUALITY-CONTROL TESTING

The AEC device should provide consistent exposures to the image receptor for variations in technique factors, patient thicknesses, and detector selection. Several aspects of the AEC performance can be monitored by imaging a homogeneous patient equivalent phantom plus additional thickness plates.

Consistency of exposures with varying mA, kVp, part thicknesses, and detector selection can be evaluated individually and in combination by imaging a patient equivalent phantom and measuring the resultant milliroentgen (mR) exposure and pixel brightness levels. Reproducibility of exposures for a given set of exposure factors and selected detector should result in mR readings within 5%, and pixel brightness levels for areas within the displayed imaged should be within 30%.

The radiographer must use AEC accurately, regardless of the type of image receptor used. Failure to do so can result in overexposure of the patient or production of a poor-quality image. It cannot be overstated that, when using digital image receptors, the radiographer must be very conscientious about preventing excessive radiation exposure to the patient. If a high amount of radiation reaches the digital image receptor, the image will probably appear diagnostic, but the patient receives unnecessary exposure.

During computer processing, image brightness can be adjusted after underexposure; however, there may be an increase in the visibility of quantum noise. The radiographer must monitor the exposure indicator as a means of detecting AEC malfunctions for digital image receptors.

The response of the AEC device when changing exposure variables and their effect on exposure time and brightness on the area of interest are stated in Table 13.1.

| Table 13.1 | Digital Imaging and AEC |

An upright PA chest examination performed using the following factors produces an optimal image:

| | |
|---|---|
| Flat-panel detector | AEC with 2 outer detectors |
| 120 kVp | Upright Bucky |
| 400 mA | 0 (normal) density control |

Assuming all other factors remain the same, unless indicated, how would the following changes affect the response of the AEC device and image quality?

| CHANGE | EFFECT ON EXPOSURE TIME | EFFECT ON BRIGHTNESS IN AREA OF INTEREST | EXPLANATION |
|---|---|---|---|
| CR image receptor | No effect | No effect | The AEC is calibrated to the flat panel detector. The exposure ends when the exposure is sufficient for the IR, which is suboptimal for the CR image receptor. The computer maintains the brightness, but quantum noise is apparent because of underexposure of the imaging plate. |
| Center detector selected | Increased | No effect | Because the thoracic spine lies over the center detector, the IR receives more exposure than is needed. The mAs and exposure indicator will reflect an increase in exposure to the image receptor. The computer maintains the brightness, but the image contrast is decreased because of excessive scatter, and the patient is overexposed. |
| 70 kVp | Increased | No effect | The length of exposure to the IR will be increased, resulting in an increase in the actual mAs to maintain the exposure to the IR. However, the subject contrast is increased because of the lower kVp. |
| 100 mA | Increased | No effect | The length of exposure is increased to maintain exposure to the IR. |
| −2 Density control | Decreased | No effect | Changing the exposure adjustment button changes the setting of the AEC so it turns off the exposure much sooner. The mAs and exposure indicator will reflect a decrease in exposure to the IR. The computer maintains the brightness, but quantum noise is apparent because of underexposure of the IR. |

| Table 13.1 | Digital Imaging and AEC—cont'd | | |
|---|---|---|---|
| CHANGE | EFFECT ON EXPOSURE TIME | EFFECT ON BRIGHTNESS IN AREA OF INTEREST | EXPLANATION |
| Selecting the table Bucky setting but still using the upright Bucky | Increased | No effect | Excessive radiation reaches the IR because the detectors in the table Bucky are unable to terminate the exposure. The mAs and exposure indicator will reflect an increase in exposure to the IR. The computer maintains the brightness, but the image contrast is decreased because of excessive scatter, and the patient is overexposed. |
| Patient has cardiac pacemaker positioned over detector | Increased | No effect | The detector that is behind the pacemaker takes a long time to turn the exposure off because the radiation must pass through the pacemaker. The mAs and exposure indicator will reflect an increase in exposure to the IR. The computer maintains the brightness, but the image contrast is decreased because of excessive scatter, and the patient is overexposed. |

*AEC,* Automatic exposure control; *CR,* computed radiography; *IR,* imaging receptor; *kVp,* kilovoltage peak; *mA,* milliamperage; *mAs,* milliamperage/second; *PA,* posteroanterior.

 **Critical Concept**

**Digital Image Receptors and the Automatic Exposure Control Response**

When using digital image receptors, the radiographer must be very conscientious about preventing excessive radiation exposure to the patient.

## EXPOSURE TECHNIQUE CHARTS

The radiographer has the primary task of selecting the exposure factors that produce a quality radiographic image. Many variables affect the production of a quality image. Knowledge of these factors and of the qualities inherent in a diagnostic radiographic image helps the radiographer select exposure factors for a particular radiographic examination. Exposure technique charts are useful tools that help the radiographer select a manual exposure technique or use AEC regardless of the type of IR.

**Exposure technique charts** are preestablished guidelines used by the radiographer to select standardized manual or AEC exposure factors for each type of radiographic examination. Exposure technique charts standardize the selection of exposure factors for the typical patient so that the quality of radiographic images is consistent. Additional information such as collimation, AEC detector selection, and the acceptable range for the exposure indicator can be included in the technique chart.

For each radiographic procedure, the radiographer consults the technique chart for the recommended exposure variables—kVp, mAs (or AEC detectors), type of IR, grid, and SID. Based on the thickness of the anatomic part, the radiographer selects the exposure factors presented in the technique chart. For example, if a patient is scheduled for a routine abdominal examination, the radiographer positions the patient and aligns the central ray (CR) to the patient and IR, measures the abdomen (for a manual technique), and consults the chart for the predetermined standardized exposure variables including the appropriate combination of AEC detectors.

Because many factors affect the selection of appropriate exposure factors, technique charts are instrumental in the production of consistent-quality images, reduction in repeat radiographic studies, and reduction in patient exposure. The proper development and use of technique charts are keys to the selection of appropriate exposure factors.

 **Critical Concept**

**Exposure Technique Charts and Radiographic Quality**

A properly designed and used technique chart standardizes the selection of exposure factors to help the radiographer consistently produce quality radiographs while minimizing patient exposure.

Exposure technique charts are important for digital imaging, because digital systems have a wide dynamic range and can compensate for exposure technique errors. Technique charts should be developed and used with all types of radiographic imaging systems to maintain patient radiation exposure at a level as low as reasonably achievable.

### CONDITIONS

A technique chart presents exposure factors used for a specific examination based on the type of radiographic equipment. Technique charts help ensure that consistent image quality is achieved throughout the entire diagnostic radiology department; they also decrease the number of repeat radiographic studies needed and therefore decrease patient exposure.

Technique charts do not replace the critical thinking skills required of the radiographer. The radiographer must continue to use individual judgment and discretion in properly selecting exposure factors for each patient and type of examination. The radiographer's primary task is to produce diagnostic-quality images while delivering the least amount of radiation exposure to patients. Technique charts are designed for the average or typical patient and do not account for unusual circumstances. Patient variability in terms of body build, physical condition, or the presence of a pathologic condition requires the radiographer to problem-solve when selecting exposure factors. These atypical conditions require accurate patient assessment and appropriate exposure technique adjustment by the radiographer.

A technique chart should be established for each x-ray tube, even if a single generator is used for more than one tube. For example, if a radiographic room has two x-ray tubes, one for a radiographic table and one for an upright Bucky unit, each tube should have its own technique chart because of possible inherent differences in the exposure output produced by each tube. Each mobile radiographic unit must also have its own technique chart.

For technique charts to be effective tools in producing consistent-quality images, departmental standards for radiographic quality should be established. In addition, standardization of exposure factors and the use of accessory devices are needed. For example, the adult knee can be radiographed adequately with or without the use of a grid. Although both radiographic images might be acceptable, departmental standards may specify that the knee be radiographed with the use of a grid. These types of decisions should be made before technique chart development takes place so departmental standards can be clarified. Technique charts are then constructed using these standards, and radiographers should adhere to the departmental standards.

For technique charts to be effective, the radiographic system must operate properly. A comprehensive and effective quality-control program for all radiographic equipment ensures monitoring of any variability in the equipment's performance.

Accurate measurement of part thickness is a critical condition for the effective use of technique charts. The measured part thickness determines the selected kVp and mAs (when using manual exposure techniques) for the radiographic examination. If the part is measured inaccurately, incorrect exposure factors may be selected. Measurement of part thickness must be standardized throughout the radiology department.

**Calipers** are devices that measure part thickness and should be readily accessible in every radiographic room (Fig. 13.10). In addition, the technique chart should specify the exact location for measuring part thickness. Part measurement may be performed at the location of the CR midpoint or the thickest portion of the area to be radiographed. Errors in part thickness

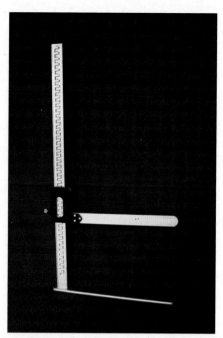

**Fig. 13.10 Calipers.** A caliper is used to measure part thickness.

measurement are one of the more common mistakes made when one is consulting technique charts.

Because the range of exposures needed to produce a quality digital image is wider (wide exposure latitude), precise measurement of the anatomic part is not critical. Although the technique charts discussed in this chapter use patient measurement to determine the exposure factors to be selected, categorizing the typical patient according to size (small, medium, and large) should be sufficient when using digital IRs.

## DESIGN CHARACTERISTICS

Technique charts can vary widely in terms of their design, but they share some common characteristics. The primary exposure factors of kVp and mAs and common accessory devices used, such as IR type and a grid, are included regardless of the type of technique chart used.

## TYPES OF TECHNIQUE CHARTS

Two primary types of exposure technique charts exist: variable kVp-fixed mAs and fixed kVp-variable mAs. Each type of chart has different characteristics, and both have advantages and disadvantages.

### Variable kVp-Fixed mAs Technique Chart

The **variable kVp-fixed mAs technique chart** is based on the concept that kVp can be increased as the anatomic part size increases. Specifically, the baseline kVp is increased by 2 for every 1-cm increase in part thickness, whereas the mAs is maintained (Table 13.2). The baseline kVp is the original kVp predetermined for the anatomic area to be radiographed. The baseline kVp is then adjusted for changes in part thickness.

## Table 13.2 Variable kVp-Fixed mAs Technique Chart

| ANATOMIC PART | KNEE | IMAGE RECEPTOR | COMPUTED RADIOGRAPHY |
|---|---|---|---|
| Projection | AP | Tabletop/Bucky | Bucky |
| Measuring point | Midpatella | Grid ratio | 12:1 |
| SID | 40 inches | Focal spot size | Small |
| | cm | kVp | mAs |
| | 10 | 63 | 8 |
| | 11 | 65 | 8 |
| | 12 | 67 | 8 |
| | 13 | 69 | 8 |
| | 14 | 71 | 8 |
| | 15 | 73 | 8 |
| | 16 | 75 | 8 |
| | 17 | 77 | 8 |
| | 18 | 79 | 8 |

*AP,* Anteroposterior; *SID,* source-to-image receptor distance.

Accurate measurement of part thickness is critical to the effective use of this type of technique chart. Part thickness must be measured accurately to ensure that the 2-kVp adjustment is applied appropriately. The radiographer consults the technique chart and prepares the exposure factors specified for the type of radiographic examination (i.e., mAs, SID, grid use, and type of IR). The anatomic part is measured accurately, and the kVp is adjusted appropriately. For example, a standard exposure technique for a patient's knee measuring 10 cm (4 inches) is 63 kVp at 8 mAs, digital radiographic (DR) IR, and use of a 12:1 table Bucky grid. A patient with a knee measuring 15 cm (6 inches) then requires a change only in the kVp from 63 to 73 (2 kVp change for every 1-cm change in part thickness).

### ! Critical Concept

#### Variable kVp-Fixed mAs Technique Chart

The variable kVp chart adjusts the kVp for changes in part thickness while maintaining a fixed mAs.

The baseline kVp for each anatomic area has not been standardized. Historically, a variety of methods have been used to determine the baseline kVp. The goal is to determine a kVp that adequately penetrates the anatomic part when using a 2-kVp adjustment for every 1-cm change in tissue thickness. The baseline kVp can be determined experimentally with the use of radiographic phantoms (patient equivalent devices).

Developing a variable kVp technique chart that can be used effectively throughout the kVp range has proved problematic. In addition, technological advances in imaging receptors may challenge the applicability of the variable kVp-fixed mAs type technique chart.

In general, changing the kVp for variations in part thickness may be ineffective throughout the entire range of radiographic examinations. A variable kVp-fixed mAs chart may be most effective with pediatric patients or when small extremities, such as hands, toes, and feet, are being imaged. At low kVp, small changes in kVp may be more effective than changing the mAs.

This type of chart has the advantage of being easy to formulate because making kVp changes to compensate for different part sizes is simple. However, because kVp is variable, subject contrast may vary as well, and these types of charts tend to be less accurate for part size extremes (very thin and very thick part thicknesses). In addition, adequate penetration of the part is not necessarily ensured.

### Fixed kVp-Variable mAs Technique Chart

The fixed kVp-variable mAs technique chart (Table 13.3) uses the concept of selecting an optimal kVp that is required for the radiographic examination and adjusting the mAs for variations in part thickness. Optimal kVp can be described as the kVp that is high enough to ensure penetration of the part but not too high to diminish subject contrast. For this type of chart, the optimal kVp for each part is indicated, and mAs is varied as a function of part thickness.

### ! Critical Concept

#### Fixed kVp Peak-Variable mAs Technique Charts

Fixed kVp-variable mAs technique charts identify optimal kVp values and alter the mAs for variations in part thickness.

Optimal kVp required for each anatomic area have not been standardized. Although charts identifying common kVp for different anatomic areas can be found, experienced radiographers tend to develop their own optimal kVp. The goal is to determine the kVp that will penetrate the part without compromising subject contrast; however, digital computer processing provides the opportunity to vary the image contrast displayed. Specifying the optimal kVp used

## Table 13.3 Fixed kVp-Variable mAs Technique Chart

| ANATOMIC PART | KNEE | IMAGE RECEPTOR | COMPUTED RADIOGRAPHY |
|---|---|---|---|
| Projection | AP | Tabletop/Bucky | Bucky |
| Measuring point | Midpatella | Grid ratio | 12:1 |
| SID | 40 inches | Focal spot size | Small |
| | cm | kVp | mAs |
| | 10-13 | 73 | 4 |
| | 14-17 | 73 | 8 |
| | 18-21 | 73 | 16 |

*AP,* Anteroposterior; *SID,* source-to-image receptor distance.

in a fixed kVp-variable mAs technique chart encourages all radiographers to adhere to the departmental standards.

Once optimal kVp are established, fixed kVp-variable mAs technique charts alter the mAs for variations in thickness of the anatomic part. Because x-rays are attenuated exponentially, a general guideline is that for every 4- to 5-cm change in part thickness, the mAs should be adjusted by a factor of 2. Using the previous example for a patient's knee measuring 10 cm (4 inches) and an optimal kVp, the exposure technique is 73 kVp at 4 mAs, DR IR with a 12:1 table Bucky grid. A patient with a knee measuring 15 cm (6 inches) requires a change only in the mAs, from 4 to 8 (a 5-cm [2-inch] increase in part thickness requires a doubling of the mAs).

Accurate measurement of the anatomic part is important but is less critical compared with the precision needed with variable kVp charts. An advantage of fixed kVp-variable mAs technique charts is that patient groups can be formed around 4- to 5-cm (1.6- to 2-inch) changes. Patient thickness groups can be created instead of listing thickness changes in increments of 1 cm.

Alternatively, patients can be grouped by size (such as small, medium, large, extra-large) or actual weight ranges in pounds (such as 100-130 pounds), and therefore measuring the thickness would not be required. In addition, using consistently higher "optimal" kVp ranges with digital imaging systems can reduce the variability among exposure techniques for the same or similar anatomic region. The fixed kVp-variable mAs technique chart has the advantages of easier use, more consistency in the production of quality radiographic images, greater assurance of adequate penetration of all anatomic parts, uniform subject contrast, and increased accuracy with extreme variation in size of the anatomic part.

## EXPOSURE TECHNIQUE CHART DEVELOPMENT

Radiographers can develop effective technique charts that assist in exposure technique selection. The steps involved in technique chart development are similar, regardless of the design of the technique chart. The primary tools needed are radiographic phantoms, calipers for accurate measurement, and a calculator. Once diagnostic images are produced using these phantoms, exposure techniques can be extrapolated (mathematically estimated) for imaging other similar anatomic areas.

A critical component in technique chart development is to determine the minimum kVp that adequately penetrates the anatomic part to be radiographed. One method available is to use the concept of **comparative anatomy**, which can assist the radiographer in determining minimum kVp. This concept states that different parts of the same size can be radiographed by use of

the same exposure factors, provided that the minimum kVp needed to penetrate the part is used in each case. For example, a radiographer knows what exposure factors to use with a particular radiographic unit for a knee that measures 10 cm (4 inches) in the anteroposterior (AP) aspect, but he or she is now confronted with radiographing a shoulder. The radiographer measures the shoulder in the AP aspect and determines that it measures 10 cm (4 inches). The radiographer does not have a technique for a shoulder for this radiographic unit. The concept of comparative anatomy states that the shoulder in this case can be radiographed successfully using the same technique that the radiographer has used for the 10-cm (4-inch) knee if the minimum kVp to penetrate the part has been used for the shoulder and knee.

The stages for development of exposure technique charts are similar regardless of the type of chart. Patient-equivalent phantoms for sample anatomic areas provide a means for establishing standardized exposure factors. The concept of comparative anatomy helps the radiographer extrapolate exposure techniques for similar anatomic areas. After the initial development of an exposure technique chart, the chart must be tested for accuracy and revised if necessary.

Poor radiographic quality may result when the exposure technique chart is not used properly. Radiographers need to problem-solve by evaluating the numerous exposure variables that could have contributed to a poor-quality image before assuming the chart is ineffective.

A commitment by management and staff to use exposure technique charts is critical to the consistent production of quality radiographic images. Well-developed technique charts are of little use if radiographers choose not to consult them.

 **Critical Concept**

**Exposure Technique Charts**

A commitment by management and staff to use exposure technique charts is critical to the consistent production of quality radiographic images. Well-developed technique charts are of little use if radiographers choose not to consult them.

## SPECIAL CONSIDERATIONS

Appropriate exposure factor selection and its modification for variability in the patient are critical to the production of a quality radiographic image. Thus, the radiographer must be able to recognize a multitude of patient and equipment variables and have a thorough understanding of how these variables affect the resulting image in order to make adjustments to produce a quality radiographic image.

## Pediatric Patients

Pediatric patients are a technical challenge for radiographers for many reasons. Because of their smaller size, they require lower kVp and mAs values compared with adults.

Pediatric chest radiography requires the radiographer to choose fast exposure times to stop diaphragm motion in patients who cannot or will not voluntarily suspend their breathing. A fast exposure time may eliminate the possibility of using AEC systems for pediatric chest radiography. Owing to their small size, the pediatric patient may not adequately cover the AEC detectors, and therefore, a manual exposure technique should be used.

Exposure factors used for the adult skull can be used for pediatric patients aged 6 years and older, because the bone density of these children has developed to an adult level. However, exposure factors must be modified for patients younger than 6 years. It is recommended for the radiographer to decrease the kVp by at least 15% to compensate for this lack of bone density. In addition, one should limit the use of grids whenever possible since grid use requires an increase in mAs. Radiographic examination of all other parts of pediatric patients' anatomy requires an adjustment in exposure techniques.

Because pediatric patients are more sensitive to ionizing radiation and have a longer life span than adults, it is even more critical to monitor the exposure indicator during digital imaging to minimize unnecessary radiation exposure.

## Geriatric Patients

Aging patients may experience physical changes such as limitations in hearing, vision, and balance. Additionally, their skin is thinner and more easily torn or bruised. Psychological changes in the mental state of geriatric patients may affect their ability to follow instructions during imaging procedures. The radiographer should be prepared to provide enhanced patient care in terms of additional time for the imaging procedure, and sensitivity to patient comfort by using a table pad, positioning sponges, and blankets for warmth. Radiographers should also ensure the safety of geriatric patients during transport on and off the table and when positioning patients during the procedure.

Exposure techniques may need to be decreased for patients who appear thin and frail. Tissues may be lower in subject contrast and therefore require decreased kVp, which results in higher subject contrast. To eliminate motion, it is recommended for the radiographer to accordingly adjust the mA and exposure time.

## Bariatric Patients

Imaging patients categorized as obese are more commonplace in radiology. Bariatric surgery is becoming more routine and therefore imaging procedures may be needed both before and after surgery. Bariatric patients bring unique challenges in terms of their weight and body diameter.

Important issues to consider when imaging bariatric patients include the table weight limit and the size (aperture) diameter of fluoroscopic imaging equipment. Bariatric patients need an increase in both kVp and mAs values to produce diagnostic images. In addition, the use of a grid is important to reduce the scatter radiation from reaching the image receptor, which would decrease image contrast. Depending on the imaging procedure performed, bariatric patients may need to be imaged in halves or quadrants owing to the size limitation of the image receptor.

## Projections and Positions

Different radiographic projections and patient positions of the same anatomic part often require modification of exposure factors. For example, an oblique position of the lumbar spine requires more exposure than an AP projection because of an increase in the amount of tissue that the primary beam must pass through. However, an oblique ankle requires slightly less exposure than the AP for comparable exposure to the IR.

General guidelines, based on variations in radiographic projection or patient position, can be followed to change exposure factors. Compared with an AP projection, an increase or decrease in the amount of tissue should determine any changes in exposure factors for oblique and lateral patient positions.

## Casts and Splints

Casts and splints can be produced with materials that attenuate x-rays differently. Selecting appropriate exposure factors can be challenging because of the wide variation of materials used for these devices. The radiographer should pay close attention to both the type of material and how the cast or splint is used.

*Casts.* Casts can be made of either fiberglass or plaster. Fiberglass generally requires no change in exposure factors from the values used for the same anatomic part without a cast.

Plaster presents a problem in terms of exposure factors. Plaster casts require an increase in exposure factors compared with imaging the same part without a cast. However, the method and amount of increase in exposure has not been standardized.

Exposure factor adjustments made for cast materials may be based on the part thickness using a technique chart. For example, if an AP ankle measured through the CR is 4 inches (10 cm) without the cast and 8 inches (20 cm) with the cast, the radiographer simply increases the exposure technique to that of an ankle measuring 8 inches (20 cm) to obtain an acceptable radiograph.

*Splints.* Splints present less of a challenge for the determination of appropriate exposure factors than casts. Inflatable (air) and fiberglass splints do not require any increase in exposure. Wood, aluminum, and solid plastic splints may require that exposure factors be increased, but only if they are in the path of the primary beam. For example, if two pieces of wood are bound to the sides of a lower leg, no increase in exposure is necessary for an AP projection, because the splint is not in the path of the primary beam and does not interfere with the radiographic image. Using the same example, if a lateral projection is produced, the splint is in the path of the primary beam and interferes with the radiographic imaging of the part. This necessitates an increase in exposure technique to produce a properly exposed radiograph.

## Pathologic Conditions

Pathologic conditions that can alter the absorption characteristics of the anatomic part being examined are divided into two categories. *Additive diseases* are diseases or conditions that increase the absorption characteristics of the part, making the part more difficult to penetrate. *Destructive diseases* are those diseases or conditions that decrease the absorption characteristics of the part, making the part less difficult to penetrate. Table 13.4 presents a list of additive and destructive diseases. Additive diseases decrease the amount of x-rays that transmit through the part to the image receptor, while destructive diseases increase the amount of x-rays which transmit to the image receptor. Generally,

| Table 13.4 | Some Common Additive and Destructive Diseases and Conditions by Anatomic Area | |
|---|---|
| **ADDITIVE CONDITIONS** | **DESTRUCTIVE CONDITIONS** |
| **Abdomen** | |
| Aortic aneurysm | Bowel obstruction |
| Ascites | Free air |
| Cirrhosis | |
| Hypertrophy of some organs (e.g., splenomegaly) | |
| **Chest** | |
| Atelectasis | Emphysema |
| Congestive heart failure | Pneumothorax |
| Malignancy | |
| Pleural effusion | |
| Pneumonia | |
| **Skeleton** | |
| Hydrocephalus | Gout |
| Metastases (osteoblastic) | Metastases (osteolytic) |
| Osteochondroma (exostoses) | Multiple myeloma |
| Paget disease (late stage) | Paget disease (early stage) |
| **Nonspecific sites** | |
| Abscess | Atrophy |
| Edema | Emaciation |
| Sclerosis | Malnutrition |

it is necessary to increase the kVp when radiographing parts that have been affected by additive diseases and to decrease the kVp when radiographing parts affected by destructive diseases.

However, it is not necessary to compensate for all additive and destructive diseases. It is often desirable to image diseases with exposure factors that would normally be used for a specific anatomic part so that the effect of that disease on that part can be visualized clearly.

When it is necessary or desirable to compensate for additive or destructive diseases or conditions, it is best to make changes in the kVp. Changing the kVp is fundamentally correct because the kVp affects the penetrating ability of the primary beam, and it is the penetrability of the anatomic part that is affected by these specific diseases and conditions. It is not possible to state an exact amount or percentage of kVp that should be changed because the state or severity of the disease or condition is different with each patient. However, a minimum change of 15% in kVp is recommended. There are some instances in which a change in mAs may be more appropriate to the type of pathologic condition. For example, if the anatomic area has significant increases in gas, such as in bowel obstruction, a large decrease in mAs is best.

## Soft Tissue

Objects such as small pieces of wood, glass, or swallowed bones are difficult to visualize radiographically using the normal exposure factors for a specific anatomic part. Several situations in which a soft tissue technique (decreased mAs) may be needed are visualization of the larynx in a young child with the croup, possible foreign body obstruction in the throat, and foreign body location in the extremities (Fig. 13.11). However, digital imaging systems allow visualization of soft tissues without changing the exposure technique.

## Contrast Media

A **contrast medium** (also called *contrast agent*) is used when imaging anatomic tissues that have low subject contrast. A contrast medium is a substance that can be instilled into the body by injection or ingestion. The type of contrast media used changes the absorption characteristics of the tissues by either increasing or decreasing the attenuation of the x-ray beam. Positive contrast agents, such as barium (atomic number of 56) and iodine (atomic number of 53), have a high atomic number and absorb more x-rays (increase attenuation) than the surrounding tissue (Fig. 13.12). Negative contrast agents, such as air (atomic number of 8), decrease the attenuation of the x-ray beam and transmit more radiation than the surrounding tissue (Fig. 13.13). Positive contrast agents produce more brightness than the adjacent tissues. Negative contrast agents produce less brightness than the adjacent tissues.

Even though negative contrast agents decrease the attenuation characteristics of the part being examined, their use does not require a change in exposure factors.

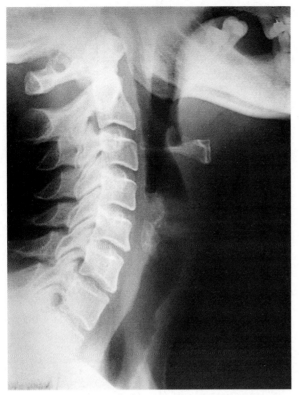

Fig. 13.11 **Soft Tissue Imaging.** Lateral soft tissue neck image. (Courtesy Frank E: *Merrill's atlas of radiographic positioning and procedures,* ed 12, St Louis, 2012, Mosby.)

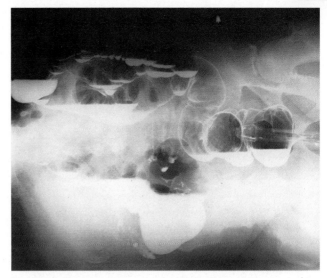

Fig. 13.13 **Negative Contrast Agents.** Radiographic image showing decreased brightness because of the decrease in x-ray beam attenuation by use of a negative contrast agent. (Courtesy Fauber TL: *Radiographic imaging and exposure,* ed 3, St Louis, 2009, Mosby.)

Negative contrast agents can also be used in conjunction with positive contrast agents. Positive contrast media studies require an increase in exposure factors compared with imaging the same part without a positive contrast medium.

The use of a contrast agent is an effective method of increasing the subject contrast when imaging areas of low subject contrast.

The quality of the radiographic image depends on a multitude of variables. Knowledge of these variables and their radiographic effect assists the radiographer in selecting exposure techniques to produce quality radiographic images.

### On the Spot

- AEC systems are designed to produce sufficient radiation exposure to the image receptor to produce a quality radiographic image.
- AEC uses detectors (typically ionization type) that measure the amount of radiation exiting the patient and terminate the exposure when it reaches a preset amount; this amount corresponds to that needed to produce an image of diagnostic quality.
- The kVp selected must penetrate the part and produce the desired subject contrast. Increasing or decreasing the kVp causes the exposure time to be decreased or increased accordingly.
- Changing the mA, when the option is available, causes the exposure time to decrease or increase accordingly.
- For AEC to work accurately, the x-ray beam must be centered precisely on the anatomic area of interest, the correct detectors must be selected, and the anatomic part must cover the dimension of the detectors.
- The mAs readout informs the radiographer of the total radiation exposure used for the procedure.
- Other AEC features that can be manipulated include exposure adjustment controls that allow for increased or

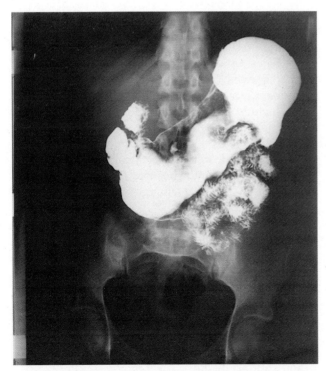

Fig. 13.12 **Positive Contrast Agents.** Radiographic image showing increased brightness because of the increase in x-ray beam attenuation by use of a positive contrast agent. (Courtesy Fauber TL: *Radiographic imaging and exposure,* ed 3, St Louis, 2009, Mosby.)

decreased exposure to the image receptor and the backup time (or backup mAs), which provides a safety mechanism preventing the exposure from exceeding a set amount.
- Limitations of AEC systems are that they are typically calibrated to only one type of image receptor and that the minimum response time may be longer than the exposure needed.
- Anatomically programmed radiography is another exposure system that allows selection of a specific body part and position, resulting in display of preprogrammed exposure factors. These factors may include AEC information.
- Quality control is important in monitoring the performance of the AEC system. Reproducibility of exposures for a given set of exposure factors and selected detector should result in mR readings within 5%, and pixel brightness levels for areas within the displayed image should be within 30%.
- Exposure technique charts standardize the selection of exposure factors for the typical patient so that the quality of radiographic images is consistent.
- Exposure factors may need to be modified for pediatric, geriatric, and bariatric patients, and varying projections and positions, casts and splints, contrast media, and pathologic conditions.

## CRITICAL THINKING QUESTIONS

1. Given so many patient and exposure factor variables, how can exposure time be automatically controlled to produce sufficient radiation exposure to the image receptor?
2. What are the advantages and disadvantages of using AEC and anatomically programmed radiography?

## REVIEW QUESTIONS

1. Automatic exposure control (AEC) devices work by measuring _____.
   a. attenuation of primary radiation by the patient
   b. radiation that exits the patient
   c. radiation that is absorbed by the patient
   d. radiation exiting the tube
2. Which exposure system operates by ionizing air that creates an electrical charge?
   a. Anatomically programmed radiography
   b. Phototimer
   c. Ionization chamber
   d. None of the above
3. During operation of the AEC device, the time of exposure:
   a. is inversely related to the intensity of the exit radiation.
   b. is directly related to the intensity of the exit radiation.
   c. has an inverse squared relationship to the exit radiation.
   d. has no relationship to the intensity of the exit radiation.

4. What factors are important when using automatic exposure control (AEC) devices?
   1. detector selection
   2. centering part to detector
   3. back-up mAs, if set
   a. 1 and 2 only
   b. 1 and 3 only
   c. 2 and 3 only
   d. 1, 2, and 3
5. Increasing patient thickness while using an AEC device would result in:
   a. increased exposure time.
   b. decreased brightness.
   c. decreased mAs readout.
   d. increased image contrast.
6. Which detector or combination of detectors is best for a right hip examination?
   a. Center
   b. Left
   c. Right
   d. Right and left
7. What is the primary goal of exposure technique charts?
   a. Extend life of x-ray tube
   b. Improve radiographer's accuracy
   c. Consistency in image quality
   d. Increase patient work flow
8. What type of exposure technique system uses a fixed mAs regardless of patient thickness?
   a. Fixed kVp
   b. Variable kVp
   c. Preprogrammed
   d. AEC
9. Of the following, which is most important when using a technique chart?
   a. Same radiographer revises chart
   b. Same chart used for all x-ray tubes
   c. Accurately measure patient
   d. Include a patient history
10. An advantage of the variable kVp technique chart is that it:
    a. produces lower-contrast images.
    b. reduces patient exposure.
    c. makes a 2-kVp change sufficient with any kVp.
    d. makes smaller technique changes possible.
11. Which of the following special considerations may require a decrease in mAs?
    a. Bariatric patient
    b. Soft tissue examination
    c. Pediatric patient
    d. b and c only.
12. Which of the following special considerations may require an increase in mAs?
    a. Contrast media
    b. Bariatric patient
    c. Tissue edema
    d. All of the above

# Image Evaluation

## Objectives

- Define image evaluation in radiography.
- Describe various sources of errors that cause repeat images.
- Analyze radiographic images for diagnostic quality.
- Describe a repeat analysis and its impact on a radiology department.

- Explain the potential benefits of performing a repeat analysis.
- Define quality assurance (QA) and quality control (QC).
- Describe common QC tests in radiography and the radiographer's role in QC testing.

## Key Terms

| | | |
|---|---|---|
| Image artifact | Quality assurance (QA) | Repeat analysis |
| Image evaluation | Quality control (QC) | Repeat exposure |

## INTRODUCTION

Evaluating images is a primary job responsibility of the radiographer. Radiographers must determine if images are of sufficient diagnostic quality to submit for interpretation by a radiologist. This analysis includes recognizing whether specific image evaluation criteria are met. If one or more of these criteria are not met to a certain standard, the radiographer may need to repeat the projection. Repeat imaging increases patient exposure and slows patient workflow in the diagnostic radiology department. Radiographers who critically evaluate images consistently provide high-quality images to radiologists for interpretation (including pathology identification), which improves patient diagnoses and treatment. Radiology departments can contribute to improving image quality, reducing unnecessary patient exposure, and increasing workflow by conducting reject image analyses and quality-control testing.

## IMAGE EVALUATION

### IMAGE EVALUATION PROCESS

In radiography, **image evaluation** is the process of systematically and critically evaluating an image to determine whether it meets the minimum criteria of diagnostic quality to submit for interpretation. Radiographers should evaluate images with a systematic approach to ensure any errors are identified. If an error causes the need for a repeat exposure, technologists must know how to correct the error so a quality repeat image is produced. This typically includes five steps.

1. The radiographer must identify whether the specific criteria are met.
2. The radiographer must identify the cause(s) of why any criteria were not met.
3. The radiographer must determine if the image must be repeated or can be submitted for interpretation.
4. If the image must be repeated, the radiographer must decide what adjustment(s) are needed to produce an image that will meet the evaluation criteria.
5. The radiographer repeats the projection and evaluates it to ensure all image evaluation criteria are met.

> **! Critical Concept**
>
> **Systematic Image Evaluation Process**
>
> Radiographers should evaluate images through a systematic method to ensure any errors are identified and corrected for repeat exposures.

| Table 14.1 | | PACEMAC Method of Image Evaluation |
|---|---|---|
| P | Positioning | Is the patient positioning in a true AP/PA/lateral? For oblique positions, is the patient rotated the correct amount? |
| A | Anatomy | Is all the required anatomy included in the image? Does anatomy display acceptable spatial resolution and minimal distortion? Was there any residual "ghost" anatomy from the previous exposure? |
| C | Centering | Is the central ray properly aligned to the part and the receptor? Was the Bucky mechanism in the detent position? |
| E | Exposure | Does the exposure indicator fall within the acceptable range? Or does it indicate the receptor was underexposed or overexposed? |
| M | Marker | Was the correct lead marker placed in the exposure field? Does the marker superimpose relevant anatomy or pathology? |
| A | Artifacts | Are there any patient, detector, processing, or exposure artifacts present? Does any artifact obstruct visualization of relevant anatomy or pathology? |
| C | Collimation | Is the collimated exposure field appropriate for the imaged part? Did poor collimation cause fogging from excessive scatter radiation? |

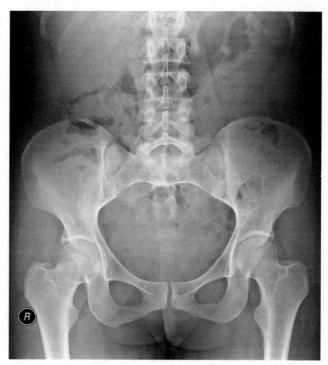

Fig. 14.1 During evaluation with the PACEMAC method, the radiographer detected multiple errors.

One example of an image evaluation method is PACEMAC. Each letter of the PACEMAC acronym represents criteria for evaluating images. Radiographers can analyze images using the principles in Table 14.1.

Figure 14.1 is a sample image(s) evaluated with the PACEMAC method.

## Positioning

- The patient appears to be properly positioned in the supine position. The spinous processes are centered within the vertebral bodies.

## Anatomy

- *The superior portion of the left kidney is clipped off the image.* The remainder of the relevant anatomy is included in the image.

## Centering

- *The x-ray beam was not centered to the anatomy of interest. This error resulted in clipping of the superior portion of the left kidney and irradiation of anatomy below the pubic symphysis.*

## Exposure

- The image appears to be appropriately exposed. The radiographer should ensure the exposure indicator is within the acceptable range.

## Marker

- *A right-side marker was annotated onto the image. The radiographer either did not place a lead marker or placed it outside the exposure field.*

## Artifacts

- No obvious patient or processing artifacts appear on the image.

## Collimation

- The collimated exposure field appears appropriate in size.

At times, technologists may only detect a single error with a radiographic image. At first glance, the image in Figure 14.2 appears perfect with no errors. However, the radiographer recognized the exposure indicator was outside the acceptable range and indicated significant overexposure to the image receptor. Image processing software adjusted image brightness and contrast to display an acceptable-appearing image. However, the exposure error (likely from excessive mAs) resulted in unnecessary radiation exposure to the patient.

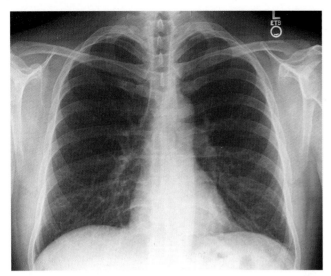

Fig. 14.2 Analysis of the image with the PACEMAC method revealed overexposure of the receptor after the exposure indicator was evaluated.

## REPEAT EXPOSURES

**Repeat exposure** refers to the necessity for taking additional images due to radiographer error. Repeat exposure is required when an image does not meet one or more of the minimum criteria to be considered diagnostically acceptable to transmit to a radiologist for interpretation. Several different errors cause technologists to repeat radiographic images. For example, incorrect positioning of the part is the most common cause for repeat exposures. A repeat exposure may be required if the part is not properly aligned (centering) to the image receptor and/or the central ray. Underexposure (resulting in excessive quantum noise) or overexposure (loss of contrast from saturation of pixels) of the image receptor can also require repeat exposure.

Image artifacts are another cause of repeat exposures. An **image artifact** is an element of an image that does not correlate to patient anatomy. An undesirable image artifact can obscure relevant anatomy and pathology. Image artifacts are classified by their source. Patient-related artifacts include jewelry and motion. Processing-related artifacts include residual or "ghost" anatomy from incomplete erasure. Detector-related artifacts include calibration issues and physical damage. In addition, artifacts can appear from the loss of a pixel, a row of pixels, a column of pixels, or an entire segment of pixels.

Other potential causes of repeat exposures include:
- Placement of a lead marker in the anatomy of interest
- Loss of spatial resolution due to patient motion
- Excessive distortion of anatomy from misalignment of the central ray, part, and image receptor
- Errors related to incorrect use of automatic exposure control (AEC)
- Grid cutoff caused by a grid-related error (off-level, etc.)

Regardless of the cause, any repeat exposure results in unnecessary radiation exposure to the patient and decreased workflow efficiency within the radiology department.

## REPEAT ANALYSIS

A **repeat analysis** (also referred to as reject analysis) is the process of analyzing a set of repeated images to determine repeat rate and categorizing the errors that caused the repeat exposures. Repeat rate is the percentage of total projections performed that required repeat imaging. Repeat rate is calculated by dividing the number of repeated projections by the total number of projections. For example, a technologist who performs 1000 projections with 50 repeats would have a repeat rate of 5%. While target repeat rates vary, a common range is 5% to 8%. Special considerations which may increase repeat rate include:
- Practice setting – Hospitals may have higher repeat rates than outpatient centers.
- Type of patient – Pediatric patients present challenges that may result in increased repeat rate.
- Type of examination – A higher repeat rate may occur with more challenging-to-perform projections or when imaging parts that require breathing techniques.
- Trainees/students – Students in an educational program tend to repeat more images as part of the learning process.

Digital radiography allows for automation of collecting and analyzing repeat exposures. Analyzing repeated images provides valuable information on technologist competency, equipment operation, and image quality standards. The analysis should calculate each technologist's repeat rate and categorize their repeated images by clinical area (room, portable, etc.) and type of error. Ideally, radiology departments should standardize reasons for repeat exposures for all radiographic units in a radiology department. The repeat analysis can then provide a framework for corrective action. The analysis can identify knowledge technologists need to acquire and skills they need to improve. For example, a radiographer may need assistance with controlling patient motion. A repeat analysis may also identify equipment operation problems which require service and repair. For instance, a radiology department may need to replace an image receptor that consistently displays undesired artifacts. Whether the repeat analysis reveals issues related to technologists or equipment, the goal is to produce quality images with acceptable repeat rates. This results in a decrease in unnecessary patient exposure and more efficient patient workflow. Ideally, radiology departments should perform repeat analyses frequently enough to identify problems before an unacceptable repeat rate occurs.

## QUALITY ASSURANCE/QUALITY CONTROL

**Quality assurance (QA)** in medical imaging is a process of collecting and evaluating data to provide a high standard of health care. QA focuses on activities and processes, evaluation of outcomes, and the establishment of policies and procedures to provide timely and acceptable diagnostic information with minimum radiation dose to patients.

All health care facilities have a QA program to ensure quality patient care and radiation safety in medical imaging. A good QA program can lower the costs of both time and money by revealing processes that can be made more efficient, drawing attention to the use of supplies and determining the repeat rates of the department as well as each technologist. These savings can be seen broadly as improved patient throughput, increased life span of the equipment, and cost savings from reduced waste of supplies.

**Quality control (QC)** is the evaluation of imaging equipment and other components used in the imaging process. This is done by establishing acceptable criteria for measuring specific areas related to the equipment, performing those measures at an agreed-on interval, documenting the results to track variances, and determining the acceptable tolerances and necessary corrective measures for tests that fall outside of the acceptable criteria. The American Society of Radiologic Technologists states: "It is a best practice in digital radiography to implement a comprehensive quality assurance program that involves aspects of quality control and continuous quality improvement, including repeat analyses that are specific to the digital imaging system."

QC is an aspect of the overall QA program of a facility or department. It is a type of preventive maintenance to ensure that all components are in good working order and can include the imaging equipment, monitors, and shielding as well as tracking repeats. As it relates to the equipment, this can include lights, audible tones, and moving parts such as the collimator. Improperly performing components can result in inefficiencies and poor image quality. Furthermore, such malfunctions could be a danger to patients, lead to a misdiagnosis, or cause delays in results and repeat images.

The technologist should become familiar with the QA program and more specifically the aspects of QC. If a radiographer recognizes a problem, they should immediately report it to the appropriate person.

The following is a list related to QC of which all technologists should develop a basic understanding.
- What tests are performed and at what interval?
- What are the acceptable and unacceptable limits for tests?
- What should be done if the test results fall outside of tolerance limits?
- Who is responsible for QC?
- What policies are related to QC?

Most imaging equipment goes through an extensive testing process once it is installed. This testing is done by a medical physicist to ensure that it is operating safely and correctly. The medical physicist will then help set the parameters for each quality-control test recommended by the manufacturer, federal, state, or institutional policy. These parameters become the criteria for the specific test, and subsequent testing should fall within the parameters that are set. Additionally, requirements are established for what to do if tests fall outside of acceptable tolerance limits. This can include repeating the test, contacting a service engineer, or discontinuing the use of the equipment altogether until it can be corrected.

The medical physicist works with the facility, department, and technologist to establish the QC for medical imaging. Quality control of some kind is performed daily, weekly, monthly, quarterly, and annually, with testing performed by the technologist or the medical physicist. Because the technologist is the primary user of the equipment, they have the best understanding of how it is performing on a daily basis. Below is an example of quality-control tests that may be completed at various intervals. Understand that not all imaging equipment has the same tests and the same interval. Quality-control tests are dependent on the manufacturer, federal, state, and local laws, institutional policies, or departmental requirements.

Quality-control tests can include:
- Daily
  - Warmup of equipment
  - Phantom Image
  - Image evaluation
- Weekly
  - Calibration
  - Visual inspection
- Monthly
  - Repeat analysis
  - Quarterly QC tests
  - Collimator test
- Annual
  - Radiation output
  - Beam filtration
  - Alignment of light and x-ray field
  - Grid uniformity
  - AEC assessment
  - Beam collimation
  - Noise and artifacts, signal-to-noise ratio (SNR)
  - Spatial resolution, modulation transfer function (MTF)
  - Contrast, contrast-to-noise ratio (CNR)
  - Image receptor, detective quantum efficiency (DQE)
  - Dose measurement
  - Electronic displays/view box luminescence
  - Personal protective equipment

Refer to Chapter 10 for information related to image display testing.

## On the Spot

- Evaluating images is a primary job responsibility of the radiographer. Radiographers must determine if images are of sufficient diagnostic quality to submit for interpretation by a radiologist.
- Radiographers should evaluate images with a systematic approach to ensure any errors are identified. If an error causes the need for a repeat exposure, technologists must know how to correct the error so a quality repeat image is produced.
- Using the PACEMAC method is one way to systematically approach image evaluation to identify and correct image errors.
- Repeat exposure is required when an image does not meet one or more of the minimum criteria to be considered diagnostically acceptable to transmit to a radiologist for interpretation. Repeat exposures result in an overall increase in patient dose.
- A repeat analysis (also referred to as reject analysis) is the process of analyzing a set of repeated images to determine repeat rate and categorizing the errors that caused the repeat exposures. Repeat rate is the percentage of total projections performed that required repeat imaging.
- Quality assurance (QA) focuses on activities and processes, evaluating outcomes, and establishing policies and procedures to provide timely and acceptable diagnostic information with minimum radiation dose to patients.
- Quality control (QC) is the evaluation of imaging equipment and other components used in the image process. It is a part of the overall QA program that focuses on the equipment and imaging chain.
- Most imaging equipment goes through an extensive testing process by a medical physicist once it is installed. This testing ensures that the equipment is operating safely and correctly. The medical physicist also helps set the parameters for each QC test recommended by the manufacturer, or federal, state, or institutional policy that then becomes the criteria for correct operation.

## DISCUSSION QUESTIONS

1. What is the value of a quality-assurance and quality-control program to the patient care process?
2. How can radiographers ensure they consistently produce diagnostic quality images with an acceptable repeat rate?

## REVIEW QUESTIONS

1. The process of systematically and critically evaluating an image to determine whether it meets the minimum criteria of diagnostic quality to submit for interpretation is:
   a. image quality.
   b. image evaluation.
   c. image interpretation.
   d. image testing.
2. The most common cause of repeat exposures is related to:
   a. part positioning.
   b. centering.
   c. the image receptor.
   d. collimation.
3. The evaluation of imaging equipment and other components used in the imaging process is:
   a. quality assurance.
   b. quality management.
   c. quality control.
   d. quality measures.
4. A radiographer who performs 2000 projections with 80 repeat exposures would have a repeat rate of:
   a. 2%.
   b. 4%.
   c. 8%.
   d. 10%.
5. What is the radiographer's first step in the image evaluation process?
   a. The radiographer must identify the cause(s) of why any criteria were not met.
   b. If the image must be repeated, the radiographer must decide what adjustment(s) are needed to produce an image that will meet the evaluation criteria.
   c. The radiographer must identify whether the specific criteria are met.
   d. The radiographer must determine if the image must be repeated or can be submitted for interpretation.
6. Which of the following are sources of image artifacts?
   a. Processing-related
   b. Detector-related
   c. Patient-related
   d. All of the above

# 15

# Fluoroscopic Imaging

## Outline

## Objectives

- Differentiate between fluoroscopic and radiographic imaging.
- Recognize the unique features of an image-intensified fluoroscopic unit and explain how the image is created and viewed.
- Explain the purpose of automatic brightness control.
- Explain the operation of an image intensifier in magnification mode and its effect on image quality and patient exposure.
- Describe the fluoroscopic viewing and recording systems and the advantages and disadvantages of each.
- Compare and contrast features of image-intensified units from digital fluoroscopic units.

- Identify the unique features of flat-panel detector fluoroscopy and their effect on image quality and patient exposure.
- Differentiate between continuous and pulsed fluoroscopy.
- Recognize the fluoroscopic features that affect patient radiation exposure.
- Identify the major areas of quality control pertaining to fluoroscopy.
- Differentiate between those quality-control processes that are the responsibility of the radiographer and those of the medical physicist.

## Key Terms

accelerating anode
air kerma
analog-to-digital converter (ADC)
automatic brightness control (ABC)
automatic exposure rate control (AERC)
brightness gain
camera tube
charge-coupled device (CCD)
continuous fluoroscopy
conversion factor

dose-area product (DAP)
dose rates
electronic magnification
electrostatic focusing lenses
fluoro loop save
flux gain
frame averaging
image intensifier
input phosphor
kerma area product (KAP)
last image hold (LIH)

magnification mode
minification gain
output phosphor
photocathode
pulse rate
pulse width
pulsed fluoroscopy
spatial resolution
virtual collimation

## INTRODUCTION

Shortly after Dr. Roentgen's discovery of x-rays and subsequent announcement, many other scientists began experimenting with this new phenomenon. Among them was the famed American inventor Thomas Edison. Among Mr. Edison's more notable inventions in this area was the first commercially available fluoroscope in 1896, although it was not in a form we would recognize today (Fig. 15.1). His fluoroscope was a calcium tungstate screen that

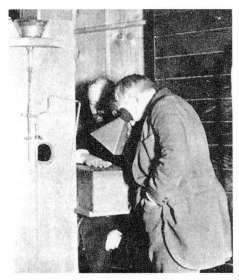

**Fig. 15.1 Thomas Edison.** Thomas Edison experimenting with the fluoroscope he designed. The subject is his assistant, Clarence Dally. (Courtesy Eisenberg RL: *Radiology: an illustrated history*, St Louis, 1992, Mosby.)

interacted with the remnant beam, producing a very faint image that one viewed while standing in the path of the x-ray beam as it exited the patient and screen. The practice of standing in the direct path of the x-ray beam meant that the dose to the operator was extremely high. Additionally, because the image was very dim, the operator had to "dark-adapt" by sitting in a darkened room for a period of time or by wearing adaptation goggles with red lenses before performing the fluoroscopic examination.

Unlike radiographic imaging that produces static radiographs of anatomic tissues, fluoroscopy's great advantage was that it allowed for imaging of the functioning or motion (dynamics) of anatomic structures. That is, the inner workings of the human body could be viewed in real time.

In the 1950s, the image intensifier was introduced into the fluoroscopic system. The image intensifier improved the process in two ways. First, it brightened the image significantly, eliminating the need to dark-adapt and improving visualization of anatomic details. Second, it allowed for a means of indirectly viewing the fluoroscopic image, first by mirror optics and later by television monitors, greatly reducing the radiation dose to the operator. This chapter discusses the image intensifier and its characteristics, viewing and recording systems, and the digital fluoroscopy process in use today.

## IMAGE INTENSIFICATION

In image-intensified fluoroscopy, the milliamperage (mA) used during imaging is considerably lower (0.5-5 mA) than that in radiographic mode, which is operated at a higher mA of 50 to 1200 mA. A low mA provides

for the increased time the image intensifier is operated. Because the time of exposure is lengthened, the control panel includes a timer that buzzes audibly when 5 minutes of x-ray fluoroscopic time has been used. Another important feature of a fluoroscopic unit is the deadman switch. The continuous x-ray beam is activated by either a hand switch on the unit or a foot pedal that must be continuously depressed for the x-rays to be produced. Releasing the pressure applied to the pedal or switch terminates the radiation exposure.

## IMAGE INTENSIFIER

The image intensifier is an electronic vacuum tube that converts the remnant beam to light, then to electrons, then back to light, increasing the light intensity in the process. It consists of five basic parts: the **input phosphor, photocathode, electrostatic focusing lenses, accelerating anode,** and **output phosphor** (Figs. 15.2 and 15.3). The image light intensities from the output phosphor are converted to an electronic video signal and sent to a television monitor for viewing. Fig. 15.4 is an example of a typical radiographic and image-intensified fluoroscopic unit. Additional filming devices, such as spot film or cine (movie film), can be attached to the fluoroscopic system to create permanent radiographic images of specific areas of interest.

The input phosphor is made of cesium iodide and is bonded to the curved surface of the intensifier tube itself. Cesium iodide absorbs the remnant x-ray photon energy and emits light in response. The photocathode is made of cesium and antimony compounds. These metals emit electrons in response to light stimulus in a process called *photoemission.* The photocathode is bonded directly to the input phosphor using a very thin adhesive layer. These layers are curved so that all the electrons emitted from the photocathode travel the same distance to the output phosphor (see Fig. 15.3). The electrostatic focusing lenses are not really lenses but are negatively charged plates along the length of the image intensifier tube. These negatively charged plates repel the electron stream, focusing it toward the small output phosphor. To set the electron stream in motion at a constant velocity, an **accelerating anode** is located at the neck of the image intensifier near the output phosphor. This accelerating anode maintains a constant potential of approximately 25 kV. The output phosphor is made of silver-activated zinc cadmium sulfide and is much smaller than the input phosphor. It is located at the opposite end of the image intensifier tube, just beyond the accelerating anode. This layer absorbs electrons and emits light in response.

The entire intensifier tube is approximately 50 cm (20 inches) in length and 15 to 58 cm (6-23 inches) in diameter (diameter depends on manufacturer and intended use). The input phosphor faces the patient and receives the x-ray exposure that constitutes the

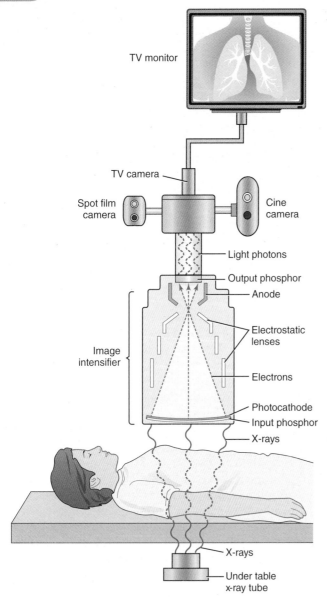

**Fig. 15.2 Fluoroscopic Chain.** The general components of the fluoroscopic chain. Note that the x-ray tube for the system is typically located under the table.

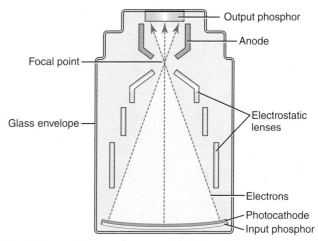

**Fig. 15.3 Image Intensifier.** The image intensifier is situated within the fluoroscopic tower and is attached to a camera tube. The method of attachment depends on the image-capture features of the system.

> ### ⊙ Critical Concept
>
> **Image Intensifier Operation**
>
> The image intensifier is an electronic vacuum tube that converts the remnant beam to light, then electrons, then back to light, increasing the light intensity in the process. The high-energy electrons that interact with the output phosphor each result in substantially more light photons than were necessary to cause their release at the photocathode, resulting in a brighter image.

## BRIGHTNESS GAIN

**Brightness gain** is an expression of the ability of an image intensifier tube to convert x-ray energy into light energy and increase the brightness of the image in the process. Traditionally, brightness gain was found by multiplying the flux gain by the minification gain. A brighter image is a result of high-energy electrons striking a small diameter output phosphor. Accelerating the electrons increases the light intensities at the output phosphor (**flux gain**). The reduction in the size of the output phosphor image compared with that of the input phosphor image also increases the light intensities (**minification gain**).

Flux gain relates to the very concept of using an image intensifier to create a brighter image by taking a few x-ray photons and converting that energy into many light photons. Flux gain is expressed as the ratio of the number of light photons at the output phosphor to the number of light photons emitted by the input phosphor and represents the intensifier tube's conversion efficiency. *Minification gain* is an expression of the degree to which the image is minified (made smaller) from input phosphor to output phosphor. This characteristic makes the image appear brighter because the same number of electrons is being concentrated on a smaller surface area. It is found by dividing the square of the diameter of

remnant beam. The x-rays are absorbed by the input phosphor and light is emitted in response, proportional to the percentage of x-ray absorption. This light immediately exposes the photocathode, which in turn emits electrons in proportion to the light intensity. The ratio of light to electron emission is not one-to-one. It takes many light photons to result in the emission of one electron. The resultant electrons are accelerated toward the output phosphor by the accelerating anode and "focused" toward the output phosphor by the electrostatic focusing lenses. These high-energy electrons result in many light photons being emitted from the output phosphor. Each electron results in substantially more light photons than was necessary to cause its release. The result of this process is an increase in image brightness.

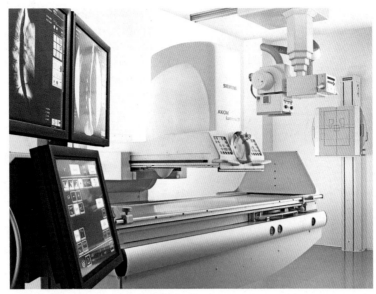

Fig. 15.4 A typical radiographic and image-intensified fluoroscopic unit. (Courtesy Siemens Healthcare, Malvern, Penn.)

the input phosphor by the square of the diameter of the output phosphor.

Generally, the input phosphors are 15 to 30 cm (6-12 inches) and the output phosphor is usually 2.5 cm (1 inch).

Although the term *brightness gain* continues to be used, it is now common practice to express this increase in brightness with the term *conversion factor*. The International Commission on Radiation Units and Measurements now recommends the use of the conversion factor to quantify the increase in brightness created by an image intensifier. **Conversion factor** is an expression of the luminance at the output phosphor divided by the input exposure rate, and its unit of measure is the candela per square meter per milliroentgen per second ($cd/m^2/mR/s$). The numeric conversion factor value is roughly equal to 1% of the brightness gain value. The higher the conversion factor or brightness gain value, the greater the efficiency of the image intensifier. See Box 15.1 for brightness gain and conversion factor formulas.

## Box 15.1 Brightness Gain and Conversion Factor Formulas

Brightness gain = Minification gain × Flux gain

$$\text{Flux gain} = \frac{\text{number of output light photons}}{\text{number of input x-ray photons}}$$

$$\textbf{Minification gain} = \left(\frac{d_i}{d_0}\right)^2$$

$$\text{Conversion factor} = \frac{\text{Output phosphor illumination (cd/m}^2\text{)}}{\text{input exposure rate (mR/s)}}$$

### ! Critical Concept

#### Brightness Gain and Conversion Factor

Brightness gain is an expression of the ability of an image intensifier to convert x-ray energy into light energy and increase brightness in the process. It is now more common to express this as *conversion factor*, which is an expression of the luminance at the output phosphor divided by the input exposure rate.

Regardless of whether the term *brightness gain* or the term *conversion factor* is used to express the increase in brightness, the ability of the image intensifier to increase brightness deteriorates with the age of the tube. The radiographer should be aware that, as the image intensifier ages, more radiation is necessary to produce the same level of output brightness, translating to an ever-increasing patient dose.

### ! Critical Concept

#### Patient Exposure and Age of the Image Intensifier

As an image intensifier ages, the exposure to the patient increases to maintain brightness. The radiographer should be alert to this trend.

### AUTOMATIC BRIGHTNESS CONTROL

The radiographer must also be familiar with **automatic brightness control (ABC)**, a function of the fluoroscopic unit that maintains the overall appearance of the intensified image (radiographic contrast and brightness) by automatically adjusting the kilovoltage peak (kVp), milliamperage (mA), or both. The ABC (also known as automatic brightness stabilization [ABS]) generally operates by monitoring either the current through the image intensifier or the output phosphor intensity and adjusting the exposure factor(s) if the monitored value falls below preset levels. The fluoroscopic unit allows the operator to select a desired brightness level, and this level is subsequently maintained by the ABC. The ABC is a little slow in its response to changes in patient tissue thickness and tissue density as the fluoroscopy tower is moved about over the patient. This is visible to the radiographer as a lag in image brightness on the monitor as the tower is moved.

 **Critical Concept**

**Automatic Brightness Control**

Automatic brightness control (ABC) maintains the overall appearance of the intensified image (radiographic contrast and brightness) by automatically adjusting the kilovoltage peak (kVp), milliamperage (mA), or both. The ABC (also known as automatic brightness stabilization [ABS]) generally operates either by monitoring the current through the image intensifier or the output phosphor intensity and adjusting the exposure factor(s) if the monitored value falls below preset levels.

## MAGNIFICATION MODE

Another function of some image intensifiers is multifield mode or magnification mode. Most image intensifiers in use today have this capability. When operated in **magnification mode**, the voltage to the electrostatic focusing lenses is increased. This increase tightens the diameter of the electron stream, and the focal point is shifted farther from the output phosphor (Fig. 15.5). The effect is that only those electrons from the center area of the input phosphor interact with the output phosphor and contribute to the image, giving the appearance of magnification. For example, a 30/23/15-cm (12/9/6-inch) trifocus image intensifier can be operated in any of those three modes. When operated in the 23-cm (9-inch) mode, only the electrons from the center 23 cm (9 inches) of the input phosphor

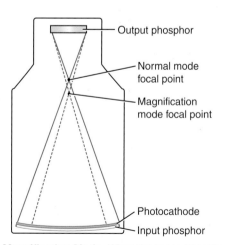

Fig. 15.5 **Magnification Mode.** When the image intensifier is operated in magnification mode, the voltage on the electrostatic focusing lenses is increased, narrowing the diameter of the electron stream and shifting the focal point farther from the output phosphor, resulting in a magnified image.

interact with the output phosphor; those about the periphery will miss and not contribute to the image. The same is true of the 15-cm (6-inch) mode. Selecting magnification mode automatically adjusts x-ray beam collimation to match the displayed tissue image and avoids irradiating tissue that does not appear in the image. The degree of magnification (magnification factor [MF]) may be found by dividing the full-size input diameter by the selected input diameter. For example: MF $30 \div 15 = 2 \times$ magnification.

 **Critical Concept**

**Magnification Mode**

When operated in magnification mode, the voltage to the electrostatic focusing lenses is increased. This increase tightens the diameter of the electron stream, and the focal point is shifted farther from the output phosphor so that only those electrons from the center area of the input phosphor interact with the output phosphor, giving the appearance of magnification.

This magnification improves the operator's ability to see small structures (spatial resolution, discussed shortly) but at the expense of increasing patient dose. Recall that remnant x-ray photons are converted to light and then to electrons and are focused on the output phosphor. If fewer electrons are incident on the output phosphor, the output intensity decreases. To compensate, more x-ray photons are needed at the beginning of the process to produce more light, resulting in more electrons emitted from the photocathode. The ABC automatically increases x-ray exposure to achieve this. Again, with an increase in x-rays comes an increase in patient dose.

 **Critical Concept**

**Magnification Mode and Patient Dose**

Operating the image intensifier in one of the magnification modes will increase the operator's ability to see small structures, but at the price of increasing radiation dose to the patient.

Magnification modes improve **spatial resolution**, which refers to the smallest structure that may be detected in an image. Spatial resolution is measured in line pairs per millimeter (Lp/mm), and typical fluoroscopic systems have spatial resolution capabilities of 4 to 6 Lp/mm but depend greatly on the rest of the imaging chain (i.e., the viewing and recording systems).

Distortion is also an issue with image-intensified fluoroscopy. In radiography, distortion is a misrepresentation of the true size or shape of an object. In the case of image-intensified fluoroscopy, shape distortion can be a problem. In image-intensified fluoroscopy, distortion is a result of inaccurate control or focusing of the electrons released at the periphery of

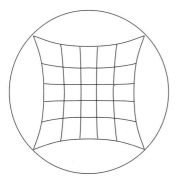

Image displaying
"pincushion" distortion

**Fig. 15.6 Pincushion Distortion.** Appearance of the pincushion effect. The circle represents the television monitor display, and the grid
represents the effect on the image.

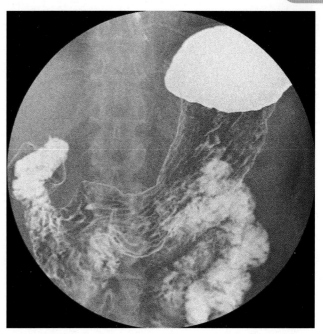

**Fig. 15.7 Quantum Noise.** If too few x-rays exit the patient and expose the input phosphor, not enough light will be produced, decreasing the number of electrons released by the photocathode to interact
with the output phosphor. A "grainy" or "noisy" image results. (Courtesy Bontrager K, Lampignano J: *Textbook of radiographic positioning
and related anatomy,* ed 7, St Louis, 2009, Mosby.)

the photocathode and the curved shape of the photocathode. The combined result is an unequal magnification (distortion) of the image, creating what is called a
"pincushion appearance" (Fig. 15.6). This problem also
causes a loss of brightness around the periphery of the
image, which is referred to as *vignetting*.

One last factor to consider with image intensifiers
is noise. Image noise results when insufficient information is present to create the image. In the case of
image-intensified fluoroscopy, this lack of image-forming information ultimately is a result of an insufficient
quantity of x-rays. If too few x-rays exit the patient
and expose the input phosphor, not enough light is
produced, which decreases the number of electrons
released by the photocathode to interact with the output phosphor. This results in a "grainy" or "noisy"
image (Fig. 15.7). Although other factors in the fluoroscopic chain may contribute to noise, the solution
generally comes back to increasing the mA (quantity
of radiation). For image-intensified fluoroscopy, this is
a small increase in mA because these systems operate
at 2 to 5 mA. Because older image intensifier units are
operated as **continuous fluoroscopy**, to minimize radiation dose the operator should intermittently pulse the
x-ray beam by activating the exposure switch on and
off rapidly. See Table 15.1 for fluoroscopic equipment
inspection checklist.

### ! Critical Concept

**Intermittent Fluoroscopy**

Because older image intensifier units are operated as continuous fluoroscopy, to minimize radiation dose the operator
should intermittently pulse the x-ray beam by activating the
exposure switch on and off rapidly.

## VIEWING SYSTEMS

The original image intensifiers produced an image that
was viewed using a mirror optics system, something
akin to a sophisticated way of looking at the output
phosphor with a "rearview mirror." Although it did

| Table 15.1 | Fluoroscopic Equipment Inspection Checklist | |
|---|---|---|
| **INSPECT** | **ENSURE THAT** | |
| Bucky slot cover | When the Bucky is parked at the foot of the table, the metal cover should expand and cover the entire opening. | |
| Protective curtain | The curtain should be in good condition and move freely into place when the tower is moved to the operating position. | |
| Tower: locks, power assist, control panel | The electromagnetic locks are in good working order, the power assist moves the tower about easily in all directions, and all control panel indicator lights are operational. | |
| Exposure switch (deadman switch) | The switch does not stick and operates the x-ray tube while in the depressed position only. (Also test the switch with the tower in the park position. It should not activate the x-ray tube while parked.) | |
| Collimator shutters | In the fully open position, the shutters should restrict the beam to the size of the input phosphor and be accurate to within ±3%. | |
| Fluoroscopic timer | Should create an audible alarm after 5 minutes of fluoroscopic "beam-on" time. | |
| Monitor brightness | While exposing a penetrometer through a fluoroscopic phantom, the monitor image is adjusted to display as many of the penetrometer steps as possible. | |
| Table tilt motion | The table tilts smoothly to its limit in both directions and the angulation indicator is operational. | |

eliminate the need for the operator to stand in the path of the x-ray beam, it was a waste of the image intensifier technology. With advancements in technology, the viewing system became a television monitor. To view the image from the output phosphor on a television monitor, it must first be converted to an electrical signal (often referred to as a *video signal*) by the television camera. Two devices are commonly used to accomplish this: the camera tube and the charge-coupled device (CCD).

## Television Cameras

Television cameras used to display intensified fluoroscopic images include the older camera tube (vidicon/Plumbicon) and the newer CCD. The camera tube is approximately 15 cm (6 inches) in length and encloses an electron gun and a photoconductive target assembly. The diameter of the tube is the same size as that of the output phosphor. The **camera tube** most often used is the *vidicon tube* (Fig. 15.8). The vidicon tube is connected to the output phosphor of the image intensifier by either a fiberoptic bundle or an optical lens system (Fig. 15.9) (discussed shortly). The vidicon tube is a diode tube contained in a glass envelope to maintain a vacuum. The cathode consists of an electron gun that provides a continuous stream of electrons and a control grid that forms the electron stream into a "beam." Around the tube are a series of

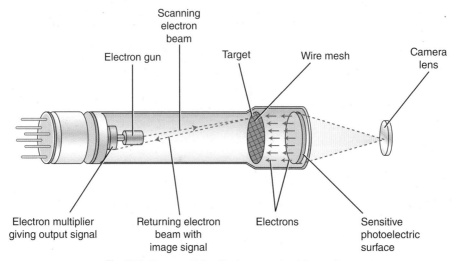

Fig. 15.8 **Camera Tube.** Basic parts of a vidicon tube.

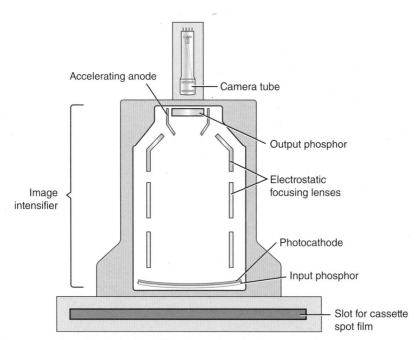

Fig. 15.9 **Camera Tube and the Image Intensifier.** The output phosphor is connected to the "photoelectric surface" end of the camera tube using a lens system or fiberoptics.

alignment, focusing, and deflection coils. These coils accelerate and precisely control the electron beam. Through the action of these coils, the beam sweeps the anode back and forth from top to bottom in a sequence known as a *raster pattern*. This sweeping motion is very fast, approximately 1,000,000 sweeps per minute. The anode of the tube consists of a face plate, a signal plate, and a target. The face plate, a thinned segment of the glass envelope positioned closest to the output phosphor of the image intensifier, allows transmission of light from the image intensifier to the camera tube. The signal plate is bonded to the face plate and is a thin layer of graphite material that conducts electricity. This metallic layer is thin enough to transmit light traveling through the face plate from the image intensifier but thick enough to conduct electricity that will be generated in the camera tube. The target layer is a photoconductive layer made of antimony trisulfide in vidicon tubes and lead oxide in plumbicon tubes. This photoconductive material will conduct the electricity if illuminated; otherwise, it acts as an insulator. Between this layer and the electron beam is another control grid that decelerates and aligns the electron beam so that it is oriented correctly when it interacts with the anode.

The electron beam is activated and begins sweeping the anode target. Light travels from the output phosphor of the image intensifier through the face plate and signal plate to the other side of the target layer. If the electron beam and light from the output phosphor are incident on the same place at the same time, electrons are transmitted through the target to the signal plate. The signal plate carries this current as an electronic signal to the television monitor, where it is reconstructed as a visible image. The process of image reconstruction is discussed shortly. If the electron beam is in a different place in its sweep than a photon of light from the output phosphor, the target acts as an insulator. This action of the target modulates the electronic signal. That is, the greater the light intensity, the greater the number of electrons transmitted and the greater the magnitude of the electronic signal to the monitor, giving variations in brightness of different parts of the television image.

### Charge-Coupled Device
The **charge-coupled device (CCD)** is a light-sensitive semiconducting device that generates an electrical charge when stimulated by light and stores this charge in a capacitor. The charge is proportional to the light intensity and is stored in rows of pixels. The CCD is a series of metal oxide semiconductor capacitors, with each capacitor representing a pixel. Each pixel is composed of photosensitive material that dislodges electrons when stimulated by light photons. To digitize the charge from this device, the electrodes between each pixel, called *row gates*, are charged in sequence, moving

the signal down the row, where it is transferred into the capacitors. From the capacitors, the charge is sent as an electronic signal to the television monitor. In this way, each pixel is individually "read" and sent to the television monitor (Fig. 15.10).

Compared with the vidicon-type camera tube, the CCD is read out by the charge in each pixel, whereas the vidicon is read out by an electronic beam. CCD TV cameras have some advantages over the camera tubes in that they are more sensitive to a wider range of light intensities and show no geometric distortion of the fluoroscopic display image. The CCD is smaller in size than the vidicon camera tube and works well in digital imaging.

**Critical Concept**

**Television Cameras and the Television Monitor**

The camera tube and CCD are devices that convert the image from the intensifier's output phosphor to an electronic signal that can be reconstructed on the television monitor.

*Coupling of Devices to the Image Intensifier.* As mentioned earlier, the camera tube or CCD may be coupled to the output phosphor of the image intensifier by either a fiberoptic bundle or optical lens system. The fiberoptic bundle is simply a bundle of very thin optical glass filaments. This system is very durable and simple in design but does not allow for spot filming.

The optical lens system is a series of optical lenses that focus the image from the output phosphor on the camera tube. When spot filming is desired, a beam-splitting mirror (a partially silvered mirror that allows some light to pass through and reflects some in a different direction) is moved into the path of the output image and diverts some of the light to the desired spot-filming device (e.g., photospot, cine camera) (see Fig. 15.11). This system, although allowing for spot filming of this type, is more susceptible to rough handling, which may cause maladjustment of the mirror and lenses and result in a blurred image.

### Television Monitor
The purpose of the television monitor is to convert the electronic signal from the camera tube or CCD back into a visible image. In older image-intensified units, this monitor was a cathode ray tube that consisted of an electron gun with a control grid, focusing and deflecting coils, an anode, and a fluorescent screen (Fig. 15.12). The electron gun is modulated (controlled) by the signal from the camera tube or CCD. That is, the television monitor electron gun is moving in the same pattern as the camera tube (or signal from the CCD), and electrons emitted from it are in proportion to the signal intensity. The control grid forms the electrons into a beam that is controlled by the focusing and deflecting coils and directed to the fluorescent

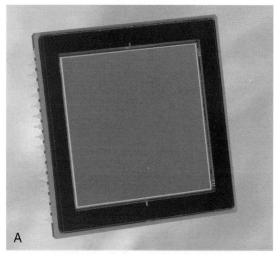

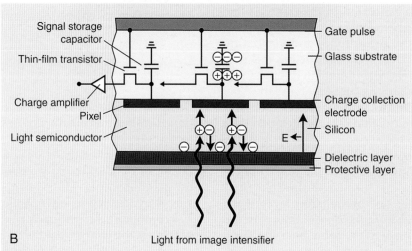

Fig. 15.10 **(A) The charge-coupled device (CCD).** (B) The CCD is a light-sensitive semiconducting device that generates an electrical charge when stimulated by light and stores this charge in a capacitor until the charge is sent as an electronic signal to the TV monitor. (A courtesy Carter CE, Veale BL: *Digital radiography and PACS*, St Louis, 2007, Mosby; B courtesy Bushong SC: *Radiologic science for technologists*, ed 11, St Louis, 2017, Mosby.)

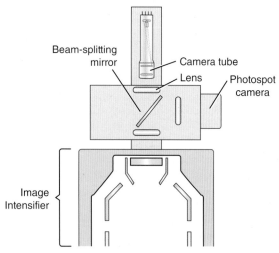

Fig. 15.11 **Beam-Splitting Mirror.** If the image intensifier is equipped with a spot filming device, the beam-splitting mirror diverts some of the light to the device for obtaining images.

screen. The beam sweeps the screen in the same raster pattern described in the discussion of the camera tube. In essence, the television monitor is reconstructing the image from the output phosphor as a visible image. The image is created on the fluorescent screen one line at a time starting in the upper left-hand corner and moving to the right (active trace). It then blanks (turns off) and returns to the left side (horizontal retrace). This process continues to the bottom of the screen. It then returns to the top (vertical retrace) and begins again by placing a line between each of the previous lines. This action creates a television frame. Typical television monitors are called *525-line systems* because the traces create a 525-line frame. High-resolution monitors have 1024 lines per frame. However, the monitor continues to be the weak link in terms of resolution of the fluoroscopic chain. The image intensifier can resolve approximately 5 Lp/mm, whereas the monitor can display only 1 to 2 Lp/mm.

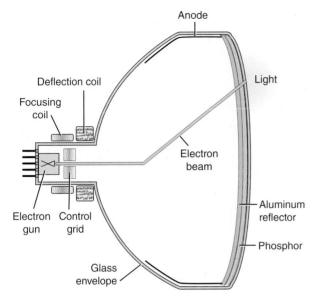

**Fig. 15.12 Television Monitor.** The general parts of the television monitor. Note that the electron gun of the monitor is modulated by the camera tube attached to the image intensifier.

## RECORDING SYSTEMS

### Film Cameras

Film cameras (sometimes called *photospot cameras*) have been a mainstay of image intensified fluoroscopy (refer back to Fig. 15.11). They most commonly use 105-mm "chip" film or 70-mm roll film. The photospot camera is also a static imaging system used with an optical lens system incorporating a beam-splitting mirror. When the spot-film exposure switch is pressed, the beam-splitting mirror is moved into place, diverting some of the beam toward the photospot camera and exposing the film. This device uses the visible light image from the output phosphor of the image intensifier and exposes the 105-mm (or 70-mm) film photographically, much like a 35-mm film camera used in photography. This system allows for very fast imaging

of up to 12 frames per second, and because it is "photographing" the image from the output phosphor of the image intensifier, it requires approximately half the radiation dose of the cassette spot-filming system.

## DIGITAL FLUOROSCOPY

Like image-intensified fluoroscopy, digital fluoroscopy has evolved over time. The early versions of digital fluoroscopy used the conventional fluoroscopic chain but added an **analog-to-digital converter (ADC)** and computer between the camera tube and the monitor (Fig. 15.13). An ADC is a device that takes the video (analog) signal and divides it into a series of bits (1s and 0s) that the computer "understands." The number of bits the signal is divided into determines the contrast resolution (number of gray shades) of the system. The ADC is necessary for the computer to process and display the image. Once in digital form, the image can be postprocessed and stored in that format or printed onto film using a dry laser printer.

The incorporation of a CCD into this setup further improved digital fluoroscopy. The CCD eliminated some of the problems associated with the camera tube. The CCD is more light-sensitive (higher detective quantum efficiency [DQE]) and exhibits less noise and no spatial distortion. It also has a higher spatial resolution and requires less radiation in the system, reducing patient dose.

### FLAT-PANEL DETECTOR FLUOROSCOPY

A more recent advance in digital fluoroscopy is the introduction of a flat-panel detector in place of an image intensifier (Fig. 15.14). Two forms of flat-panel detectors may be used for fluoroscopic applications: the cesium iodide amorphous silicon indirect-capture detector and the amorphous selenium direct-capture detector.

Currently, the most commonly used flat-panel detector for fluoroscopic application is the cesium

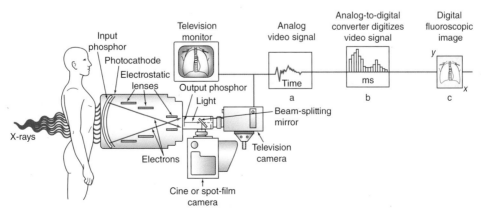

**Fig. 15.13 Analog and Digital Signals in Fluoroscopy.** The video signal from the television camera is analog, where the voltage signal continuously varies. This analog signal is sampled (a), producing a stepped representation of the analog video signal (b). The numerical values of each step are stored (c), producing a matrix of digital image data.

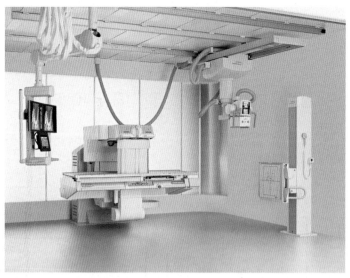

**Fig. 15.14** Digital fluoroscopy using flat-panel detector technology. (Courtesy of Siemens Medical Solutions USA, Inc.)

iodide amorphous silicon indirect-capture detector. The scintillator of this system uses cesium iodide or gadolinium oxysulfide as the phosphor. The photodetector is amorphous silicon, which is a liquid that can be painted onto a substrate (foundation or underlying layer) and is the material that makes flat-panel detectors possible. The other component is the TFT array. TFTs are electronic components layered onto a glass substrate that include the readout, charge collector, and light-sensitive elements. The panel is configured into a network of pixels (or detector elements [DELs]) covered by the scintillator plate, with each pixel containing a photodetector and a TFT. With this system, x-ray energy is absorbed by the scintillator and converted to light energy. This light is then absorbed by the photodetectors and converted to electric charges. These electric charges are in turn captured and transmitted by the TFT array to the monitor for display.

Flat-panel detectors are very popular in interventional and cardiology applications and gaining ground in general fluoroscopy. They are much lighter and more compact, they produce a digital signal directly (no need for a camera tube or ADC), and—because it is a digital system producing a digital signal, absent of the electronic components of the image intensifier system—there is less electronic noise. Detector array sizes are currently available in sizes of 25 × 25 cm to 40 × 40 cm (10 × 10 inches to 16 × 16 inches).

Although the cesium iodide amorphous silicon indirect-capture detector is essentially the same as that for digital radiography, there are a few differences for use as a dynamic digital detector in digital fluoroscopy applications. In general, dynamic versions of these detectors must respond in rapid sequences to create a dynamic image. Current dynamic versions are capable of up to 60 frames per second. To accomplish this, rapid readout speeds (how quickly the active matrix processes the image data) are necessary. The design is

a two-dimensional rectilinear array of pixels that can be electronically processed line by line in a fraction of a second. Furthermore, for fluoroscopic applications, very low-noise flat-panel detector systems are needed. Fluoroscopy generally operates at a low-dose output, so any operational noise degrades the fluoroscopic image, making noise a greater factor in detectors used for this application. Application-specific integrated circuits are used to minimize noise and amplify signal from the active matrix. These circuits are particularly important in fluoroscopic applications because they minimize noise, maximize readout speed, and allow for switching from low-dose to high-dose inputs (for static imaging). Another consideration with the low-dose fluoroscopic applications is the need to maintain a large fill factor (the area of each pixel that is sensitive to x-ray detection materials). With general radiography that uses a larger dose output, this is generally not a problem, but it becomes a problem with fluoroscopic applications, particularly with indirect-capture detectors. Other features such as a light-emitting diode array "backlighting system" have also been incorporated to erase the detector between frames to prevent "ghosting" caused by any residual exposure charge from the previous frame.

### ! Critical Concept

**Flat-Panel Detectors for Dynamic Imaging**

Fluoroscopic versions of flat-panel detectors must respond in rapid sequences to create dynamic images, must maintain a large fill factor to reduce image noise because of low-dose fluoroscopic applications, and must erase the detector between frames to prevent "ghosting" caused by any residual exposure charge from the previous frame.

The use of flat-panel detectors in place of an image intensifier offers several advantages. The first is a reduction in size, bulk, and weight of the fluoroscopic tower. A flat-panel detector greatly reduces all three, allowing easier manipulation of the tower, greater flexibility of movement, and greater access to the patient during the examination. A flat-panel detector with a 30 × 40 cm (12 × 16 inch) active area occupies less than 25% of the volume of a 30-cm (12-inch) image intensifier tube and less than 15% of the volume of a 40-cm (16-inch) image intensifier tube. The flat-panel detectors also replace the spot filming and other recording devices. They operate in radiographic mode (50–1200 mA) so that, in many cases, additional radiographic images are not needed. The images, both dynamic and static, are recorded by the system and can be readily archived with the patient record in a picture archiving and communication system (PACS). The images produced are very large data files; spot images can be 8 MB or larger and dynamic images as large as 240 MB per second. Furthermore, flat-panel detectors do not degrade with age; are more durable; present a rectangular field providing more information; and have better contrast resolution, higher DQE, wider dynamic range, and all the postprocessing options common to digital images. The spatial resolution of flat-panel detectors is higher than that of image-intensified systems (2.5–3.2 Lp/mm versus 1–2 Lp/mm). Finally, flat-panel detectors do not exhibit most image artifacts seen with image intensifiers. Flat-panel detectors have an operational dynamic range 60 times larger than that of image intensifier systems and because of this do not exhibit veiling glare. Because the DELs of a flat-panel detector are arranged in a grid pattern (uniform columns and rows), they do not exhibit the pincushion and S distortion artifacts. Vignetting (unequal brightness) and defocusing artifacts are also eliminated with flat-panel detectors. They do all of this with as much as a 50% lower radiation dose to the patient, while operating at much higher mA settings than image-intensified fluoroscopy systems (50–1200 mA).

Like image-intensified fluoroscopic units, the use of a "deadman" exposure switch (one that turns the exposure off when the switch is released) has long been a part of all fluoroscopy systems.

**Critical Concept**

**Digital Fluoroscopic Systems**

The use of flat-panel detectors in place of an image intensifier offers several advantages such as a reduction in the size, bulk, and weight of the fluoroscopic tower, allowing for easier manipulation of the tower and greater access to the patient during the examination. The flat-panel detectors also replace the spot filming and other recording devices, and because they can operate in radiographic mode, in many cases additional radiographic images are not needed. The images, both dynamic and static, can also be readily archived with the patient record in a PACS.

## FLUOROSCOPIC FEATURES

Modern fluoroscopic equipment offers several features that affect the quality of the fluoroscopic image and radiation dose to the patient. There are several controls and settings, both on the control console and tower, which allow adjustment of the radiation output and image quality. To begin, the consideration for selecting kVp is the same as for general radiography. Recall that the higher the kVp, the higher the maximum and average energies of the x-ray beam. Here too, most of the x-ray beam will be Bremsstrahlung, and the average energy of the beam will be one-third of the kVp selected. Using higher kVp settings (appropriate for the examination) will result in a higher energy beam and lower patient dose.

Collimation of the fluoroscopic beam reduces the field size exposing the patient. Fully open, the unit will expose the patient to a beam adequate to cover the full size of the image intensifier or detector. With the newest units, lines will appear on the **last image hold (LIH)** displayed on the monitor, indicating the position of the collimator plates. This allows the collimator to be further adjusted without exposing the patient to additional radiation (**virtual collimation**). The collimator should be adjusted to eliminate all anatomic structures not necessary to the examination being performed. Collimation changes the field of view (FOV) displayed, but it does not magnify the image (Fig. 15.15). By reducing

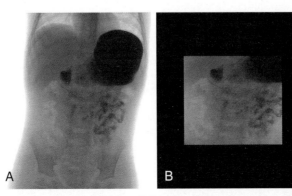

**Fig. 15.15 Collimation and FOV. (A)** Full field of view (FOV) image without collimation. **(B)** Smaller field of view (FOV) with increased collimation. Note the anatomy visualized is not magnified.

the area of tissue being exposed, overall patient dose is reduced.

**Frame averaging** is an operation that reduces overall patient dose and image noise by averaging multiple image frames together. Because the combining of frames reduces noise, less radiation is needed to maintain image quality; however, spatial resolution will be decreased.

The option to include the grid is also a control feature. The grid will reduce the amount of scatter reaching the image intensifier or detector and improve image quality. But because it also removes some useful radiation from the remnant beam, mA (quantity of radiation) must be increased to maintain overall exposure to the image intensifier or detector. In general, its use increases radiation dose to the patient. The decision to use it should be based on the examination and the anatomic area's capacity to produce scatter radiation. The abdomen, for example, will produce more scatter radiation, and the grid should be selected, whereas extremities or pediatric patients may not require its use.

Modern fluoroscopic units also allow for the selection and interchangeability of added filtration thickness or material. The operation of this control may entail the substitution of filters of different thicknesses or switching of filtration material. The typical material used for beam filtration is aluminum, which has an atomic number ideally suited to removing low-energy x-ray photons. It is important to remove these low-energy photons from the beam before they can expose the patient and contribute only to patient dose. This filtration acts to increase the average energy of the beam by removing low-energy photons. Higher-atomic-number materials such as copper are used in some units and may be selected when additional filtration and beam hardening are desired.

 **Make the Physics Connection**

**Chapter 6**

An increase in tube filtration causes a decrease in x-ray beam quantity and an increase in quality. With the low-energy photons removed, the average energy is higher.

Anatomic programs are also available on modern fluoroscopic units. These programs are preset fluoroscopic examination settings established and programmed into the unit at the time of manufacture or at the time of installation as dictated by the facility. Each preset will display a predetermined set of exposure factors, filter thickness and type, etc., just as presets do on radiographic units. Along this same line are the default settings on the unit. These defaults are intended to be "ideal" or "standard" values for minimizing dose and maximizing image quality. They are not strict rules of operation and should be changed depending on circumstances and the examination to be performed. The operator should evaluate the default settings when they appear on the control panel or tower to be sure they match the examination and patient (e.g., size, pediatric versus adult, pathology, anatomy of interest).

 **Critical Concept**

**Fluoroscopic Features**

Use of virtual collimation during last image hold (LIH), frame averaging, and added filtration will reduce patient dose, whereas use of a grid will increase patient dose.

## Automatic Exposure Rate Control

Like automatic brightness control (ABC) used in older image intensified units, **automatic exposure rate control (AERC)** serves a similar function in modern fluoroscopy. AERC automatically adjusts the tube current (mA), voltage (kVp), filtration, and pulse width to maintain radiation exposure to the flat-panel detector. A variety of variables during a fluoroscopic examination can result in changes in the radiation exposure reaching the flat-panel detector. Changes in patient thickness, tissue attenuation, object-to-image receptor distance (OID), collimation, and FOV may require an increase or decrease in the radiation reaching the detector.

 **Critical Concept**

**Automatic Exposure Rate Control (AERC)**

AERC automatically adjusts the tube current (mA), voltage (kVp), filtration, and pulse width to maintain radiation exposure to the flat-panel detector. Changes in patient thickness, tissue attenuation, OID, collimation, and FOV may require an increase or decrease in the radiation reaching the detector.

## Magnification

**Electronic magnification** is the selection of a smaller FOV. When a smaller FOV is selected, an area smaller than the size of the detector is exposed by the x-ray beam, but the area is enlarged to fill the display monitor area, which magnifies the anatomic structures (Fig. 15.16). Similar to intensified fluoroscopy, flat-panel detectors provide several different magnification modes. However, the spatial resolution of flat-panel detectors is the same for all FOV options and the patient radiation dose is not significantly increased provided binning (process of grouping and averaging adjacent DELs) is not used. When binning is used, for a smaller FOV, spatial resolution will be increased and noise is increased, resulting in increased radiation exposure to reduce the noise. However, the increase in radiation dose is less compared with magnification during image-intensified fluoroscopy. The largest FOV should be used whenever possible to reduce patient radiation dose along with increased collimation to reduce irradiation of unnecessary patient tissues.

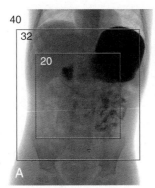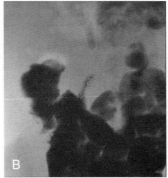

40
32
20
A                    B

Fig. 15.16 **Electronic Magnification. (A)** Full field of view (FOV) image. **(B)** Electronic magnification mode results in a magnified image displayed.

## Pulsed Fluoroscopy

An operational feature of modern fluoroscopy units is using a pulsed beam technology to reduce radiation output necessary for the fluoroscopic image and radiation dose. This is termed **pulsed fluoroscopy** and is simply a design of the unit that rapidly turns the x-ray beam on and off during operation. This operation introduces two concepts necessary to understand its value: pulse rate and pulse width. **Pulse rate** refers to how many pulses occur per second of operation (how many exposures occur per second). **Pulse width** refers to the length of each pulse (how long each exposure lasts). The operator can select pulse rates generally from 1 pulse per second to 30 pulses per second. Pulse widths are generally less than 6 ms for pediatrics and less than 10 ms for adults. If the unit is operated at 30 pulses per second, the radiation dose is no different than that in the older form of operation (continuous fluoroscopy). However, if operated at pulse rates below 30, a radiation dose reduction is realized (see Fig. 15.17).

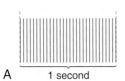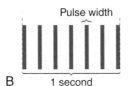

Pulse width
A    1 second    B    1 second

Fig. 15.17 **Continuous Versus Pulsed Fluoroscopy. (A)** Continuous fluoroscopy produces 30 images (frames) during a period of 1 second. **(B)** Pulsed fluoroscopy can vary the number of images (frames) per second. This example has 7 frames per second. Note the change in the pulse width. (B courtesy Fauber TL: *Radiographic imaging and exposure*, ed 6, St. Louis, 2022, Elsevier, Inc.)

## Dose Rates

Most fluoroscopic units today allow for the selection of **dose rates**. The dose rate setting may be labeled as low, medium, or high (or icons may be used to imply the same). These settings change the dose generally by 50% (medium is 50% of high and low is 50% of medium). These selections control the radiation dose rate at the detector. As with radiography, the operator should select the dose rate depending on the examination to be performed. For example, differentiation of soft tissue structures with lower subject contrast requires a higher dose rate, whereas barium studies (higher subject contrast) require a comparatively lower dose rate.

## Image Recording

A sequence of digital radiographic images can be recorded per second with flat-panel detector fluoroscopy, which reduces the need for follow-up radiographic images. These radiographic images have improved quality compared with fluoroscopic images; however, patient radiation exposure is significantly increased. Use of features such as LIH or last frame hold, along with **fluoro loop save**, will save single images or a fluoroscopic sequence loop to memory. These fluoroscopic images can be postprocessed and maintained in the patient's permanent record.

## Critical Concept
### Image Recording

Use of features such as LIH or last frame hold along with fluoro loop save will save single fluoroscopic images or a fluoroscopic sequence loop to memory. These features reduce patient radiation exposure compared with producing digital radiographic images.

## DOSE MONITORING

**Air kerma** (kinetic energy released in matter) specifies the intensity of x-rays at a given point in air at a known distance from the focal spot or source of x-rays, and the cumulative or total air kerma will be monitored during the fluoroscopic procedure. An important quality-control check is the maximum air kerma rate for fluoroscopy is 10 R/min or 88 mGy/min. Other dose displays such as DAP and KAP provide indicators of patient radiation risk and should be documented in the patient's record. **Dose-area product (DAP)** meters measure exposure in air, (followed by a computation to estimate absorbed dose to the patient)and are required on all new fluoroscopes in the United States. **Kerma area product (KAP)** is the same as DAP and is the product of the total air kerma and the area of the x-ray beam at the entrance of the patient. Units of DAP/KAP are expressed in micro- or milli-gray per area squared but can vary by manufacturer (see Box 15.2). In addition to dose displays, the total amount of fluoroscopic time for the procedure must be documented in the patient's record.

| Box 15.2 | Dose Measures as Indicators of Patient Radiation Risk |
|---|---|

**DOSE MONITORING**
**Air kerma**—Kinetic energy released in mass; specifies the intensity of x-rays at a given point in air at a known distance from the source of x-rays.
   Cumulative (total) air kerma
   Maximum air kerma rate for fluoroscopy is 10 R/min or 88 mGy/min
   **Kerma area product (KAP)** also known as dose area product (DAP) is the product of cumulative air kerma and the area of the x-ray beam at the entrance of the patient.
   Dose monitoring units may vary by manufacturer:

$$1\,\mu Gy\text{-}m^2 = 1\,cGy\text{-}cm^2 = 10\,mGy\text{-}cm$$

$$1\,centi = 10\,milli = 10,000\,micro$$

$$1\,centimeter\ squared\ (cm^2) = 0.0001\,m^2$$

## Critical Concept
### Dose Monitoring

Air kerma (kinetic **e**nergy **r**eleased in **m**atter) specifies the intensity of x-rays at a given point in air at a known distance from the focal spot or source of x-rays, and the cumulative or total air kerma will be monitored during the fluoroscopic procedure. Other dose displays such as DAP and KAP provide indicators of patient radiation risk and should be documented in the patient's record.

## VIEWING SYSTEMS

Advancements in monitors have improved the quality of the displayed fluoroscopic image. These improved display monitors are currently used with both image intensified units and digital fluoroscopic units (Fig. 15.18).

### Liquid Crystal Display Monitors

Liquid crystal display (LCD) monitors are one of the modern display monitor options. LCD monitors offer superior resolution and brightness over television monitors. They work in a completely different way than television monitors. LCD monitors comprise several layers (Fig. 15.19). The heart of the LCD is the liquid crystal layer, which is sandwiched between polarizing layers that contain nematic liquid crystals. These crystals are typically rod shaped, semiliquid, and can change the direction of light (unpolarized electromagnetic radiation (EMR) waves traveling in two planes) that passes through them. The crystals exist in an unorganized "twisted" state. When an electric current is applied, the crystals organize or "untwist." In the untwisted state, they organize into configurations that will block or allow light to pass through depending on the polarizing filters. The polarized layers on each side are oriented at a 90-degree angle to each other so that light that may be able to pass through one would be at the wrong orientation to pass through the other. When electric current is applied to the liquid crystal layer, the "untwisting" changes orientation of light passing through (polarizing the EMR waves to travel in one plane) the back layer and allows it to pass through the front. A thin-film transistor (TFT) panel is located behind the liquid crystal layer. The number of TFTs is equal to the number of pixels displayed. The TFTs control the current to each pixel and switch it on or off by causing the liquid crystals to twist or untwist. A monochromatic LCD monitor will display the light as shades of gray. A color LCD monitor has a color filter layer added to display shades of color. The intensity of light is controlled by the current to the crystals, which is controlled by the TFTs. This in turn determines the shade of gray (if monochromatic) or shade of color (if a color monitor).

### Plasma Monitors

Plasma monitors may also be an option for display monitors. Plasma monitors are very similar in

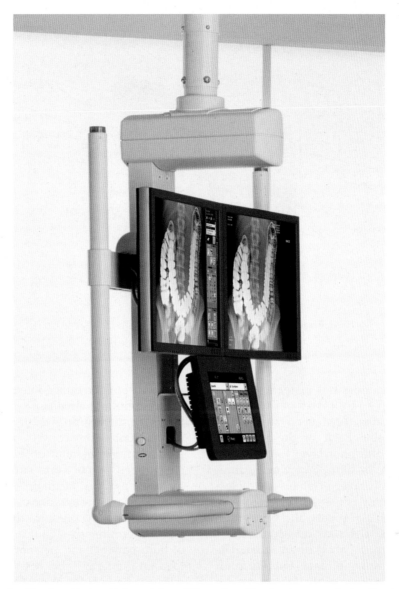

Fig. 15.18 **Display Monitor.** Modern high-resolution LCD monitor with a touch screen display. (Courtesy of Siemens Medical Solutions USA, Inc.)

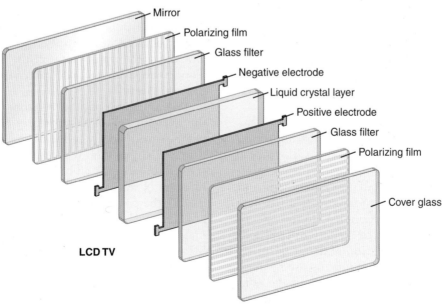

Fig. 15.19 **LCD Monitor.** The layers and components of a liquid crystal display monitor.

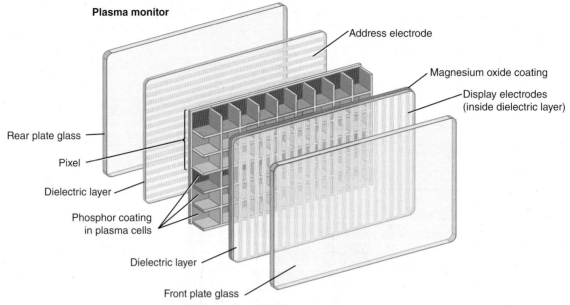

**Plasma monitor**

Address electrode

Magnesium oxide coating

Display electrodes
(inside dielectric layer)

Rear plate glass

Pixel

Dielectric layer

Phosphor coating
in plasma cells

Dielectric layer

Front plate glass

Fig. 15.20 **Plasma Monitor.** The layers and components of a plasma monitor.

construction to LCD monitors but instead of a liquid crystal layer they have a thin layer of pixels (Fig. 15.20). Each pixel contains three neon and xenon gas-filled cells (subpixels). Each of these cells is coated with a different phosphor layer formula that will produce red, green, or blue light when stimulated. On each side of this layer of pixels are dielectric layers. When electricity is passed between these dielectric layers through the pixels, the gas within is ionized. The liberated electrons release ultraviolet radiation to return to the shell of an atom. The ultraviolet radiation in turn stimulates the phosphor coating in the cell, producing visible light of a color corresponding to the phosphor formula. The current through the pixels (and subpixels) is modulated by the electrodes several thousand times per second, thereby controlling the intensity of light produced. This control and modulation process makes it possible for plasma monitors to produce billions of different shades of color.

## MINIMIZING RADIATION EXPOSURE

Minimizing radiation exposure is just as important during fluoroscopic imaging as it is with radiographic imaging. It is the fluoroscopic operator's responsibility to be knowledgeable about the equipment and methods to reduce patient radiation dose. A few methods of minimizing radiation dose to the patient during fluoroscopic procedures include intermittent fluoroscopy, collimation, omission of the grid during fluoroscopy, added filtration, minimal use of the magnification feature, and the use of the last image hold where the x-ray exposure is not activated while the operator reviews the image.

Because older image-intensified fluoroscopic units use a continuous stream of x-rays, the exposure should be intermittently pulsed by the operator. The use of intermittent fluoroscopy by the operator will reduce patient and personnel dose. This has long been an encouraged practice and simply refers to the operator using as little "beam-on" time as possible to make the necessary observations and complete the examination. Applying pressure to the exposure switch or pedal intermittently significantly reduces the exposure of both patients and personnel and reduces the heat load on the x-ray tube. Recall that fluoroscopy is the primary contributor to occupational exposure and, in recent years, with the very complex interventional procedures, a potentially high source of patient exposure. Modern image-intensified and digital fluoroscopy use a controlled pulsed x-ray exposure, and the operator is not required to intermittently release the pressure. Operating the fluoroscope in the lowest pulse mode along with a lower dose rate will minimize patient radiation dose.

The collimator should be adjusted to only include the relevant anatomic structures for the examination being performed. By reducing the area of tissue being exposed, collimation will reduce overall patient dose. If the fluoroscopic unit has features such as virtual collimation (x-ray field size can be adjusted without irradiating the patient) and the ability to save a sequence of fluoroscopic images without acquiring radiographic images, patient exposure will be further decreased. Increasing collimation and decreasing the number of acquired (radiographic) images will reduce patient exposure.

In general, using a grid increases radiation dose to the patient. The decision to use it should be based on the examination and the anatomic area's capacity to produce scatter radiation. Modern fluoroscopic units also allow for the selection and interchangeability of added filtration thickness or material. It is important to remove these unwanted photons from the beam before they can expose the patient and contribute only to patient dose.

The use of preset or default settings is available to minimize patient dose and maximize image quality. The operator should evaluate the default settings when they appear on the control panel or tower to be sure they match the examination and patient (e.g., size, pediatric versus adult, pathology, anatomy of interest). Time, distance, and shielding are the standard radiation safety practices used during fluoroscopic imaging. Reducing the x-ray exposure time reduces the exposure to the patient and any personnel remaining in the room. The control panel timer produces an audible noise when 5 minutes of x-ray fluoroscopic time have been used. It is the operator's responsibility to minimize x-ray fluoroscopy time, and the radiographer should document the total amount of x-ray fluoroscopic time used during the procedure. Modern fluoroscopic units provide dose monitoring in addition to the cumulative fluoroscopic timer. The DAP/KAP and cumulative air kerma provide radiation exposure data and need to be recorded in the patient's medical record. If these dose-monitoring systems are not available, then the cumulative exposure time and number of acquired images need to be documented. In addition, the intensity of the x-ray exposure at the tabletop should not exceed 10 R per minute (88 mGy per minute) for units equipped with ABC/AERC. Whenever the patient's exposure is reduced, personnel exposure is also reduced.

The source-to-skin distance (SSD) should be no less than 38 cm (15 inches) for stationary fluoroscopic units and no less than 30 cm (12 inches) on a mobile C-arm fluoroscopic unit. Increasing the SSD and decreasing the distance between the patient and the detector (OID) will decrease patient exposure. Varying the patient's position during fluoroscopy will spread the radiation to different areas of the skin, thereby reducing the overall skin exposure. Personnel other than the operator should increase their distance from the patient to reduce exposure to scatter radiation because scatter originates from the patient.

In addition to all personnel in the room wearing lead aprons (recommended 0.5 mm of lead equivalent), two additional types of shielding are required during fluoroscopy. Because the Bucky tray is positioned at the end of the table for operation of the under-the-table x-ray tube, a Bucky slot cover with at least 0.25 mm of lead equivalent should automatically cover the opened space at the side of the table. In addition, a protective lead curtain with at least 0.25 mm of lead equivalent must be placed between the patient and the operator to reduce exposure to the operator (see Table 15.2).

| Table 15.2 | Methods of Reducing Patient and Personnel Exposure During Fluoroscopy |
|---|---|

- Operating the fluoroscopic exposure intermittently or in the lowest pulsed mode, along with a lower dose rate and the use of last image hold, will minimize patient radiation dose.
- Evaluate and use preset or default settings available to minimize patient dose.
- Reducing the amount of x-ray fluoroscopic time reduces patient and personnel exposure.
- Increase collimation with virtual collimation, remove the grid, and minimize the use of magnification.
- Monitor and document the amount of total x-ray fluoroscopic time displayed in 5-minute increments on the control panel in addition to the number of acquired radiographic images. If provided, cumulative radiation dose data should be recorded.
- The intensity of x-ray exposure at the tabletop should not exceed 10 R/min (88 mGy/min) for units equipped with ABC/AERC.
- The SSD should be not less than 38 cm (15 in) for stationary fluoroscopic units and not less than 30 cm (12 in) on mobile C-arm fluoroscopic units.
- Personnel in the fluoroscopic room during procedures should increase their distance from the patient to reduce exposure to scatter radiation.
- Personnel should wear appropriate lead shielding during fluoroscopic procedures.
- The Bucky slot cover must contain at least 0.25 mm of lead-equivalent shielding and cover the opened space on the side of the table.
- A protective curtain placed between the patient and operator must have at least 0.25 mm of lead equivalent.

*ABS,* Automatic brightness stabilization; *AERC,* automatic exposure rate control; *SSD,* source-to-skin distance.

## QUALITY CONTROL

Quality-control programs are vitally important for all ionizing radiation-producing equipment to monitor equipment performance and minimize patient dose. Fluoroscopic equipment is used extensively in health care and contributes significantly to the radiation dose received by the general population. Federal guidelines regarding fluoroscopic equipment may be found in Title 21 of the Code of Federal Regulations Part 1020 (21 CFR 1020) subchapter J. Quality control is a team effort among the radiographer, radiologist, and medical physicist. The role of the radiologist is generally one of supervision of the whole quality-control program and process. The radiographer's role is more that of a facilitator in the process, and the medical physicist has primary responsibility for performance testing and interpretation. Although some data may be collected, and some monitoring performed by a radiographer, performance tests and their interpretation are carried out by a medical physicist. That said, the radiographer should be familiar with the monitoring and testing necessary to ensure that the fluoroscopic unit is operating correctly. The

## Table 15.3 Quality Control (QC) Specific to Fluoroscopic Equipment

| QC TEST | DESCRIPTION |
|---|---|
| Fluoroscopic system resolution | Tests the system's ability to display details of small objects (high-contrast resolution) and larger objects (low-contrast resolution). |
| Fluoroscopic automatic exposure rate control (AERC) performance | Evaluates image quality for changes in exposure parameters such as high dose rate, pulsed modes, and field of view (FOV). |
| Fluoroscopic phantom image quality | Evaluates the quality of the displayed fluoroscopic image, including image distortion or lag. |
| Fluoroscopic exposure rates | Measures the intensity of the x-ray beam. Fluoroscopic exposure rate should not exceed 10 R/min for units with ABC/AERC systems. |
| Fluoroscopic alignment test | Ensures the radiation beam aligns with the center of the image intensifier/detector within 2% of the SID. |
| Patient dose monitoring system calibration (if present) | Evaluates proper function of patient dose monitoring systems such as DAP/KAP meters. |
| Digital monitor performance | Evaluates the display characteristics of the monitor (described in Chapter 10) |

*ABS,* Automatic brightness stabilization; *AERC,* automatic exposure rate control; *DAP,* dose-area product; *KAP,* Kerma area product; *SID,* source-to-image receptor distance.

radiographer, in particular a quality-control radiographer, may be responsible for the operational inspection of the equipment. This inspection should be conducted using a checklist of the items found in Table 15.2 and conducted at least every 6 months. This radiographer may also be responsible for an inspection of the fluoroscopic suite itself to examine the general physical condition of the room, unit, supporting electrical cables, and control booth, noting any wear or deteriorating condition. This inspection of the physical condition should be placed on the same schedule and conducted along with the operational inspection.

The other important part of the quality-control program is the performance inspection and testing of the equipment. Although a quality-control radiographer may perform some of these tests, an appropriately trained and licensed medical physicist should conduct and interpret this portion of the program and oversee the entire quality-control monitoring program. Quality-control tests specific to fluoroscopic equipment can be found in Table 15.3.

 **On the Spot**

- Thomas Edison is credited with inventing the first commercially available fluoroscope. Many improvements have been made to the concept, and it was the introduction of the image intensifier that greatly advanced the system.
- The image intensifier is an electronic vacuum tube that consists of five basic parts: the input phosphor, photocathode, electrostatic focusing lenses, accelerating anode, and output phosphor. It converts the remnant beam to light, then electrons, then back to light, which increases the light intensity in the process.
- Brightness gain is an expression of the ability of an image intensifier tube to convert x-ray energy into light energy and increase the brightness of the image in the process. It is determined by multiplying the flux gain by the minification gain.
- Flux gain is expressed as the ratio of the number of light photons at the output phosphor to the number of light photons emitted at the input phosphor, and *minification gain* is an expression of the degree to which the image is minified (made smaller) from input phosphor to output phosphor.
- ABC is a function of the fluoroscopic unit that maintains the overall appearance of the fluoroscopic image (radiographic contrast and brightness) by automatically adjusting the kVp, mA, or both, either by monitoring the current through the image intensifier or the output phosphor intensity and adjusting the exposure factor(s) if the monitored value falls below preset levels.
- When an image intensifier is operated in magnification mode, the voltage to the electrostatic focusing lenses is increased, which reduces the diameter of the electron stream, shifting the focal point farther from the output phosphor and giving the appearance of magnification while improving spatial resolution. This also causes an increase in radiation dose to the patient.
- Distortion—particularly the pincushion effect, unequal brightness (vignetting), and image noise—are common problems with image-intensified fluoroscopy.
- The camera tube is one method of coupling the image intensifier to a television monitor. The vidicon tube is connected to the output phosphor of the image intensifier by either a fiberoptic bundle or an optical lens system. The electron beam is activated and begins sweeping the anode target. If the electron beam and light from the output phosphor are incident on the same place at the same time, electrons are transmitted through the target to the signal plate, which carries this current as an electronic signal to the television monitor, where it is reconstructed as a visible image.
- The CCD is another method of coupling the image intensifier to the television monitor. It is a light-sensitive semiconducting device that generates an electrical charge when stimulated by light and stores this charge in a capacitor. To digitize the charge from this device, the gates of each pixel are charged in sequence, moving the signal down the row, where it is transferred into a capacitor. From the capacitors, the charge is sent as an electronic signal to the television monitor.

- The purpose of the television monitor is to convert the electronic signal from the camera tube or CCD back into a visible image. In essence, the television monitor is reconstructing the image from the output phosphor as a visible image on the fluorescent screen by way of the camera tube or CCD.
- Photospot filming is another method of recording static images during intensified fluoroscopic examinations, but this method is actually "photographing" the image off of the output phosphor via a beam-splitting mirror.
- The early versions of digital fluoroscopy used the image-intensified fluoroscopic chain but added an ADC and computer between the camera tube and the monitor. The ADC is necessary for the computer to process and display the image. Once in digital form, the image can be postprocessed and stored in that format or printed onto film using a dry laser printer, for example.
- Fluoroscopic versions of flat-panel detectors must respond in rapid sequences to create dynamic images, must maintain a large fill factor to reduce image noise due to low-dose fluoroscopic applications, and must erase the detector between frames to prevent "ghosting" caused by any residual exposure charge from the previous frame.
- The use of flat-panel detectors in place of an image intensifier offers several advantages such as a reduction in size, bulk, and weight of the fluoroscopic tower, allowing for easier manipulation of the tower and greater access to the patient during the examination. The flat-panel detectors also replace the other recording devices, and because they are capable of operating in radiographic mode, in many cases additional radiographic images are not needed. The images, both dynamic and static, can also be readily archived with the patient record in a PACS.
- Modern fluoroscopic units have features such as automatic exposure rate control, the ability to select dose rates, virtual collimation, filtration change, the ability to select a predetermined set of exposure factors, pulsed fluoroscopy, frame averaging, electronic magnification, fluoro loop save, and dose monitoring.
- LCD and plasma monitors are modern display monitor options. They offer superior resolution and brightness over television monitors and work in a completely different way than television monitors.
- Quality control is a team effort between the radiographer, radiologist, and medical physicist. Although some data may be collected and some monitoring performed by a radiographer, performance tests and their interpretation are carried out by a medical physicist. That said, the radiographer should be familiar with the monitoring and testing necessary to ensure that the fluoroscopic unit is operating correctly.

## CRITICAL THINKING QUESTIONS

1. Describe the function of a flat-panel detector as it relates to patient dose reduction.
2. Your patient wants to know how a fluoroscope works and whether they should be concerned about their radiation exposure. How would you answer the patient?

## REVIEW QUESTIONS

1. Which of the following is composed of cesium iodide?
   a. Conventional fluoroscopic screen
   b. Intensifier input phosphor
   c. Intensifier output phosphor
   d. Intensifier photocathode
2. Which of the following are negatively charged electrodes plated on the inner surface of the glass envelope of the image intensifier?
   a. Photocathode
   b. Electrostatic focusing lenses
   c. Input phosphor
   d. Output phosphor
3. Which of the following emits electrons in response to light stimulus?
   a. Conventional fluoroscopic screen
   b. Intensified input phosphor
   c. Intensified output phosphor
   d. Intensified photocathode
4. What part of the image intensifier will attract the electrons and increase their kinetic energy?
   a. Input phosphor
   b. Output phosphor
   c. Electrostatic focusing lenses
   d. Accelerating anode
5. Which of the following will occur if voltage to the electrostatic focusing lenses is increased?
   a. Inversion of the image
   b. Reversal of the image
   c. Minification of the image
   d. Magnification of the image
6. What portion of the TV camera tube will conduct only when illuminated?
   a. Electron gun
   b. Target layer
   c. Signal plate
   d. Face plate
7. A signal is received by the display monitor from which part of the TV camera tube?
   a. Electron gun
   b. Target
   c. Signal plate
   d. Face plate
8. Which display monitor design used nematic liquid crystals?
   a. LCD
   b. Plasma
   c. Television (CRT)
   d. These gases are not used in monitors.
9. Which of the following is within the spatial resolution range of a flat-panel detector?
   a. 1.0 Lp/mm
   b. 2.0 Lp/mm
   c. 3.0 Lp/mm
   d. 4.0 Lp/mm

10. The maximum air kerma rate for fluoroscopy is:
    a. 2 R/min.
    b. 6 R/min.
    c. 10 R/min.
    d. 14 R/min.
11. The ratio of the number of light photons at the output phosphor to the number at the input phosphor equals:
    a. brightness gain.
    b. flux gain.
    c. minification gain.
    d. magnification gain.
12. What fluoroscopic operation is defined as the number of exposures per second?
    a. Frame averaging
    b. Pulse width
    c. Pulse rate
    d. Dose rates

13. The ability to adjust the collimator without exposing the patient to additional radiation is known as:
    a. frame averaging.
    b. air kerma.
    c. virtual collimation.
    d. electrostatic focusing lens.
14. What fluoroscopic feature defines the exposure length of time during pulsed fluoroscopy?
    a. Dose rates
    b. Pulse width
    c. Pulse rate
    d. Flux gain
15. Which fluoroscopic feature will minimize patient radiation exposure?
    a. Frame averaging
    b. Last image hold
    c. Fluoro loop save
    d. All the above

# Additional Equipment

## Outline

## Objectives

- Explain the need for digital subtraction techniques during interventional fluoroscopic procedures.
- Differentiate between radiographic and fluoroscopic mobile equipment.
- State the purpose of dedicated units and identify their unique features.
- Explain the principles of linear tomography.
- Recognize the variations required in exposure technique factors for mobile and dedicated units and linear tomography.

## Key Terms

bone densitometry
C-arm
dedicated units
digital breast tomosynthesis (DBT)
digital subtraction techniques
focal plane

fulcrum
linear tomography
mammography
mini C-arm
mobile equipment
object plane

O-arm
osteoporosis
panoramic x-ray (panorex)
pivot point
road mapping
tomographic angle

## INTRODUCTION

A variety of specialized equipment are used in imaging that either improves visualization or provides important information about anatomic tissue. Radiographers need to be familiar with the unique features of the specialized equipment used in the radiology department. Additional education and training may be required to operate the specialized equipment in a safe and competent manner.

## INTERVENTIONAL FLUOROSCOPY

Fluoroscopic units used in interventional radiology have unique features such as biplane technology for image-guided therapy procedures along with full control of the imaging equipment at the table without sterility breaks (Fig. 16.1). In addition to the features available on routine diagnostic digital fluoroscopic units, interventional fluoroscopic units such as those used in cardiac imaging need the ability to create cine fluoroscopic images at 60 frames per second and digital subtraction techniques. **Digital subtraction techniques** (Fig. 16.2) increase the visibility of vasculature by creating images precontrast, postcontrast, and the subtracted image. The precontrast image is the mask image that will be subtracted from the postcontrast image. This results in an image with just the contrast-filled vasculature. The overlying structures such as bone and soft tissue are removed from the subtracted image, so the vasculature is better visualized. **Road mapping** (Fig. 16.3) is another digital subtraction technique that uses the maximum contrast-filled image as a mask that can be subtracted from precontrast images. This technique provides a better method to navigate the catheter or wire through tortuous vessels. Without the road

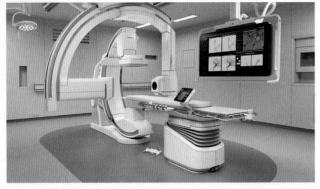

**Fig. 16.1 Bi-Plane C-arm Interventional Fluoroscopic Unit Used for Image-Guided Therapy.** (Courtesy Philips Healthcare. All rights reserved.)

mapping technique, it would be more difficult to anticipate the twists and turns of the small vessel to maneuver the catheter or wire for placement in the vessel.

Depending on the type of interventional or complex procedure, significant advancements in fluoroscopic equipment will continue in an effort to assist the physicians and technologists in the successful completion of both diagnostic and therapeutic procedures. Additional training and experience is necessary for the interventional technologist to assist the physician in completion of a variety of complex procedures while being mindful of the need for specialized patient care, equipment operation, and monitoring patient radiation dose.

---

### ⚠ Critical Concept

**Digital Subtraction Techniques**

Digital subtraction techniques create mask images that can be subtracted from images with maximum contrast-filled vessels. The overlying structures such as bone and soft tissue are removed from the subtracted image, so the vasculature is better visualized. Road mapping is another digital subtraction technique that uses the maximum contrast-filled image as a mask that can be subtracted from precontrast images. This technique provides a better method to navigate the catheter or wire through tortuous vessels.

---

## MOBILE EQUIPMENT

**Mobile equipment** can be radiographic or fluoroscopic units that are transportable to the patient's bedside or the operating room. Patients imaged with a mobile unit are not capable of being imaged in the radiology department because of a condition or a circumstance such as undergoing surgery. To operate a mobile unit safely, the radiographer must be aware of its unique features.

### RADIOGRAPHIC UNITS

Mobile x-ray units can be smaller, light-duty or full-power units that are transported on wheels (Fig. 16.4). These mobile units may be transported with or without the use of motors. Mobile units can be categorized in several ways depending on the design of the generator: direct power, battery power, capacitor discharge, or high frequency. Mobile units operated by plugging into a wall outlet for direct power may experience fluctuations in voltage, which affects the radiation output. Battery-operated units provide more consistent radiation output, similar to a three-phase generator, but need to be recharged. Capacitor discharge units must be plugged into a wall outlet during operation but produce consistent radiation output, similar to that of a single-phase generator. High-frequency units produce a consistent radiation output and are lightweight but must be plugged into a wall outlet during operation.

Exposure techniques can therefore vary greatly depending on the type of mobile unit and its radiation output for a selected exposure technique. Additionally, care must be taken in manipulating the unit at the patient's bedside to avoid any damage to the mobile unit or bedside patient care equipment. A radiography suite is a "controlled" and shielded environment specially designed for radiographic imaging. In a mobile environment, however, radiographers must take responsibility for radiation protection for themselves, the patient, and other individuals within close

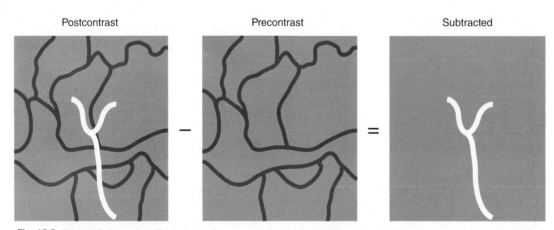

Postcontrast        Precontrast        Subtracted

**Fig. 16.2 Digital Subtraction Technique.** A precontrast mask image is subtracted from the maximum contrast-filled image. The subtracted image shows the contrast-filled vasculature without the superimposition of the bone and soft tissues.

Roadmap mask                Live fluoro                Live fluoro with roadmap

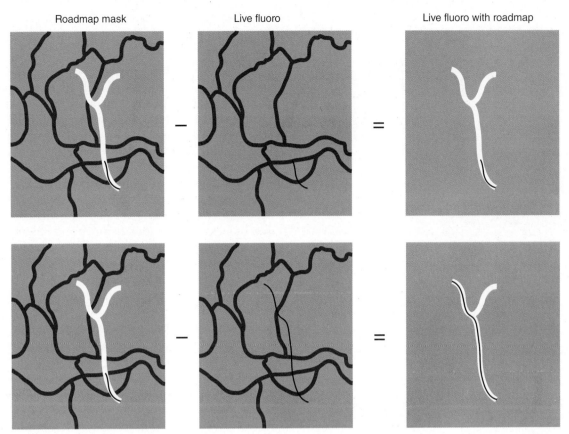

Fig. 16.3 **Road Mapping Digital Subtraction Technique.** Two mask images are used for subtraction. A precontrast image and a maximum contrast image mask are subtracted during live fluoro that results in the contrast-filled vasculature images used to navigate the catheter or wire through tortuous vasculature.

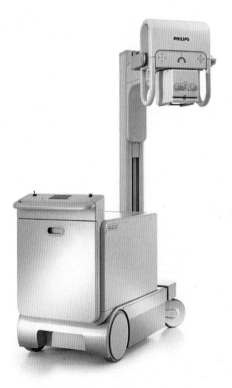

Fig. 16.4 **Radiographic Mobile Unit.** A mobile x-ray unit. (Courtesy Philips Healthcare, Andover, Mass.)

proximity. Radiographers should wear a lead apron during the radiation exposure and stand as far from the patient and x-ray tube as possible (at least 6 feet). Shielding of the patient and other individuals who must remain in the room should be performed as in the radiology department.

Imaging patients using a mobile x-ray unit presents many challenges. Radiographers need to carefully assess the patient's condition to determine the appropriate alignment of the x-ray tube, patient, and image receptor. The tube-head assembly is freely adjustable, and the radiographer must take care to create the correct tube-part-receptor orientation, which is more readily established in a radiographic suite. The ability to obtain a standard source-to-image receptor distance (SID), use a grid, and operate an automatic exposure control (AEC) device (if available) may be jeopardized during mobile imaging. Obstacles (patient care equipment), patient condition, and the physical room environment may greatly limit or alter the radiographer's options for obtaining what are otherwise routine images. It is imperative that the radiographer be able to adjust the equipment to maintain proper alignment of the tube and image receptor to achieve a diagnostic-quality image at the patient's bedside; therefore,

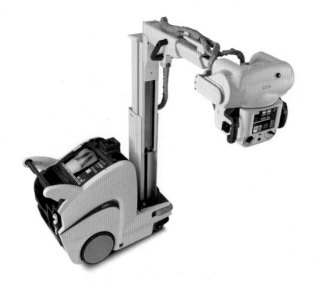

Fig. 16.5 **Direct Radiography (DR) Mobile Unit.** (Courtesy Carestream Health, Inc.)

additional training and experience is warranted before attempting mobile imaging.

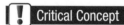

### Critical Concept

**Mobile Radiographic Imaging**

Mobile x-ray units can vary in the radiation output for a given exposure technique. In addition, care must be exercised in transporting and manipulating the mobile unit at the patient's bedside. It takes additional training and experience to align the x-ray tube, patient, and image receptor to achieve a diagnostic-quality radiographic image at a patient's bedside.

Newer mobile x-ray units are more compact and easier to maneuver. The direct radiography (DR) mobile x-ray units include wireless detectors and touch screen display and can deliver images faster for diagnostic interpretation and to picture archiving and communication system (PACS) (Fig. 16.5).

## FLUOROSCOPIC UNITS

**C-arm** mobile units have fluoroscopic capabilities that are typically used in the operating room when imaging is necessary during surgical procedures. Display monitors are also included, which offer both static and dynamic imaging during the procedure. Because it is a fluoroscopic system, many of the features of a fixed fluoroscopic unit are also made available with a C-arm. A C-arm unit is designed with an x-ray tube and image intensifier or flat-panel detector (FPD) attached in a C configuration (Fig. 16.6 and Fig. 16.7). As a result, the unit can be positioned in a variety of planes, enabling viewing from different perspectives. Generally, three sets of locks are provided to move and hold the C-arm in place. One set moves the entire "C" toward or away from the base (the equivalent of moving a table side to side). Another set allows the pivot of the "C" about its axis (the equivalent of angling a general radiographic tube head assembly). The last set allows the "C" to slide along its arc (the equivalent of moving the patient from anteroposterior or posteroanterior to oblique to lateral without having to move the patient).

Generally, the x-ray tube should be positioned under the patient and the image intensifier or FPD above the patient. Positioning the C-arm in this manner during the imaging procedure reduces the radiation exposure to the operator. Because the C-arm uses fluoroscopy, standard radiation exposure techniques and safety practices used during fluoroscopy in the radiology department must also be adhered to during operation of a C-arm unit. The radiographer should also pay attention to the distance between the patient and x-ray tube and to total fluoroscopy time. The minimum source to skin distance for mobile C-arm units is 30 cm. Here, too, fluoroscopy is being used in an "uncontrolled" environment, and it is the radiographer's responsibility to monitor and apply radiation safety measures.

Significant advancements have been made with C-arm type fluoroscopic units used for a variety of

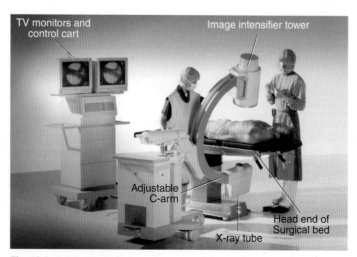

Fig. 16.6 **C-Arm Mobile Unit.** (Courtesy Philips Healthcare, Andover, Mass.)

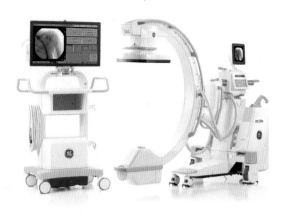

**Fig. 16.7 OEC Elite CFD C-arm Unit.** (Courtesy GE Healthcare © General Electric Company.)

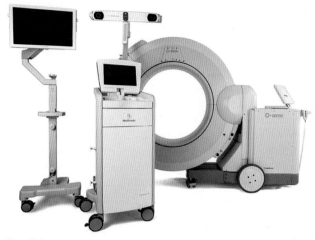

**Fig. 16.9 O-arm Unit.** (Courtesy Lampignano: *Bontrager's textbook of radiographic positioning and related anatomy,* ed 9, St Louis, 2018, Elsevier.)

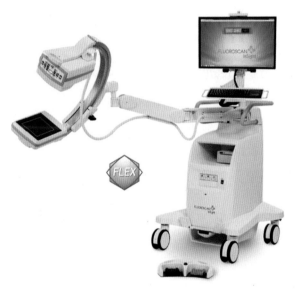

**Fig. 16.8 Mini C-arm Unit.** (Courtesy of HOLOGIC, Inc. and affiliates.)

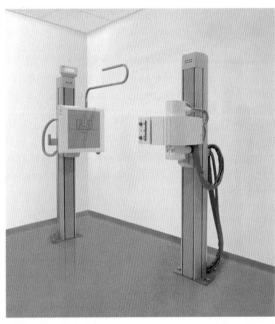

**Fig. 16.10 Dedicated Chest Unit.** (Courtesy Siemens Healthcare, Malvern, Penn.)

anatomic areas. For example, the **mini C-arm** (Fig. 16.8) provides a lower dose rate and greater equipment flexibility while providing quality images of extremities. The mini C-arm is available with flat-panel detector fluoroscopy, rotating detectors, both full field of view and magnification modes, and a touch-screen display.

Surgical procedures have multiple imaging needs and the **O-arm** system (Fig. 16.9) can provide both static and dynamic images along with two-dimensional (2D) and three-dimensional (3D) images. Equipment movement is motor controlled, the gantry opens for easy patient access laterally, and specialized draping is used to maintain sterility when the gantry is closed. Fluoroscopic and radiographic images are obtained with flat-panel detector technology, which allows the surgeon to assess the outcome of the procedure before closing the patient.

## DEDICATED UNITS

Radiographic units designed for specific imaging procedures are classified as **dedicated units**. Although dedicated units may have limited applicability, radiographers must be familiar with these specialized radiographic systems.

### CHEST

A dedicated chest unit is designed to image the thorax in the upright position. The Bucky mechanism is attached to an x-ray tube that can be moved vertically to adjust to the height of the patient (Fig. 16.10). The image receptor is fixed and prepares the digital image receptor for the next exposure. Digital chest units send image data to a computer for processing and then display the images on a monitor. The control panel is more compact than the panel of a standard radiographic x-ray unit and displays fewer automatic preprogrammed radiographic exposure factor selections. A dedicated chest unit has limited capabilities but can image patients more quickly and efficiently. In addition, a dedicated chest unit eliminates the need for the radiographer to leave the room for image processing. These units are typically found where a very large volume of chest radiography is performed. The application of such units is to improve workflow and patient care by standardizing and simplifying a routine process (e.g., posteroanterior (PA) and lateral chest x-rays).

## PANORAMIC X-RAY

A **panoramic x-ray (panorex)** unit is designed to image curved surfaces, typically the mandible and teeth. The unit moves the x-ray tube and image receptor around the stationary patient (Fig. 16.11). The x-ray beam is well collimated to the most central portion of the beam. Long exposure times are required to achieve the desired effect. The control panel has limited milliamperage (mA) and kilovoltage peak (kVp) values available for selection. The panorex provides a high-quality image of a large surface area and is generally used for imaging of the mandible. The curved nature of this bone makes imaging difficult, and using a panorex "straightens" this bone, laying it out to appear flat on the image receptor. Although such units may have specialized application in general radiography for imaging the mandible, they are most often found in dental offices.

## BONE DENSITOMETRY

**Bone densitometry** is a specialized procedure using ionizing radiation to provide information on the condition of the skeletal bones. Bone densitometry can determine whether a patient's bone mineral density or mass is normal or low, typically for evaluation of **osteoporosis**. Osteoporosis is a bone disease in which the bones become thinner and more porous and therefore are susceptible to fractures. Because x-rays are attenuated by anatomic tissues and their attenuation can be measured, structural changes in the bones can be evaluated to assess mineral content and the density of bones.

The most common bone densitometry procedure is dual-energy x-ray absorptiometry (DXA) (Fig. 16.12). The anatomic regions are scanned with two different x-ray energies to isolate bone from soft tissue attenuation. Typically, the lower spine and hips are scanned. However, if scanning the lower spine and hips are not possible the forearm can used. The amount of x-ray photons that pass through the patient depends on the amount of bone mineral density; the denser the bone, the fewer photons are transmitted. Because bone attenuates the x-ray beam more than soft tissue, information about the condition of bone tissue can be extracted and computed.

The DXA detectors absorb the x-ray photons, process and measure the data, and then send the data to a computer for data analysis. The x-ray photons measured at both high and low energies are compared with the standards for young, healthy adults. If the data indicate there is bone mineral or density loss, the patient may be diagnosed with osteoporosis.

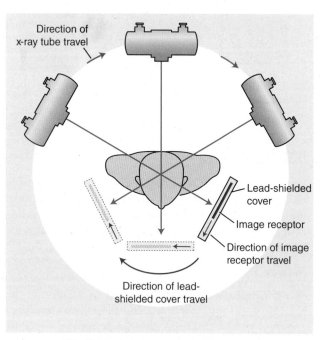

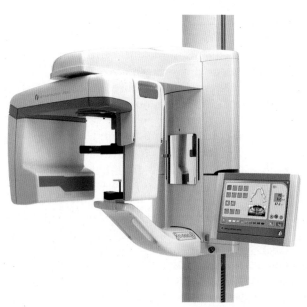

**Fig. 16.11 Panoramic X-ray Unit.** The unit moves the x-ray tube and image receptor around the stationary patient. (Courtesy Instrumentarium Dental.)

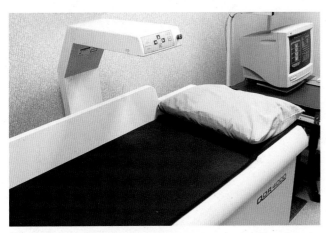

Fig. 16.12 **Bone Densitometry.** A dual-energy x-ray absorptiometry bone densitometry unit.

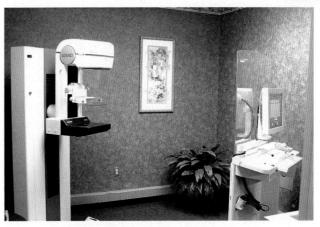

Fig. 16.13 **Mammographic Unit.** A digital mammographic unit.

Data analysis includes a T-score, which indicates the number of standard deviations the individual measurement is from the data mean for a population sample of young, healthy adults. Additionally, a Z-score compares the individual measurement with a data mean for a population of similarly aged individuals. The T-score primarily indicates fracture risk, whereas the Z-score may signify the need to evaluate the patient for secondary causes of osteoporosis.

DXA equipment and data analysis vary by manufacturer and as a result cannot be compared.

 **Critical Concept**

### Dual-Energy X-Ray Absorptiometry

The most common bone densitometry procedure is DXA. The anatomic regions, typically the lower spine and hips, are scanned with two different x-ray energies to isolate bone from soft tissue attenuation. Because bone attenuates the x-ray beam more than soft tissue, information about the structural changes in the bones can be evaluated to calculate the bone mineral density used for diagnosis of osteoporosis.

Advancements in the imaging technology to assess bone health and fracture risk include improved x-ray generators for the dual-energy x-ray production and digital detectors that increase the signal-to-noise ratio (SNR) and provide better imaging of obese patients. In addition, advanced postprocessing software can provide additional quantitative analysis from DXA scans. Newer technologies such as quantitative computed tomography (QCT) produce 3D scanning that provides more data on bone health and risk for fractures, and dedicated QCT scanners are becoming available for extremities.

Patients must be imaged using the same equipment, and positioning is critical to achieving accurate information. Radiographers and physicians must be highly skilled in achieving consistent information during bone densitometry.

## MAMMOGRAPHY

**Mammography** is a specialized radiographic imaging procedure of the breast (Fig. 16.13). Because the breast is composed of soft tissues that attenuate the x-ray beam similarly (low-subject contrast), specialized equipment and techniques must be used to best visualize its structures. There are several important features of a dedicated mammographic x-ray unit that make it uniquely qualified to image the breast tissue. In addition, exposure technique factors and imaging principles play an important role in producing quality mammograms.

### Unique Features

The fundamental principles of using ionizing radiation to image the breast are the same for mammography as in conventional imaging. However, special features of the dedicated equipment are important to achieve high-quality breast imaging. A low-kilovoltage exposure technique is necessary to image tissue having low subject contrast. A low kVp (24-34 kVp) increases the subject contrast to better visualize the similarly composed tissues of the breast. Because the kVp range for mammography is low, increased milliamperage/second (mAs) is required. Therefore, radiation exposure to the breast is increased.

Mammography uses a much lower kVp range, and therefore the mammographic x-ray tube is constructed of a different target material to produce more x-ray photons in the desired kVp range. Common mammographic target materials are molybdenum and rhodium and tungsten. At low kVp, the x-ray emission spectra from molybdenum or rhodium contain more low-energy x-rays that are better suited for breast imaging.

Operating a mammographic x-ray tube at a low kVp with the anode composed of molybdenum and rhodium provides x-ray photons with the energy levels (emission spectrum) that best visualize the breast. In addition, the tube filter is composed of molybdenum and rhodium, rhodium and silver, or just rhodium or aluminum to absorb the lowest and highest wavelengths, so the remaining x-ray energies will best visualize breast tissue. The window or exit port for the radiation is composed of beryllium, which will allow the desired longer x-ray wavelengths to exit the tube. The focal spot size needed to provide excellent spatial resolution is much smaller than conventional radiography, typically in the 0.1- to 0.3-mm range. The SID is constant and most mammography units range from 65 cm to 70 cm.

Dedicated mammography units include the use of grids, AEC devices, and digital image receptors. However, these are designed differently for imaging the breast tissue. A lower-ratio linear grid with a lower frequency is best for breast imaging. The AEC device operates similarly as in conventional radiography but must be more accurate for breast imaging in terms of reproducibility to provide consistent exposure to the image receptor (IR).

Full-field digital mammography uses image receptors similar to routine digital imaging yet require increased spatial and contrast resolution. Important advantages of digital image receptors in mammography include improved digital uniformity; improved SNR and contrast to noise ratio (CNR); and reduction of image artifacts, postprocessing capabilities, and the ability to store images in a PACS.

Dedicated mammography units have special features that allow compression and magnification of the breast. Compression of the breast makes the tissue thickness and density more uniform and reduces scatter production to improve contrast. In addition, compression places the tissue structures closer to the image receptor, which improves spatial resolution. Magnification techniques may be required to visualize small structures such as lesions or microcalcifications. The radiation dose to the breast tissue is increased during magnification techniques.

**Digital breast tomosynthesis (DBT)** is an advanced imaging technique available in many breast imaging centers. DBT is also known as 3D mammography and is similar to computed tomography (CT), discussed in Chapter 17. Although conventional 2D mammography continues to be the most common procedure for imaging the breast, it is believed that DBT improves the detection of abnormal tissue and reduces the incidence of false positives (identifying normal tissue as abnormal). Abnormal breast tissue can be superimposed by normal tissue and therefore difficult to visualize, especially for breasts classified as dense. Dense breasts have increased fibroglandular tissue compared with the amount of fatty tissue. Fat is more translucent and when imaged, easier to penetrate. The fibroglandular tissue is denser than fat and therefore more difficult to penetrate when imaged and appears opaque compared with fatty tissue.

In DBT, the x-ray tube moves over the compressed breast in an arc from one side to the other and creates multiple images of the breast from different angles

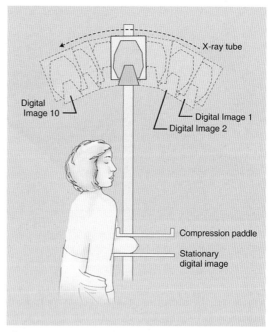

**Fig. 16.14 Digital Breast Tomosynthesis.** (Courtesy Bushong SC: *Radiologic science for technologists*, ed 11, St Louis, 2017, Mosby.)

(Fig. 16.14). These multiple images are reconstructed (synthesized) in the computer to create a set of 3D images. Like CT, the images are viewed as slices of tissue throughout the breast. These 3D images improve the ability to detect abnormal tissue superimposed with normal tissue. The angle of the arc and number of exposures vary depending on the vendor.

Because multiple images are created during 3D imaging, specialized DBT systems are needed and can vary in features, such as the length of the x-ray tube motion or tomographic angle, use of a stationary image receptor or some IR movement during the radiation exposure, and the number of images created, just to name a few. The radiation dose to the breast is slightly greater for 3D imaging compared with 2D imaging but within established limits. The specialized digital image receptors must have high detective quantum efficiency (DQE) because of the lower exposures used for each of the multiple images.

> **⚠ Critical Concepts**
>
> **Dedicated Mammography Units**
>
> Unique features of a dedicated mammography unit include the ability to produce low kVp photons by using a tube anode constructed of molybdenum and rhodium, a molybdenum- or rhodium-composed tube filter, a beryllium port window, smaller focal spot sizes for improved resolution, set SID, compression for imaging a more uniform breast, and the ability to magnify areas of the breast. DBT, also known as 3D mammography, is an advanced imaging technique available in many breast imaging centers. These 3D images improve the ability to detect abnormal tissue superimposed with normal tissue.

# LINEAR TOMOGRAPHY

A major limitation of general radiography is that 3D objects are imaged in only two dimensions. Anatomic areas of interest may be superimposed on top of one another and therefore not well visualized. **Linear tomography** is an imaging procedure using movement of the x-ray tube and image receptor in opposing directions to create images of structures in a focal plane by blurring the anatomy located above and below the plane of interest. The greater the amount of blurring of the objects above and below, the more visible is the area of interest.

Computed tomography has replaced most all the procedures that used tomography. The most common application today is in conjunction with contrast-enhanced studies of the kidneys. However, linear tomography may still be used in some imaging facilities, and the fundamentals of tomography are important to understand. Inexpensive equipment can be added to the conventional x-ray unit to perform linear tomography (Fig. 16.15). It requires a rod attached to the x-ray tube and Bucky, a motor to move the x-ray tube, and the ability to adjust the height of the area of interest either by moving the patient up or down or by changing the fulcrum (pivot point).

The basic principle of operation is that when the x-ray tube travels in an arc trajectory in one direction and the image receptor travels in the opposite direction, blurring of objects occurs above and below a fixed pivot point, or fulcrum (Fig. 16.16). Anatomic areas above and below this fixed point are less visible because of motion unsharpness or blur. Several features are important to create a quality tomographic image.

## TOMOGRAPHIC ANGLE

The **tomographic angle** is the arc created during total movement of the x-ray tube. The amount of blur created in the image is directly related to the tomographic angle. However, the thickness of the section is inversely related to the tomographic angle.

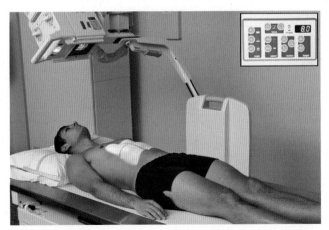

Fig. 16.15 **Linear Tomographic Unit.** (Courtesy Bontrager K: *Bontrager's textbook of radiographic positioning and techniques*, ed 8, St Louis, 2013, Mosby.)

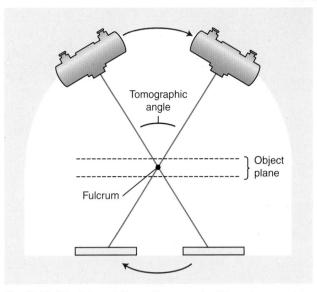

Fig. 16.16 **Principles of Linear Tomography.** When the x-ray tube travels in an arc trajectory in one direction and the image receptor travels in the opposite direction, blurring of objects occurs above and below the fulcrum.

## FULCRUM

During movement of the x-ray tube and image receptor, there is a fixed point known as the **pivot point** or **fulcrum**. The fulcrum lies within the plane of the anatomic area to be imaged. Depending on the type of tomographic system, the fulcrum can be fixed or adjustable.

### Critical Concept

**Pivot Point or Fulcrum**

During movement of the x-ray tube and image receptor, there is a fixed or pivot point that lies in the plane of interest. Depending on the type of system, the height of the fulcrum can be changed by moving the patient up and down or moving the pivot point up or down.

In a system with a fixed fulcrum, the patient is moved up or down to place the area of interest at the level of the fulcrum. In a system using an adjustable fulcrum, the patient remains fixed and the fulcrum or pivot point is moved up or down.

## FOCAL PLANE

The plane in which the area of interest lies is known as the **focal plane** or **object plane**. This plane lies at the level of the fulcrum. The structures in this plane are sharper because objects above and below are blurred as a result of the motion of the x-ray tube and image receptor. The thickness or width of the focal plane, referred to as *sections*, is determined by the tomographic angle, and they are inversely related (Fig. 16.17). The smaller the tomographic angle, the greater is the thickness of the focal plane. For a larger tomographic angle, the thickness or width of the section is decreased.

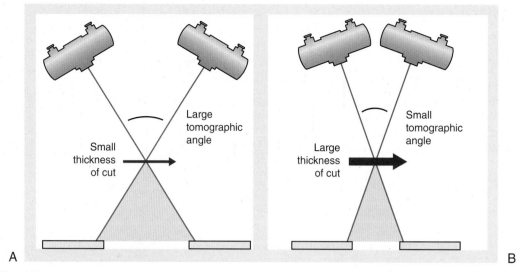

**Fig. 16.17 Focal Plane.** The thickness of a section is determined by the tomographic angle, and they are inversely related. For a larger tomographic angle, the thickness of the section is decreased **(A)**. The smaller the tomographic angle, the greater the thickness of the focal plane **(B)**.

### ! Critical Concept

#### Amplitude, Blur, and Focal Plane

The tomographic angle determines the amount of blur created in the image. Increasing the tomographic angle increases the amount of blur, and decreasing the tomographic angle decreases the amount of blur. The tomographic angle determines the thickness of the focal plane visualized. Increasing the tomographic angle decreases the thickness of the focal plane, and decreasing the tomographic angle increases the thickness of the focal plane.

## EXPOSURE TECHNIQUE

To achieve the required blurring during tomography, the exposure time must be increased. An exposure time that is too short does not allow for complete blurring, and an exposure time that is too long causes unnecessary exposure to the patient. A low mA should be selected to allow for the necessary increase in exposure time. The kVp is still selected based on the region of interest. Overall, patients receive increased radiation exposure during tomographic procedures. Proper shielding, restricting the field size, and minimizing repeats are important considerations in minimizing patient dose during tomography.

Because the x-ray tube and image receptor move in only one direction during linear tomography, it has limitations. The tomographic angle has a limited range of movement, and this affects the ability to obtain a thin focal plane. To achieve maximum blurring, the area of interest should be perpendicular to the direction of the movement. Linear tomography results in structures imaged that are parallel to the motion and therefore are distorted by elongation, which can appear as streaks. Before the use of CT, different types of motions, such

as hypocycloidal, circular, and elliptical, were used to overcome the limitations of linear tomography.

### On the Spot

- Fluoroscopic units used in interventional radiology have unique features such as biplane technology for image-guided therapy procedures. Digital subtraction techniques are used to improve visualization of the contrast-filled vessels and to assist in maneuvering the catheter or wire into tortuous vessels.
- Mobile radiographic and fluoroscopic units may be used to image patients when they are unable to travel to the radiology department. Radiation output may be more variable for mobile units.
- Dedicated units, such as chest, panorex, bone densitometry, and mammography, are types of imaging equipment designed for specific purposes and anatomic regions.
- During bone densitometry, the lower spine and hips are scanned with two different x-ray energy levels to isolate bone from soft tissue attenuation. Because bone attenuates the x-ray beam more than soft tissue, information about the structural changes in the bones can be evaluated to calculate bone mineral density, which aids the diagnosis of osteoporosis.
- Because the breast is a low subject-contrast tissue, a low kVp (22–28 kVp) is needed to visualize the similarly composed structures. Mammographic x-ray tubes are constructed to produce x-ray photons with low energy to increase contrast resolution. The focal spot sizes are 0.1 to 0.3 mm to increase spatial resolution.
- Compression of the breast is necessary during mammography to make the thickness and exposure to the IR more uniform, decrease scatter production, and increase spatial resolution.
- Digital breast tomosynthesis (DBT) is 3D imaging of the breast that improves visualization of abnormal tissue

superimposed by normal tissue. Multiple low-dose images are created as the x-ray tube moves across the breast. The images are reconstructed or synthesized by the computer to create a series of image slices throughout the breast.

- Linear tomography is an imaging technique used to blur anatomy located above and below the area of interest.
- The tomographic angle is directly related to the amount of blurring and is inversely related to the thickness of the focal plane.
- The height of the pivot point or fulcrum is adjusted to be located within the plane of interest.

## CRITICAL THINKING QUESTIONS

1. Why is a variety of specialized imaging equipment necessary in diagnostic radiology?
2. How is exposure technique selection affected when using specialized imaging equipment?

## REVIEW QUESTIONS

1. Which of the following creates images of an anatomic area within a plane while blurring structures above and below?
   a. Panorex
   b. DXA
   c. C-arm fluoroscopy
   d. Linear tomography
2. What type of mobile x-ray generator produces the least consistent radiation output?
   a. High frequency
   b. Direct power
   c. Battery power
   d. Capacitor discharge
3. What is an advantage of C-arm fluoroscopy compared with traditional image-intensified fluoroscopy in a standard x-ray room?
   a. The x-ray tube can be positioned under the patient.
   b. It provides dynamic imaging.
   c. It monitors total fluoroscopy time.
   d. It allows imaging in a variety of planes.
4. What disease process can be evaluated using bone densitometry?
   a. Atelectasis
   b. Osteoporosis
   c. Myeloma
   d. Ascites
5. In mammography, because the breast has _____ subject contrast, it is necessary to use a _____ kilovoltage exposure technique.
   a. high, high
   b. low, high
   c. high, low
   d. low, low

6. During DXA scanning, the T-score indicates the number of standard deviations the individual measurement is from the data mean for a population sample of _____.
   a. similarly aged individuals
   b. a wide range of age groups
   c. young healthy adults
   d. older healthy adults
7. What anatomic area is typically imaged with a panoramic x-ray unit?
   a. Mandible
   b. Chest
   c. Breast
   d. Kidneys
8. What feature of a dedicated mammographic unit will even out the breast tissue thickness?
   a. Molybdenum anode
   b. Compression
   c. AEC
   d. Lower ratio grid
9. Which of the following is a specialized procedure that produces a series of 3-D images to better visualize abnormal tissue superimposed by normal tissue?
   a. Digital subtraction
   b. Mini C-arm
   c. Digital breast tomosynthesis
   d. Panorex
10. During linear tomography, the amount of blur created in the image is directly related to the:
    a. pivot point.
    b. object plane.
    c. tomographic angle.
    d. length of exposure time.
11. During linear tomography, a smaller tomographic angle will create:
    a. increased amount of blur.
    b. decreased focal plane thickness.
    c. increased focal plane thickness.
    d. no change in amount of blur.
12. What technique creates an image mask of maximum contrast-filled vasculature for subtraction to assist in maneuvering a catheter or wire through a tortuous vessel?
    a. O-arm
    b. Digital breast tomosynthesis
    c. Linear tomography
    d. Road mapping

## Outline

## Objectives

- Identify the major developments in computed tomography (CT) technology, including the five generations of CT equipment, spiral CT, and multislice CT, and explain their effect on CT imaging.
- Describe the components of the CT imaging system and explain their functions.
- Differentiate between raw and image data.
- Identify the characteristics of the CT image, including *matrix*, *pixel*, and *voxel*.
- Describe the reconstruction process, following the conversion of raw data to image data.
- Differentiate between linear attenuation coefficients and CT numbers.
- Based on the Hounsfield scale, identify the CT numbers associated with water, air, and bone.
- Identify equipment associated with CT studies.
- Describe factors that are set within an examination protocol.

- Describe common postprocessing methods.
- Explain how window width (WW) and window level (WL) settings determine which pixels in the CT image will be white, black, or a shade of gray.
- Explain how WW and WL settings affect the image contrast and brightness.
- Describe CT image quality characteristics; identify how image settings affect the quality and their associated trade-offs.
- Identify artifacts associated with CT imaging and explain how they can be reduced or eliminated.
- Identify CT quality-control tests and their purpose.
- Discuss how radiation protection can be practiced for CT imaging, including methods for protecting the patient and others remaining in the room.
- Describe dose notifications and alerts and when they may be used in clinical practice.

## Key Terms

adaptive statistical iterative reconstruction (ASIR)

algorithm

annotation

array processor

artificial intelligence (AI)

automatic tube current modulation (ATCM)

beam-hardening artifact

bowtie filter

cone beam

contrast resolution

CT Dose Index in a volume (CTDI$_{vol}$)

CT number

CT table

data acquisition system (DAS)

deep learning (DL)

deep learning reconstruction (DLR)

detector array

display field of view (DFOV)

dose alert value

dose descriptor

dose length product (DLP)

dose notification value

dose optimization

dose report

edge-enhancement filter

electron-beam computed tomography (EBCT)

fan-beam geometry

filtered back projection (FBP)

gantry

generations

Hounsfield unit

image data

linear attenuation coefficient

machine learning (ML)

matrix

multiplanar reformation (MPR)

## Key Terms—cont'd

| | | |
|---|---|---|
| multiple scan average dose (MSAD) | profile | spatial resolution |
| multislice computed tomography (MSCT) | quantum noise | spiral (helical) CT |
| | raw data | streak artifact |
| partial-volume artifact | rays | view |
| photon-counting computed tomography (PCCT) | region of interest (ROI) | voxel |
| | ring artifact | voxel volume |
| pitch | scan field of view (SFOV) | windowing |
| pixel | scintillation-type detector | window level (WL) |
| postpatient collimator | slip-ring technology | window width (WW) |
| prepatient collimator | smoothing filter | Z-axis |

## INTRODUCTION

**Computed tomography (CT)** is an imaging modality that uses an x-ray beam, computer, and equipment configuration to allow cross-sectional images of the body. Introduced in the early 1970s, CT quickly revolutionized the field of medical imaging. Taking advantage of the development of faster and more powerful computers, CT combines a tightly collimated x-ray beam and detectors that rotate around the patient. X-ray transmission values are measured multiple times as the tube circles the patient, and signal data are digitized and sent to the computer (Fig. 17.1). Following a large number of calculations, a cross-sectional axial image is reconstructed and displayed. Not only does the resulting image demonstrate minimal superimposition of anatomic structures, but also the image data are based on the attenuation characteristics of the anatomy being imaged, and the image display can be adjusted to distinguish tissues that have x-ray attenuations that differ only slightly (Fig. 17.2).

A little more than 40 years later, today's CT imaging process is extremely fast and produces images with remarkable detail, not only in transverse (head-to-foot) slices but also reformatted in coronal (front-to-back), sagittal (side-to-side), and three-dimensional images. CT studies of the head, chest, abdomen, and pelvis are now routine in every aspect of health care, including the emergency department, outpatient, and inpatient imaging. CT is used to enhance positron emission tomography (PET) and single-photon emission computed tomography (SPECT) nuclear medicine studies. CT is also the mainstay of radiation therapy treatment planning. Although CT continues to expand its role in medicine, it is not without drawbacks. Patient radiation dose, especially to children, is an important issue that must continually be addressed. For these reasons, radiographers must have a basic understanding of how CT works and its advantages and issues.

## DEVELOPMENT

In the early 1970s, Godfrey Hounsfield, using mathematic formulas developed by Alan Cormack in the

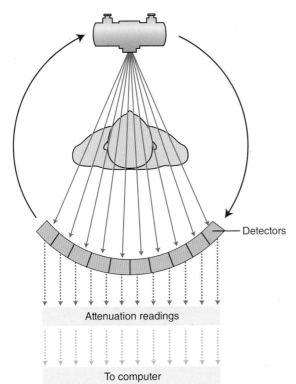

**Fig. 17.1 Computed Tomography Process.** As the x-ray tube and detectors rotate around the patient, the detectors measure the exit radiation multiple times, and the digitized attenuation readings data are sent to the computer.

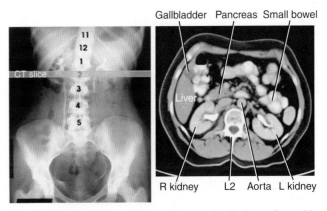

**Fig. 17.2 Cross-Sectional Slice.** Compared with the radiographic image *(left)*, the computed tomography image is able to visualize abdominal organs and structures that are more similar in tissue density. (Courtesy Bontrager KL, Lampignano JP: *Textbook of radiographic positioning and related anatomy*, ed 7, St Louis, 2010, Mosby.)

1960s, demonstrated the first CT scanner. Hounsfield's and Cormack's work in developing CT was recognized in 1979 with the Nobel Prize in Physiology or Medicine. Today's CT scanner looks significantly different from the original. The major developments in x-ray beam and detector geometry are called **generations**. Beyond these generations, additional developments have had a great influence on CT imaging. All CT systems involve an x-ray tube and detector or detectors located inside a structure called the **gantry**, which surrounds the patient. Especially for the first three generations of CT scanners, developments resulted in significant reductions in scan time.

## GENERATIONS

The first two generations of CT scanners are considered "translate-rotate" types because the x-ray beam was not wide enough to cover the entire anatomy being imaged. As seen in Fig. 17.3A, first-generation scanners had a pencil-thick x-ray beam and a single detector. The only anatomy that could be imaged was the head because it took approximately 5 minutes to collect the transmission data for one slice. While energized, the x-ray beam and detector had to travel across (translate) the head before it could rotate 1 degree and repeat the process. The x-ray beam was pulsed on and off as it moved across the head, and the transmission data were collected with parallel-beam geometry. All subsequent CT generations use **fan-beam geometry**. Second-generation CT scanners (Fig. 17.3B) had a small fan beam and detector array. The unit had only approximately 30 detectors, and the fan beam was still not wide enough to cover the anatomy, so translation was still required. However, because more anatomy was imaged at one time, the process had to be repeated only approximately 18 times. Scan time was significantly reduced to approximately 30 seconds.

Third- and fourth-generation CT scanners eliminate the need to translate because the fan beam is widened to cover any anatomic area. Both systems collect the data for one slice very quickly, in approximately 1 second or less. The major difference between the third- and fourth-generation scanners is in the detector array. Third-generation scanners (Fig. 17.3C) have a curved array of hundreds of detectors, which are located opposite the x-ray tube and rotate as the tube rotates and pulses. Fourth-generation scanners (Fig. 17.3D) have thousands of fixed detectors in a ring inside the

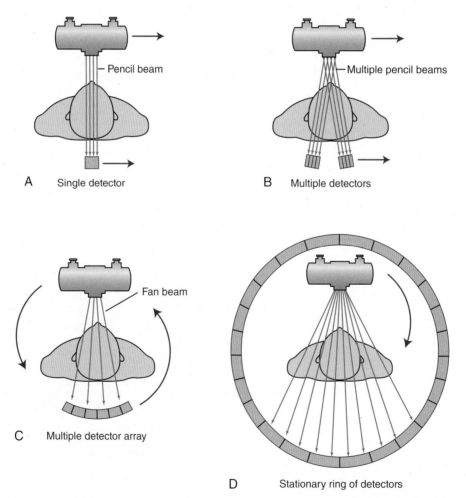

A    Single detector        Pencil beam

B    Multiple detectors        Multiple pencil beams

C    Multiple detector array        Fan beam

D    Stationary ring of detectors

**Fig. 17.3 Generations I-IV.** The first four generations of computed tomography scanning methods (first generation **[A]**, second generation **[B]**, third generation **[C]**, and fourth generation **[D]**) demonstrate how changes in the tube movement and detector configuration have evolved.

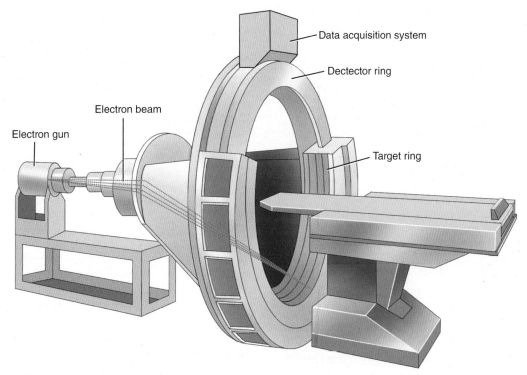

**Fig. 17.4 Electron-Beam Computed Tomography.** Considered by many to be the fifth generation of computed tomography scanners, electron-beam computed tomography uses an electron gun and tungsten arcs to allow very quick imaging times.

gantry. The tube rotates while continuously emitting radiation, but the detectors do not rotate. The primary advantage of the fourth-generation scanner is that it overcomes a specific third-generation artifact. However, most scanners in use today are based on third-generation technology.

Many consider the **electron-beam computed tomography (EBCT)** scanner to be the fifth generation (Fig. 17.4). Developed for cardiac imaging, the EBCT reduces scan time to as little as 50 ms, fast enough to image the beating heart. EBCT does not use an x-ray tube; instead, it uses a beam of electrons generated outside the gantry. Inside the gantry there are 180-degree rows of fixed detectors on one side and 180 degrees of tungsten arcs opposite. The electron beam is rapidly moved to bombard the tungsten arcs, producing an x-ray beam. The x-rays then pass through the patient, and transmission information is collected by the detectors. These units are very fast because they have no moving parts. For a number of years, they were the only scanners fast enough for cardiac imaging. However, two additional developments resulted in significant scan time reduction and minimized the use of EBCTs.

> ## ! Critical Concept
>
> ### Computed Tomography Generations
>
> CT generations represent advances in the operation of the x-ray tube and detectors, primarily to reduce scan time.

## ADDITIONAL ADVANCEMENTS

Spiral (helical) and multislice (multidetector) CT developments have had such a dramatic effect on reducing scan time and improving image quality that they are standard on modern CT units. Before the late 1980s, conventional CT studies were done in slice-by-slice mode. The patient was placed on the table and moved a certain amount into the bore of the gantry. The pulsing x-ray tube and detectors rotated 360 degrees, collecting data. Once complete, the patient and table were moved incrementally into the scanner, and the tube was rewound into its original position. The process was repeated for each slice of the procedure. In the late 1980s, CT scanners with **slip-ring technology** were introduced. Located inside the gantry, the slip-ring technology allowed the tube to continue to rotate without the need to rewind. Continuous rotation of the tube (and detectors) coupled with continuous movement of the table and patient through the gantry are the basic components of **spiral (helical) CT** (Fig. 17.5). Instead of collecting data one slice at a time, spiral CT collects the data for an entire volume of tissue (such as the head or chest) at one time. Scan time is reduced because the start and stop time of the slice-by-slice scanner is eliminated.

Another major development in CT technology is **multislice computed tomography (MSCT)**, which is used in conjunction with spiral imaging (Fig. 17.6). Instead of collecting the transmission data for one slice each time the tube rotates around the patient, MSCT collects data

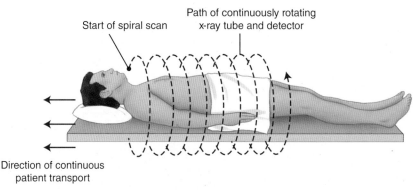

Start of spiral scan

Path of continuously rotating x-ray tube and detector

Direction of continuous patient transport

Fig. 17.5 **Spiral Computed Tomography.** As the patient moves smoothly through the gantry aperture (along the Z-axis), the tube and detectors continuously travel around the patient, creating a spiral path.

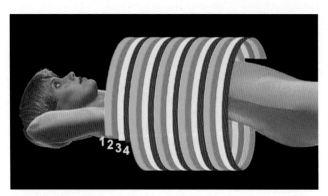

Fig. 17.6 **Multislice Spiral Computed Tomography.** In addition to the spiral method for collecting computed tomography data, having multiple rows of detectors results in four (shown here) or more slices being imaged during each revolution of the tube. (Courtesy Philips Medical Systems.)

for 4 to 320+ slices per revolution. This is accomplished by opening up the x-ray beam along the **Z-axis** (direction from head to foot) and having a detector array with 4 to 320+ rows. The number of detector rows equals the number of slices per revolution. As the number of slices being imaged per revolution increases and the x-ray beam is opened, it goes from being a fan beam to a **cone beam**. As the cone beam increases in size, the divergence of the x-rays results in increased distortion toward the top and bottom edges. However, spiral MSCT allows overall improved image quality with faster scan time and the ability to perform additional procedures such as CT angiography and cardiac imaging. Radiation dose is inversely proportional to the number of detector rows in MSCT; as the number of detector rows increases, the dose decreases because fewer rotations are needed to cover the anatomy of interest.

 **Critical Concept**

**Modern Scanners**

Today's CT system is typically a third-generation, multislice spiral scanner.

Dual-source CT (DSCT) units are advanced third-generation systems complete with two sets of tube-detector pairs. The dual acquisition systems are mounted 90 degrees apart along the rotating gantry, with one tube for high-kVp and one tube for low-kVp images. The DSCT system is known for quicker scan time and less patient dose because of its design. DSCT also has a better ability to differentiate between tissues than standard CT and is therefore receiving more clinical attention.

**Photon-counting computed tomography (PCCT)** introduces a significant advancement in CT technology. PCCT produces images with improved contrast resolution, signal-to-noise ratio, and enhanced spatial resolution (Fig. 17.7) without increasing patient dose. Whereas conventional CT scanners calculate incoming photons as a collective energy bundle measured over a given timeframe (Fig. 17.8), PCCT employs detectors that measure the charge of individual photons, eliminating the light generation phase typical of scintillation detectors (Fig. 17.9). This direct conversion from x-ray photon to electric signal increases measurement speed to a few nanoseconds from 10,000 or more for a traditional detector. The result is the measurement of the charge of each individual photon in a projection. When photon-counting technology is integrated into a CT system, this provides spectral sensitivity signal known as photon counting. The resulting images have superior detail without increasing patient dose.

As new technologies continue to be developed, improvements in image quality with reductions in scan time are the goal, as is reduced patient dose.

## IMAGE DATA PRODUCTION

A CT scanning system includes the scanning unit, the operator's console, and the computer. The major components of the scanning unit are the gantry and **CT table**, or couch (Fig. 17.10). The gantry contains the equipment that produces the data for image formation. It can be tilted and includes laser beams to determine whether the patient is accurately located in the aperture (opening) of the gantry. The CT tabletop may be flat or curved and can be raised and lowered to help the patient get on and off. It has a wide range of horizontal movement, allowing the patient to easily move

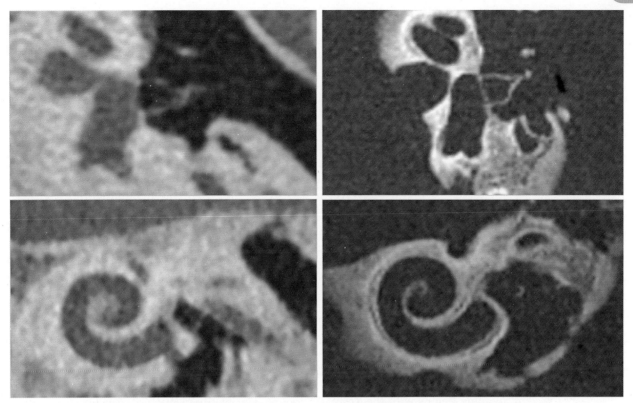

**Fig. 17.7  Improved Visualization of the Middle and Inner Ear Enabled With Photon-Counting CT.** Tiny anatomical structures of the middle and inner ear (upper row: stapes, lower row: cochlea): On the left, an image acquired with conventional CT technology; on the right, with a photon-counting CT. (Courtesy of Siemens Healthineers AG.)

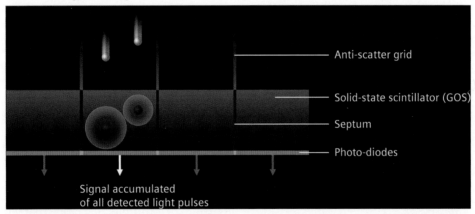

**Fig. 17.8  Functionality of a Conventional Detector.** X-rays are first converted into visible light, then detected by a photodiode. In this two-step process, the energy information, contained in the x-ray photons is lost. (Courtesy of Siemens Healthineers AG.)

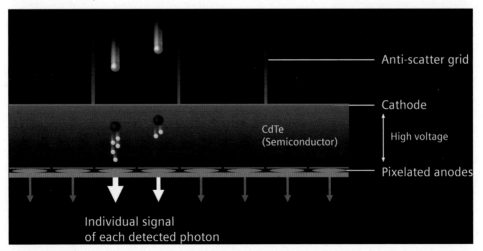

**Fig. 17.9  Functionality of a Photon-Counting Detector.** A semiconductor transforms x-rays directly to electric signals, which can be evaluated without loss of any important information. (Courtesy of Siemens Healthineers AG.)

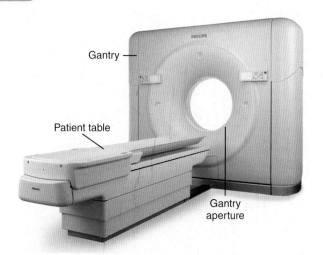

Fig. 17.10 **Computed Tomography Scanner.** The gantry, gantry aperture, and patient or computed tomography table or couch are seen here. (Courtesy Philips Medical Systems.)

through the gantry during the scan. Table movement during scanning is controlled by the protocol set at the operator's console.

The actual process of producing a CT image of a cross-sectional slice of anatomy begins with the x-ray tube and ends with a matrix of CT numbers that represent the attenuation characteristics of the anatomy being imaged. Between the two are found a generator, a filter, collimators, detectors, the data acquisition system (DAS), and the computer. Other than the computer, all are found in the CT gantry (Fig. 17.11). Together, they produce image data that can then be manipulated to demonstrate a wide spectrum of tissues.

The x-ray tube used in CT imaging is a modification of the standard tube. Because the tube is continuously pulsing and exposures are fairly lengthy, the anode must be able to withstand large amounts of heat. This is accomplished by using a larger-diameter anode that rotates very rapidly. Today's scanners use a high-frequency generator to supply electricity to the tube. With its electric current having minimal voltage ripple,

the high-frequency generator allows the production of an x-ray beam with fairly consistent energy levels. This results in more accurate, improved-quality CT data.

In addition to using a high-frequency generator, to have a high-energy x-ray beam that is as consistent as possible, the beam must be filtered. Similar to the filtration in a standard x-ray tube, placing a filter in the path of the beam attenuates lower-energy x-ray photons, resulting in an x-ray beam with a higher percentage of high-energy photons. The filter frequently used in CT is a **bowtie filter** (Fig. 17.12). Named after its shape, the bowtie filter is thinner in the center and thicker toward the periphery, where patient attenuation is less. The shape and composition of the filter creates a more uniform beam at the detectors.

Two sets of collimators serve different purposes in CT image production. The first, similar to radiography, is to limit patient exposure and reduce the amount of scatter radiation produced in the patient. This is accomplished by the **prepatient collimator**, located between the tube and patient, which limits the beam to a fan or cone shape. After the x-ray beam passes through the patient, it passes through the **postpatient collimator**, located just before the detector array. This collimator controls how much of the detector is exposed (Fig. 17.13). For single-slice CT, it controls slice thickness, whereas for MSCT it controls how many rows of detectors are being used. This collimator severely limits the amount of scatter radiation reaching the detectors, resulting in improved image contrast.

> **!  Critical Concept**
> **Collimators**
> CT uses two collimators: prepatient and postpatient. These collimators significantly reduce the amount of scatter radiation produced and that reaches the detectors, improving contrast resolution.

The **detector array** is the physical component, consisting of multiple detectors that efficiently absorbs the transmitted radiation and accurately converts it to an electrical signal. Each pulse of the tube as it rotates around the patient produces a **view**, a snapshot of all the transmission measurements from that

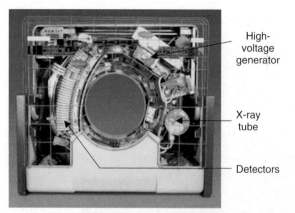

Fig. 17.11 **Inside Gantry.** Removing the computed tomography gantry cover reveals the generator, tube, and detector array. (Courtesy Philips Medical Systems.)

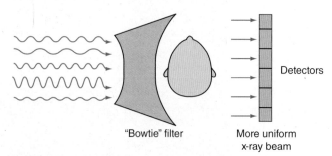

Fig. 17.12 **Bowtie Filter.** The bowtie filter removes longer-wavelength x-ray photons, resulting in more consistent energy photons reaching the detectors.

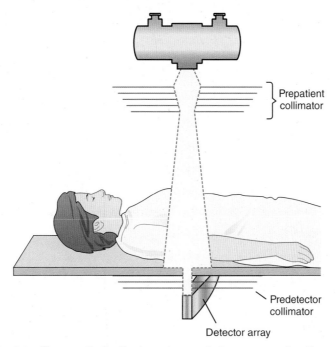

**Fig. 17.13 Collimators.** The prepatient collimator reduces patient exposure and scatter production, whereas the predetector collimator determines how much of the detector is exposed, reducing the amount of scatter contributing to the image.

location. The view is composed of **rays**, which are the parts of the x-ray beam that fall on one detector. The transmission measurement for an individual detector and the composite electrical signal may be referred to as a **profile**. Today's CT scanners use a **scintillation-type detector** coupled with a photodiode. Typically made of cadmium tungstate or a ceramic material, the scintillation detector absorbs the transmitted radiation and produces a proportional flash of light. The photodiode is a solid-state device that converts the light to a proportional electrical signal. Use of this type of detector and photodiode results in the ability to have many small detectors packed tightly together, improving the quality of the CT image. A 64-slice CT scanner has a detector array of 64 rows of 1000+ detectors (Fig. 17.14).

The last component found in the gantry is the **data acquisition system (DAS)**. The electrical signal produced by the detector-photodiode goes immediately to the DAS, which amplifies this weak signal, converts it to logarithmic data, converts it from analog to digital data, and sends it to the computer (Fig. 17.15). The logarithmic conversion of the measured electrical signal is critical to CT imaging. By knowing the original x-ray beam intensity, the intensity of the transmitted radiation (as measured by the detector), and the thickness of the part, logarithmic conversion produces attenuation information. More accurately known as the *linear attenuation coefficient* and symbolized by the Greek letter μ (mu), this information is the basic building block of the CT image. The **linear attenuation coefficient** is a measure of the probability that the x-ray beam will interact with the material it is in while traveling in a

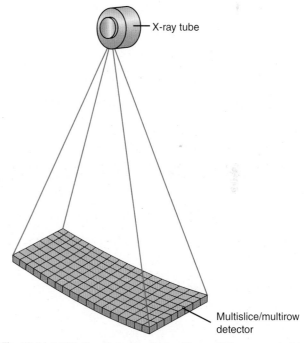

**Fig. 17.14 Multislice Detector Array.** The multislice computed tomography detector array has multiple rows of detectors, collecting data for multiple slices every tube rotation.

straight path. This value is based on both the characteristics of the material and the energy of the x-ray photons. These logarithmic data are then converted from analog (continuous) to digital (discrete) information by the analog-to-digital converter (ADC); leaving the gantry, these **raw data** are sent to the computer for image reconstruction.

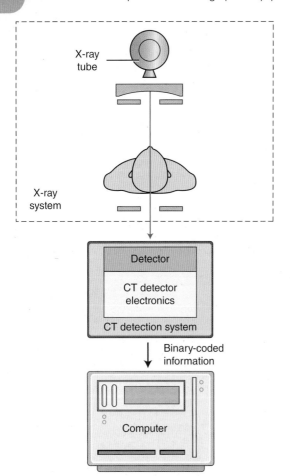

Fig. 17.15 **Raw Data.** The data acquisition system (DAS), located immediately after the detectors (in the middle section of the diagram), amplifies the electronic signal, converts it to logarithmic data, and sends it to the computer.

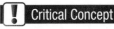

**Raw Data**

Raw data, the very large number of calculated linear attenuation coefficients of the tissue being scanned, are the basis for the CT image.

## IMAGE RECONSTRUCTION

### COMPUTED TOMOGRAPHY IMAGE CHARACTERISTICS

Similar to a digital radiographic image, the CT image can be described by a **matrix**, the number of rows and columns that make up the image. A CT image may be 512 rows × 512 columns or 1024 × 1024. Interestingly, the CT image matrix is typically smaller than the matrix for digital radiography because of the difference in the type of data used. The smallest component of the matrix and digital image is the **pixel** (picture element). In CT, each pixel is assigned a CT number, representing the attenuation characteristics of the anatomy found in the **voxel** (volume element). The voxel, determined by the size of the pixel and the thickness of

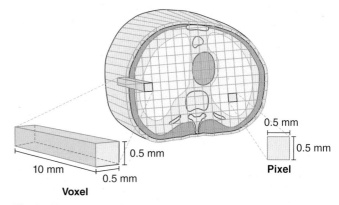

Fig. 17.16 **Pixel and Voxel.** The pixel is the smallest element of the matrix that makes up the computed tomography image. It is the two-dimensional representation of the smallest volume of tissue (voxel) of the slice being scanned.

the slice, is the actual small amount of tissue that will be represented by one pixel (Fig. 17.16). The dimensions of this small piece of tissue, the **voxel volume**, have a significant effect on image quality.

### RECONSTRUCTION PROCESS

The primary role of the CT computer is to analyze the enormous amount of raw data sent from the DAS and reconstruct it into a digital array of CT numbers (**image data**) based on the image matrix. The computer must be very fast and powerful to perform a multitude of simultaneous calculations. Many CT computers include an **array processor**, a component dedicated to performing these calculations needed for image reconstruction.

The computer takes the raw data from the DAS and, using algorithms, changes it into image data. An **algorithm** is a sequence of computer operations for accomplishing a specific task; for CT the reconstruction algorithm is key. A common reconstruction algorithm used in modern CT is **filtered back projection (FBP)** (using a computer or electronic filter). The computer must analyze all of the data for one slice of the area being imaged to determine the attenuation coefficient ($\mu$) for each voxel. Each voxel's $\mu$ is then mathematically converted to a CT number. Building on the FBP algorithm is the **adaptive statistical iterative reconstruction (ASIR)** technique. Adaptive statistical iterative reconstruction starts reconstruction after a first-pass FBP reconstruction and shortens reconstruction time while maintaining much lower image noise than if the same raw data were reconstructed with FBP alone. ASIR reduces quantum noise substantially with no effect on spatial or contrast resolution. However, FBP and ASIR are not without limitations. FBP produces images relatively quickly but requires well-conditioned, high-dose images. ASIR, on the other hand, requires far less dose than FBP but takes significantly longer. This led to research on ways to create high-quality, low-dose images at a rapid rate of speed.

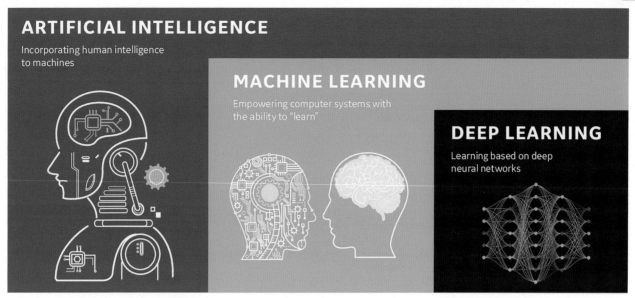

Fig. 17.17 **Artificial Intelligence.** Artificial intelligence encompasses both machine learning and deep learning. Deep learning, a subset of machine learning, uses deep neural networks to greatly enhance its accuracy.

Looking to combine the image quality and speed of FBP and ASIR, **artificial intelligence (AI)** has been integrated into the CT reconstruction process through **Machine Learning (ML)**, or more precisely, **Deep Learning (DL)** (Fig. 17.17). **Deep Learning Reconstruction (DLR)** or Deep Learning Image Reconstruction (DLIR) is a recent technological innovation that promises to transform the reconstructive process in CT imaging. DLR works on algorithms created by Convolutional Neural Networks (CNN) and Artificial Neural Networks (ANN) in image reconstruction to enhance image quality and reduce noise, thereby reducing patient dose. The CNN undergoes extensive training by comparing complex scan patterns to large datasets of pairs of low-dose and standard-dose scans. The ANN, modeled after the intricate layers of the human brain, comprises hundreds of interconnected artificial neurons that improve image reconstruction algorithms. DLR uses the information to reconstruct low-dose images with greater detail and less noise rapidly, overcoming common limitations of FBP and ASIR. The resulting images display increased clarity and detail with reduced image noise without increasing the dose to the patient.

 **Critical Concept**

**Image Reconstruction**

Image reconstruction uses the raw data from all the detected x-ray transmissions for one slice and, using the filtered back projection algorithm, calculates the linear attenuation coefficient for each voxel in the slice.

Often referred to as **Hounsfield units**, the **CT number** is related to the attenuation characteristic of the tissue in the voxel, but it is not an attenuation coefficient. By using a formula that relates the attenuation coefficient of the tissue to the attenuation coefficient of water, the CT number of water is set at zero (0).

$$\text{Hounsfield Unit} = \frac{(\mu X - \mu \,\text{Water}) \times 1000}{(\mu \,\text{Water} - \mu \,\text{Air})}$$

$\mu$ = linear attenuation coefficient

X = tissue

Any material that attenuates more x-ray photons than water has a positive CT number, and any material that attenuates fewer x-ray photons than water has a negative CT number. The Hounsfield scale provides for 2000 different CT numbers, with water being 0, bone being approximately +1000 (appearing white), and air being −1000 (appearing black) (Fig. 17.18). The end result of reconstruction is a matrix of CT numbers, the image data (Fig. 17.19).

 **Critical Concept**

**Computed Tomography Numbers**

Based on the linear attenuation coefficient, the CT number of water is mathematically calculated to be 0. All tissues with greater attenuation than water have CT numbers greater than 0, and all tissues with less attenuation than water have CT numbers less than 0.

 **Critical Concept**

**Image Data**

Image data is the matrix of CT numbers, each representing the attenuation characteristics of the tissue contained in the voxel. Although CT numbers can be assigned any shade of gray (including black or white) in the displayed image, the image data never changes.

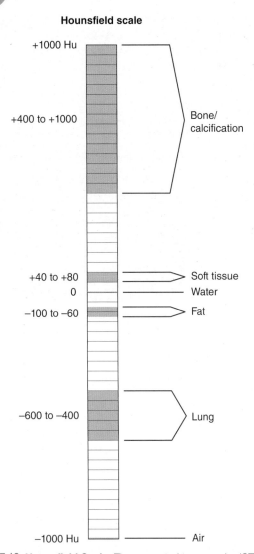

**Hounsfield scale**

+1000 Hu

+400 to +1000 — Bone/calcification

+40 to +80 — Soft tissue
0 — Water
−100 to −60 — Fat

−600 to −400 — Lung

−1000 Hu — Air

**Fig. 17.18 Hounsfield Scale.** The computed tomography (CT) numbers for a variety of tissues are identified. Based on the Hounsfield scale (±1000), note the similarity of the CT numbers of many of these tissues, slightly greater than water (0 Hounsfield units).

## IMAGING CONTROLS AND DATA STORAGE

### EQUIPMENT

The CT technologist is responsible for setting the parameters of the examination and ensuring that the study is properly saved and archived. Controls are found primarily at the operator's console but may also be found in the examination room on the gantry. Using a keyboard, mouse, and multiple monitors, the technologist selects the appropriate protocol for the requested examination and completes the scanning process (Fig. 17.20). Often the procedure involves the intravenous injection of iodinated contrast; setup then includes the operation of a power injector. The power injector allows for the injection of contrast at a specified time during the study and at a specific rate. Once the reconstructed images are displayed with shades of gray assigned to the CT numbers (based on the window settings), the technologist evaluates image quality and manipulates the image to enhance visibility of key information. Data from completed CT studies can

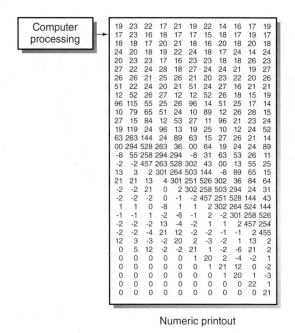

Computer processing →

Numeric printout

**Fig. 17.19 Image Data.** Image data consist of the computed tomography numbers (Hounsfield units) that have been calculated and assigned to the pixels of the image matrix. (Courtesy Seeram E: *Computed tomography*, ed 3, Philadelphia, 2009, Saunders.)

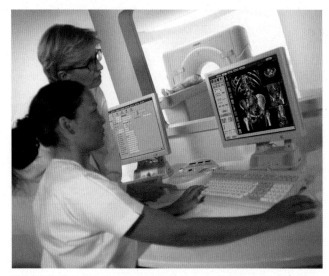

**Fig. 17.20 Operator's Console.** The operator's console includes keyboard, mouse, and multiple monitors. (Courtesy Philips Medical Systems.)

be temporarily stored on the local computer's hard drive and on large-capacity external devices for long-term storage. The technologist is responsible for accurately sending the completed studies to the picture archiving and communication system (PACS) for interpretation by the radiologist and for archiving.

### PROTOCOLS

Imaging protocols are available for many studies and include predetermined imaging settings. There may also be situations when the radiologist will need the technologist to change a protocol in response to a change in patient condition, result of a biopsy, or other recommended reason. Therefore, the technologist should be aware of what elements are involved in creating the protocol for the examination. Some of the parameters included in a protocol include milliamperage (mA), kilovolt peak (kVp), and focal spot size, similar to radiographic imaging. In addition, the CT protocol addresses slice thickness, image matrix size, **scan field of view (SFOV)**, and **display field of view (DFOV)**. The SFOV determines the actual anatomic area of interest as set by the technologist and imaged during the examination, whereas the DFOV setting controls the area of anatomy seen on the monitor. The DFOV cannot exceed the SFOV, but a DFOV that is less than the SFOV results in a magnified image.

Additional settings include scan time and image display. Scan time is affected by how fast the tube completes a 360-degree rotation and how much the tube is energized, as well as the pitch. Systems with faster tube rotation produce an image in less time, as will systems that can be set to have the tube energized and collect data during only a portion of the tube revolution (for example, a half-scan during which the tube is on and data collected over 180 degrees of the rotational arc). With spiral CT, when imaging one slice per rotation, **pitch** identifies the relationship between slice thickness and the distance the table travels every time the tube rotates (Fig. 17.21). MSCT pitch relates the beam collimation (which includes a number of slices) to the distance the table travels per rotation. Pitch ranges from 0.5 to 2. A pitch of 1 means that during each tube rotation, the table is moving the same distance as the slice thickness and collimation. A pitch greater than 1 indicates the table is moving farther than the slice thickness and collimation, resulting in a faster scan. A pitch less than 1 results in the table moving less distance than the slice thickness and collimation, so the scan takes longer and has overlapping slices. The slice overlap will also result in an increase in radiation dose. Examination protocols may also include (electronic) reconstruction filters such as edge enhancement or smoothing, and display windows such as bone or lung. Generally speaking, protocols are standardized settings but may need to be assessed and adjusted based on the individual patient.

## POSTPROCESSING

### MULTIPLE OPTIONS

Once the image data (the matrix of CT numbers) have been produced through reconstruction, postprocessing techniques allow adjustments to the image to provide additional information or allow different anatomy to be made visible. Additional information may include adding a printed comment or label to the image (**annotation**), image magnification, or selection of a **region of interest (ROI)** for statistical analysis. Using a DFOV smaller than the SFOV results in a magnified image.

**Multiplanar reformation (MPR)** can be done by the computer to display the image data in coronal, sagittal, or oblique planes (Fig. 17.22). Reformatting differs

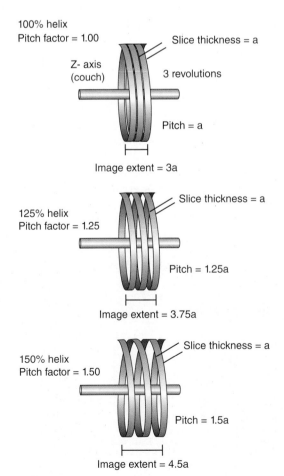

**Fig. 17.21 Pitch.** The slice thickness remains unchanged, and increasing the pitch increases the amount of tissue imaged or decreases the scan time.

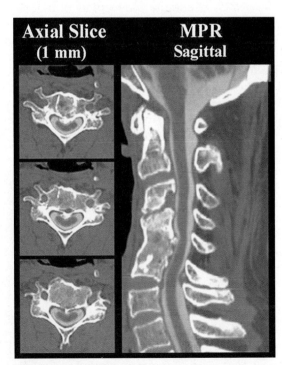

**Fig. 17.22 Multiplanar Reformation.** Multiplanar reformation (MPR) is the result of the computer using the original axial image data to produce images in other planes, such as the sagittal image seen here. (Courtesy Bontrager KL, Lampignano JP: *Textbook of radiographic positioning and related anatomy*, ed 7, St Louis, 2010, Mosby.)

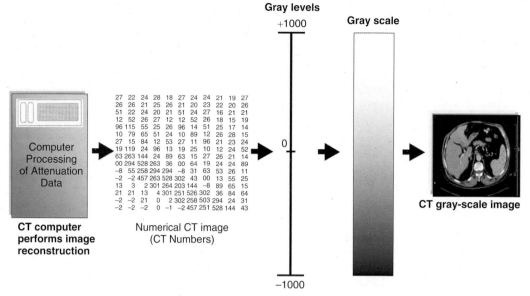

**Fig. 17.23 Image Data to Grayscale Image.** Windowing is the postprocessing technique that determines how gray levels are assigned to the image data (computed tomography number for each pixel in the matrix). (Courtesy Seeram E: *Computed tomography*, ed 3, Philadelphia, 2009, Saunders.)

from reconstruction in that the computer uses the image data that were previously reconstructed (using the filtered back-projection or iterative reconstruction algorithm) to produce these additional images. Image smoothing or **edge enhancement filters** change the appearance of the anatomy, based on the type of tissue being imaged.

## WINDOWING

The postprocessing technique of windowing allows for the display of either a wide variety of tissue types or perhaps tissues that are very similar to each other. **Windowing** includes adjusting how many CT numbers are visible in the image (**window width [WW]**) and which CT numbers are included (**window level [WL]**). The WL determines the midpoint of the range of CT numbers to be displayed. Combined, WW and WL determine which CT numbers (and the associated pixels) are visible in the image display (Fig. 17.23). For

example, an image with a WW of 400 and WL of 250 produces an image that displays pixels with CT numbers ranging from 50 to 450 (400 different numbers, 200 above and 200 below 250). All pixels with CT numbers of 50 or lower are black, whereas all pixels with CT numbers of 450 or higher are white. The pixels between these values will be a shade of gray. The images in Fig. 17.24 demonstrate the same slice of anatomy with different preset windows, changing the anatomy being displayed.

The WL is set near the CT number of the type of anatomy to be visualized. For example, because soft tissue structures have CT numbers just higher than water, the WL for soft tissue anatomy such as brain or liver is set around 30 to 60. The WW depends on how similar or dissimilar the anatomy of interest is. To visualize tissues that are very similar to each other, such as blood (CT number of approximately 20) and brain (CT number of approximately 40), the WW must be small.

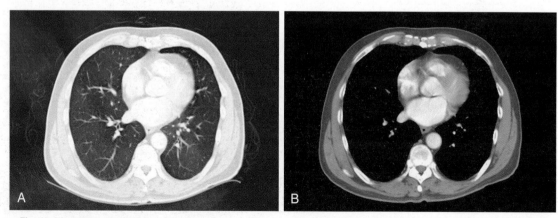

**Fig. 17.24 Different Windows.** Two images of the same computed tomography slice (without any alteration in image data) demonstrate the effect of windowing, allowing the visualization of lung tissue **(A)** using lung windows and the heart, and great vessels **(B)** using mediastinal windows. (Courtesy Bontrager KL, Lampignano JP: *Textbook of radiographic positioning and related anatomy*, ed 7, St Louis, 2010, Mosby.)

A large WW would result in an image in which brain and blood either share the same shade of gray or have shades so much alike that the human eye could not tell them apart. A wide WW is used when many different tissue types need to be seen.

It is the combination of WW and WL that determines the visibility of different tissues in the CT image. In addition, adjustment of the WW and WL affects the brightness and contrast of the image. As the WL decreases (e.g., changing from 200 to −30), the image appears brighter (more white) (Fig. 17.25). As the WW decreases (e.g., going from 800 to 80), the image demonstrates increased contrast (more black and white) (Fig. 17.26). CT WL changes affect image brightness in the opposite direction as digital radiography. As with all postprocessing techniques, the CT image data

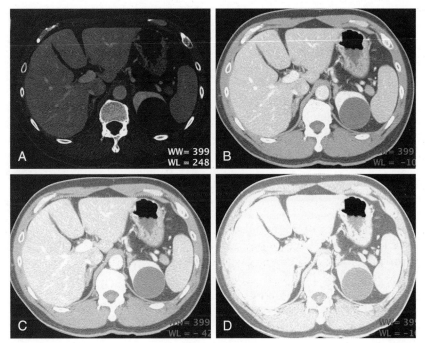

**Fig. 17.25  Effect of Changing Window Level.** Having the window width remain at 399 while reducing the window level (WL) from +248 **(A)** to −106 **(D)** demonstrates the effect of WL on image brightness. (Courtesy Seeram E: *Computed tomography*, ed 3, Philadelphia, 2009, Saunders.)

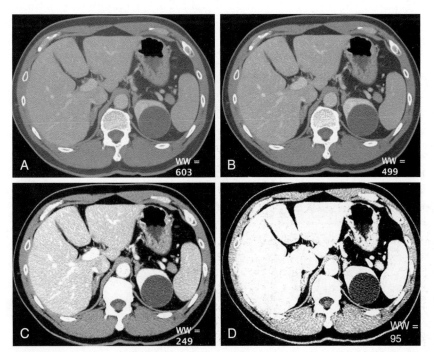

**Fig. 17.26  Effect of Changing Window Width.** Maintaining a window level of 40, narrowing the window width from 603 **(A)** to 95 **(D)** demonstrates the increase in image contrast. (Courtesy Seeram E: *Computed tomography*, ed 3, Philadelphia, 2009, Saunders.)

remain constant and, although visibility may change, no new information is present.

> **Critical Concept**
> **Windowing**
>
> Windowing, a common postprocessing technique, allows adjustment of the window width (WW) and window level (WL) to determine the shade of gray (or black or white) assigned to every CT number in the image data. Changing the WW and WL allows different tissues to be made visible.

## IMAGE QUALITY

It is the technologist's responsibility to evaluate image quality and make adjustments as appropriate. Similar to radiographic imaging, CT studies often have tradeoffs between image quality and patient radiation dose that must be considered. The primary image quality characteristics to be considered with CT include noise, spatial resolution, contrast resolution, and image artifacts.

### NOISE

In a perfect CT image of a container of water, all of the pixels would have CT numbers of 0 and be the same shade of gray. In reality, the CT numbers vary randomly, and the image is mottled or grainy. This is noise, an undesirable characteristic; the amount of noise depends on a number of factors. The equipment itself, including the detectors and electronics, contributes to noise seen in the image, but this is inherent and cannot be altered. Beyond the CT system, the technologist can influence the amount of noise and its visibility.

The major cause of noise is determined by the number of x-ray photons used to produce the image (**quantum noise**). As with radiography, the fewer the number of photons used to create the image, the greater the quantum noise (Fig. 17.27). Because the CT image is based on the photons measured by the detectors, any

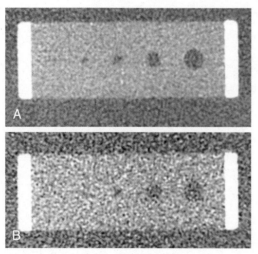

**Fig. 17.27 Noise.** An increase in quantum noise is clearly seen when the mA is reduced from 100 mA **(A)** to 50 mA **(B)**. (Courtesy Seeram E: *Computed tomography*, ed 3, Philadelphia, 2009, Saunders.)

factor that increases this measurement reduces quantum noise. This includes using a higher mA, longer rotation time, higher kVp, and a larger slice thickness. A large pixel results in decreased noise. Increasing the pitch (having the patient move through the gantry faster) reduces the number of photons used to create the image, resulting in increased noise.

The visibility of noise is strongly affected by the reconstruction filter (Fig. 17.28). Using a sharp, high-resolution or **edge-enhancement filter** makes all the information in the image appear sharper, including the noise. A **smoothing filter**, also known as a noise reduction filter, makes the noise less visible. When imaging structures with small details, such as bone, the visibility of noise is a necessary trade-off. Smoothing filters can be used when imaging soft tissue structures, because the visibility of noise more adversely affects the image, whereas a slight loss of resolution is often acceptable.

> **Critical Concept**
> **Quantum Noise**
>
> The amount of quantum noise in the CT image affects spatial resolution, contrast resolution, and patient dose. Appropriate image quality must be based on balancing these factors.

### SPATIAL RESOLUTION

CT **spatial resolution** is the ability of the image to differentiate between structures with different attenuation characteristics (CT numbers) when they are very close together. Similar to radiography, the line-pair test phantom can be used for evaluation (Fig. 17.29), and the resolution is described as line pairs per centimeter (Lp/cm) or millimeter (Lp/mm). Line-pair resolution for CT is typically 0.5 to 1 Lp/mm. A high level of spatial resolution can be achieved by having small pixels and thin slices (Fig. 17.30). The pixel size is determined by the matrix size and the field of view (FOV). As the matrix increases (more rows and columns) or the FOV decreases, the pixel size decreases. Equipment also affects spatial resolution; using a small focal spot size or having smaller detectors produces an image with increased spatial resolution.

As with noise, the reconstruction filter has a major effect on the visibility of the image sharpness. A smoothing filter smooths out edges and decreases the spatial resolution, whereas sharp- or high-resolution filters sharpen the edges and improve spatial resolution. Because these filters also affect the visibility of noise, a compromise must be made depending on the type of anatomy being imaged.

> **Critical Concept**
> **Spatial Resolution**
>
> The ability of CT images to differentiate between structures with different attenuation characteristics (CT numbers) when they are very close together.

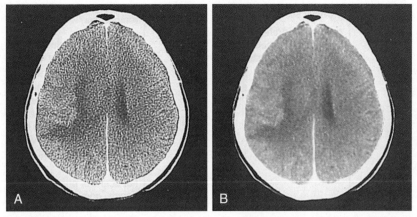

Fig. 17.28 **Filters.** The same computed tomography slice has the edge enhancement electronic filter applied **(A)** and the smoothing filter **(B)**. Notice the effect on the appearance of noise and soft tissue anatomy. (Courtesy Siemens Healthcare, Malvern, Penn.)

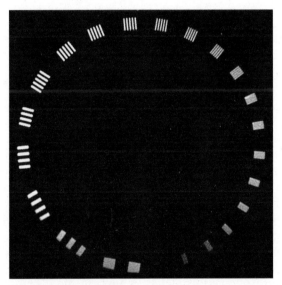

Fig. 17.29 **Spatial Resolution.** Image of a line-pair test phantom used for assessment of spatial resolution. (Courtesy Seeram E: *Computed tomography*, ed 3, Philadelphia, 2009, Saunders.)

## CONTRAST RESOLUTION

CT **contrast resolution** is the ability to discriminate between structures with very similar attenuation characteristics (CT numbers) (Fig. 17.31). Excellent contrast resolution is one of the major attributes of CT imaging. Compared with radiography, CT can differentiate between tissues that are 10 times more similar, such as ventricles compared with brain tissue. This is accomplished by having minimal scatter reach the detectors (because of very tight collimation, both pre-patient and postpatient) and by using the windowing process to visualize these small differences. Using a small WW at the appropriate WL allows structures with similar CT numbers to have visibly different shades of gray.

The limiting factor for contrast resolution is noise. Any factor that reduces the amount or visibility of noise improves contrast resolution. Therefore choice of mA, kVp, slice thickness, matrix size, FOV, and reconstruction filter affects contrast resolution.

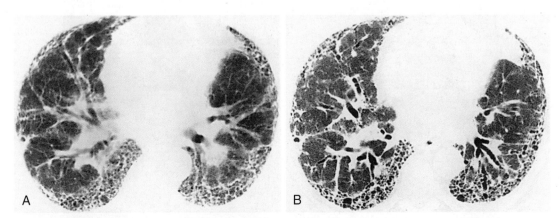

Fig. 17.30 **Effect of Changing Slice Thickness.** The effect of slice thickness is clearly shown by comparing the spatial resolution of an image of a thick 10-mm slice **(A)** and that of a thin 1.5-mm slice **(B)**. (Courtesy Mayo JR: High-resolution computed tomography, *Radiol Clin North Am* 29: 1043-1048, 1991.)

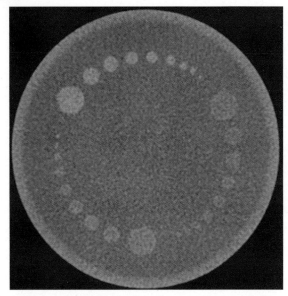

**Fig. 17.31 Low-Contrast Resolution.** Image of a low-contrast quality-control test phantom. (Courtesy Seeram E: *Computed tomography*, ed 3, Philadelphia, 2009, Saunders.)

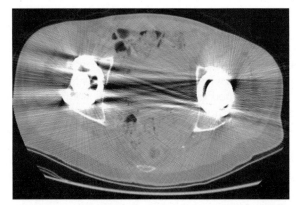

**Fig. 17.32 Streak Artifact.** Streak artifacts caused by metal prostheses are seen. (Courtesy Seeram E: *Computed tomography*, ed 3, Philadelphia, 2009, Saunders.)

 **Critical Concept**

**Contrast Resolution**

The ability of CT images to differentiate between tissues with very similar attenuation characteristics makes it an invaluable tool in diagnostic imaging.

## ARTIFACTS

The fourth component of CT image quality is artifacts. CT artifacts can be identified when the CT number in the image data does not accurately represent the attenuation characteristics of the associated anatomy. Streak, ring, shading, and partial volume are common CT artifacts. **Streak artifacts** (Fig. 17.32) are linear-shaped artifacts that are often the result of patient motion or the presence of metal in the anatomy being imaged. Immobilization, removal of metal when possible, and computer algorithms can reduce streak artifacts. **Ring artifacts** are circular-shaped artifacts that are associated with a faulty detector in third-generation scanners (this problem was eliminated in fourth-generation scanners).

Shading artifacts are common and typically are the result of the **beam-hardening artifact** (Fig. 17.33). As the x-ray beam passes through the patient, especially through bone, the lower-energy photons are filtered out, resulting in beam hardening. Because the attenuation coefficient (μ) of a material depends on the beam energy, beam hardening results in inaccurate CT numbers. This is particularly evident in head examinations. Computer algorithms can reduce beam-hardening artifacts.

**Partial-volume artifacts** arise when the voxel is so large that it contains more than one type of tissue (for example, a voxel might contain both bone and muscle). When the attenuation coefficient is calculated for this voxel (followed by determination of the CT number

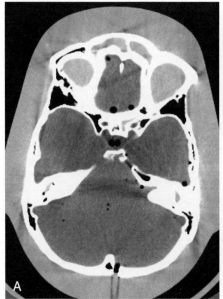 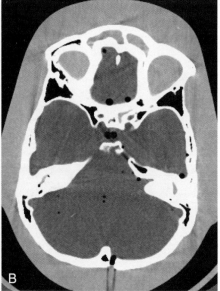

**Fig. 17.33 Beam-Hardening Artifact.** The beam-hardening artifact is seen between the petrous pyramids as a band of decreased brightness **(A)**. Algorithms have been applied to reduce the artifact **(B)**. (Courtesy Seeram E: *Computed tomography*, ed 3, Philadelphia, 2009, Saunders.)

for the pixel), it is not an accurate representation of either the bone or muscle. This artifact can be reduced by decreasing pixel size or slice thickness, resulting in a smaller voxel.

CT image quality always involves trade-offs that must be weighed in relation to the examination and the patient. Images with high spatial resolution can be produced but may be at the expense of increased noise or patient dose. High contrast resolution requires low noise, which means decreased spatial resolution or increased dose. Reducing the partial-volume artifact requires smaller voxels, necessitating increased dose or more noise. Decisions about examination protocols and their adjustments must be carefully considered.

## QUALITY CONTROL

As with radiographic x-ray equipment, CT systems require regular tube warm-up procedures, preventive maintenance, and quality-control testing to ensure the accuracy and quality of the CT image. Tube warm-up and regular maintenance should be done according to the manufacturer's directions. Specific test objects have been designed for CT quality control, evaluating a number of factors such as spatial resolution, contrast resolution, and noise. Accuracy, linearity, and uniformity are other characteristics to be assessed. When a water-filled container is imaged, a system that is accurate has the CT number in a particular spot very close to 0, whereas a system that is uniform has a variety of areas within the image, all with CT numbers very close to 0. Linearity is demonstrated when an image of a variety of materials demonstrates CT numbers consistent with the linear attenuation coefficients of those materials. There are a number of additional quality-control tests for CT systems, some of which include assessment of the accuracy of table movement, pitch, and localization devices.

Many facilities use CT performance phantoms that have been designed specifically for the scanner to conduct routine quality-control testing. These daily tests are conducted by placing the phantom at a designated area on the table and imaging it with specific parameters, taking measurements at specified areas and recording the data. The American College of Radiology (ACR) CT Accreditation Program phantom (Fig. 17.34) is designed for initial QA assessment and annual testing conducted by the physicists. As with all quality-control programs, test frequency (e.g., daily, monthly, semiannually) and acceptable standards must be set.

## RADIATION PROTECTION

Since being introduced in the 1970s, the number and type of CT procedures being performed has increased significantly each decade. Today, because of technological advances and overuse, CT examinations account for approximately one-half of the U.S. population's

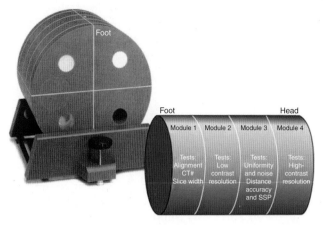

Fig. 17.34 ACR Computed Tomography (CT) Accreditation Phantom.

radiation exposure resulting from medical procedures. Questions and concerns are widespread about the radiation dose being received from these examinations, especially by children. Incidences concerning radiation overexposures have been prominent in news and media, and many health care facilities, professional organizations, and governmental agencies have responded with increased initiatives to promote radiation safety in CT imaging. It is the technologist's duty to be knowledgeable about methods available to limit dose to both the patient and others who may be in the room (Box 17.1).

ALARA is the key radiation protection principle that ensures that patient doses are kept as low as is reasonably achievable. Every exposure should have a benefit and a justification. In CT, however, the focus is on **dose optimization** as well. The CT technologist must reduce the radiation dose while maintaining the required image quality needed for making a diagnosis.

The CT technologist should ensure that patients receive the appropriate examination for their symptoms and signs. The technologist should take a thorough patient history before the ordered study to discover if there is a strict clinical indication to help eliminate unnecessary and duplicate examinations. The technologist will access the medical record to see if the patient has had any recent CT examinations and alert the ordering practitioner if necessary. Also, the technologist may need to intercede on the patient's behalf and alert the ordering practitioner if there may be a more appropriate examination or test for the indication, such as MRI or ultrasound. Although the

| **Box 17.1** Radiation Protection Practices in CT |
| --- |
| ALARA |
| Dose optimization |
| Appropriate examination |
| Appropriate protocol selection and SFOV |
| Correct patient centering |
| Out-of-plane lead shielding |

effect of these actions may seem minimal, they could potentially prevent a duplicate examination or unnecessary radiation exposure. Another method to reduce exposure is the use of immobilization devices such as straps, head holders, and IV arm boards. These prevent patient movement therefore reducing the need for repeat exposure.

Once the CT examination has been deemed appropriate, the technologist must choose the appropriate and correct protocol and technical factors to create the best image quality while limiting radiation dose to the patient. Certain technical factors, such as the mA, kVp, and pitch, directly affect patient dose. To decrease dose, the mA and kVp could be reduced and the pitch increased. However, because these factors also affect noise and contrast resolution, it is important to balance reductions in dose with appropriate image quality. **Automatic tube current modulation (ATCM)** provides ongoing adjustment of the mA based on patient size and tissue characteristics, maintaining image quality while reducing dose, especially for small patients (Fig. 17.35). ATCM can be used in three different techniques. In angular modulation (in-plane), the automatic control of the tube current is along the X-Y-axis. In longitudinal modulation (through-plane), the automatic control of the tube current is along the Z-axis. Finally, in angular-longitudinal modulation, the automatic control of the tube current is along all three axes.

Patient dose during CT imaging is complex and is expressed using different descriptors based on manufacturer and calibration phantoms. The most commonly used **dose descriptors** include the **CT Dose Index in a volume (CTDI$_{vol}$)** and **dose length product (DLP)** (Fig. 17.36). The CT dose index measures mean absorbed dose in the scanned object volume and in MSCT units is specifically called CTDI$_{vol}$ because it adjusted for weighted index and pitch. CTDI$_{vol}$ is measured in Gray (mGy, cGy). The DLP is a measurement of energy absorbed per unit of mass over a scanned

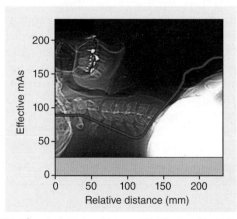

**Fig. 17.35 Automatic Tube Current Modulation (ATCM).** The mA is automatically adjusted as the patient is scanned while maintaining a uniform noise level for different thicknesses of body parts examined. This is an example of longitudinal modulation or through plane modulation.

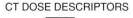

CT DOSE DESCRIPTORS

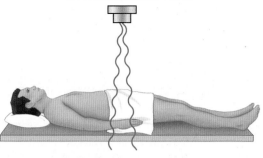

**CTDI: CT Dose Index (mGv)**
Energy absorbed per unit of mass described

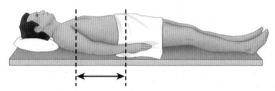

**DLP: Dose Length Product (mGv cm)**
Energy absorbed per unit of mass over a scanned length

**Fig. 17.36 CT Dose Descriptors.** CT Dose Index or CTDI is measured in mGy and is defined as the energy absorbed per unit of mass. The dose length product is measured in (mGy × centimeters) and is defined as the energy absorbed per unit of mass over a scanned length.

length (Z-axis) and can be expressed with the following formula:

$$DLP = CTDI_{vol} \times Scan\ length\ of\ exposure$$

Current CT scanners display the CTDI$_{vol}$ and DLP indices before and after the CT study is performed. This is called the **dose report** (Fig. 17.37). Required since 2002, the dose report is sent to PACS with the rest of the patient's CT study. Another dose measurement, referred to as the **multiple scan average dose (MSAD)** is the average exposure dose estimated at a central point of multiple scans during table movement. This is also measured in Gray and uses the following formula for spiral scans:

$$MSAD = \frac{1 \times CTDI}{pitch}$$

Another way to limit radiation dose to the patient is proper centering. The patient must be centered in the CT gantry isocenter for accurate imaging of the anatomy. This ensures proper dose distribution, whereas inaccurate patient centering will degrade the image quality and increase the dose to the patient (especially with ATCM). Improper centering of the patient in the gantry can lead to an increase in surface dose and the peripheral dose to the patient. Current research indicates that when using a 32-cm CTDI body phantom, a miscentering of 3 cm results in increase in doses by 18%, and miscentering of 6 cm results in increase in doses by 41%.

If the patient is centered too high in the gantry, the ATCM assumes the patient is larger and increases the

| Patient Name: | | | | Exam no: 1744 | |
|---|---|---|---|---|---|
| Accession Number: | | | | 10 Aug 2014 | |
| Patient ID: | | | | Discovery CT750 HD | |
| Exam Description: CT HALS/THORAX/ABDOMEN | | | | | |

**Dose Report**

| Series | Type | Scan Range (mm) | CTDIvol (mGy) | DLP (mGy - cm) | Phantom cm |
|---|---|---|---|---|---|
| 1 | Scout | —— | —— | —— | |
| 2 | Helical | S15.750 - I650.250 | 5.10 | 373.00 | Body 32 |
| 5 | Helical | S188.000 - I105.000 | 5.10 | 182.72 | Body 32 |

**Total Exam DLP:** 555.72

1/1

Fig. 17.37 **CT Dose Report.** This dose report is created by current CT units and display the CTDI$_{vol}$ and DLP indices before and after a CT study is performed. The dose report is sent to PACS with the rest of the patient's CT study.

technical factors used, which results in a higher dose and images with decreased quality. If the patient is centered too low in the gantry, the ATCM assumes the patient is smaller, calculates an insufficient dose, and produces images with poor image quality.

It is also necessary to position the patient correctly so that radiation is not delivered to sensitive areas. An example of this would be during pediatric head or neuro perfusion CT studies. In this situation, the technologist should position the head so that the eyes are out of the primary beam to limit dose.

Conventional radiographic shielding (lead) of radiosensitive tissues such as gonads or thyroid can be done when they are located outside of the SFOV (out-of-plane). Although the shielding may have limited value because of very tight collimation (and minimal scatter), it is recommended even if only for psychological purposes. This shielding must completely surround the patient because the tube travels in a circular motion. It is also very important that shielding not be within the SFOV so that all of the anatomy of interest is imaged and artifacts are avoided.

Thin, in-plane bismuth shields are available specifically for CT studies. They can be used to reduce exposure to the breast, thyroid, and eyes when they are within the SFOV. These shields are placed directly over the tissue and filter the beam, reducing the low-energy photons and superficial dose. The American Association of Physicists in Medicine (AAPM) recommends against using in-plane bismuth shields in lieu of other methods of radiation protection, such as proper scan length, collimation, and other methods of dose optimization.

Children require special consideration regarding radiation dose because they are more sensitive to the effects of radiation and have more years for problems to manifest. Referring physicians should be educated regarding the dose associated with CT examinations and alternative procedures, and CT examinations should use routine pediatric protocols based either on

age or weight. The Image Gently campaign was created by the Alliance for Radiation Safety in Medical Imaging to promote and improve the safety and effectiveness of medical imaging of children. Image Gently provides news and education for practitioners, technologists, and parents concerning ways to help reduce radiation dose for children.

Radiation protection of anyone who remains in the room during scanning must be considered based on time, distance, and shielding. It is important that technologists, parents, or any others who must remain in the room wear protective apparel, stand away from the gantry, and limit time in the room. Women of child-bearing age should be questioned regarding their pregnancy status.

Radiation exposure from CT studies is a major concern, particularly with respect to pediatrics. Although there is general agreement that the benefits of appropriate CT procedures far outweigh the risks, it is the responsibility of those who develop and use CT protocols to minimize the risks based on the as low as reasonably achievable (ALARA) principle.

## DOSE NOTIFICATION AND ALERTS

Beginning in 2014, the National Electrical Manufacturers Association (NEMA) requires that the XR 25 CT Dose-Check Standard software be included in all new CT scanners sold in the United States. Existing manufacturers can also make efforts to ensure that installed units also meet this radiation safety standard.

A **dose notification value** is used to trigger a message when a single planned and confirmed scan is likely to exceed a preprogrammed value (CTDI$_{vol}$ and/or DLP) (Fig. 17.38). This programmed value is set for each scan sequence in an examination. These values were set by the AAPM so that notifications would be infrequent, but they can be changed based on individual facility department preferences (Table 17.1).

A **dose alert value** is used to trigger a message when cumulative dose at a location, plus the dose for

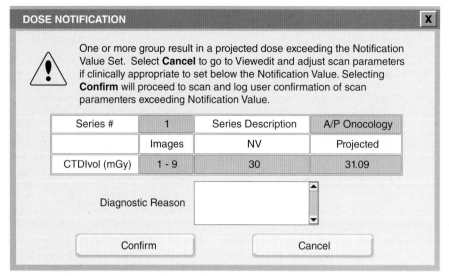

**DOSE NOTIFICATION**                                    X

⚠ One or more group result in a projected dose exceeding the Notification Value Set. Select **Cancel** to go to Viewedit and adjust scan parameters if clinically appropriate to set below the Notification Value. Selecting **Confirm** will proceed to scan and log user confirmation of scan parameters exceeding Notification Value.

| Series # | 1 | Series Description | A/P Onocology |
|---|---|---|---|
| | Images | NV | Projected |
| CTDIvol (mGy) | 1 - 9 | 30 | 31.09 |

Diagnostic Reason [        ]

[ Confirm ]          [ Cancel ]

**Fig. 17.38 CT Dose Notification Value.** This is used to trigger a message when a single planned and confirmed scan is likely to exceed a preprogrammed value (CTDI$_{vol}$ and/or DLP). These values were set by the AAPM so that notifications would be infrequent but can be changed by individual facility department preferences.

| Table 17.1 | Notification Values Recommended by the AAPM Working Group on Standardization of CT Nomenclature and Protocols |
|---|---|

| CT SCAN REGION (OF EACH INDIVIDUAL SCAN IN AN EXAMINATION) | CTDI$_{VOL}$ NOTIFICATION VALUE (mGy) |
|---|---|
| Adult head | 80 |
| Adult torso | 50 |
| Pediatric head | |
| <2 years old | 50 |
| 2-5 years old | 60 |
| Pediatric torso | |
| <10 years old (16-cm phantom)[a] | 25 |
| <10 years old (32-cm phantom)[b] | 10 |
| Brain perfusion (examination that repeatedly scans the same anatomic level to measure the flow of contrast media through the anatomy) | 600 |
| Cardiac | |
| Retrospectively gated (spiral) | 150 |
| Prospectively gated (sequential) | 50 |

[a]As of January 2011, GE, Hitachi, and Toshiba scanners use the 16-cm-diameter CDTI phantom as the basis for evaluating dose indices (CDTI$_{vol}$ and DLP) displayed and reported for pediatric body examinations.
[b]As of January 2011, Siemens and Philips scanners use the 32-cm-diameter CDTI phantom as the basis for evaluating dose indices (CDTI$_{vol}$ and DLP) displayed and reported for pediatric body examinations.
AAPM Recommendations Regarding Notification and Alert Values for CT Scanners: Guidelines for Use of the NEMA XR 25 CT Does-Check Standard," AAPM Dose Check Guidelines Version 1.0, College Park, 2011, AAPM, Table 1: https://www.aapm.org/pubs/CTProtocols/documents/NotificationLevelsStatement.pdf

the next planned and confirmed scan(s), is likely to exceed a preprogrammed value (Fig. 17.39). The value is set once and applies to all examinations in that study. This is a scanner parameter and is not protocol or sequence specific. The Food and Drug Administration-recommended default value is CTDI$_{vol}$ = 1000 mGy.

The dose notification and alert system is put into operation before patient scanning and can help protect patients from inadvertent use of excessively high CTDI$_{vol}$ and/or DLP. It is not designed to optimize dose, and these alerts do not terminate the x-ray exposure. Rather, it was designed to prevent egregious errors by the technologist or CT unit. Notifications draw attention to potentially high exposure so users can confirm that settings are appropriate. Operator education is essential, and event logs documenting exposure should be monitored by the department to ensure proper usage of the system.

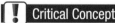 **Critical Concept**

**Patient Exposure**

Patient (especially pediatric) radiation exposure resulting from CT examinations is a significant concern and should be considered at each step of the procedure.

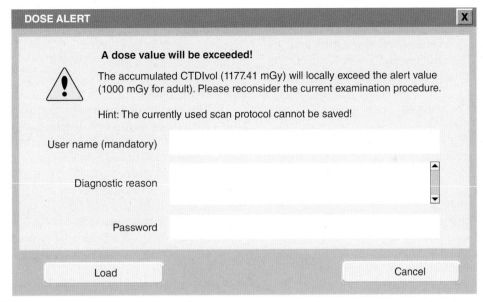

**Fig. 17.39 CT Dose Alert Value.** This is used to trigger a message when cumulative dose at a location, plus the dose for the next planned and confirmed scan(s), is likely to exceed a preprogrammed value.

## On the Spot

- CT was introduced in the 1970s and has revolutionized medical imaging by creating cross-sectional slices that are able to make similar tissues appear different.
- CT has developed through five generations of equipment, along with spiral and multislice technology, dramatically reducing scan time and improving image quality.
- Using a modified x-ray tube, high-frequency generator, two sets of collimators (producing a tightly collimated fan beam), an array of detectors, and a data acquisition system, the x-ray transmission values are measured, and linear attenuation coefficients calculated and digitized (raw data).
- Using the filtered back projection algorithm, the raw data are used to determine the linear attenuation coefficient for each voxel that will be represented by a pixel in the CT image.
- The voxel's linear attenuation coefficient is then converted to a CT number (Hounsfield unit), which describes the attenuation characteristics of the voxel's tissue relative to water. The matrix of CT numbers is the image data.
- Imaging protocols include settings for mA, kVp, slice thickness, matrix size, SFOV, DFOV, pitch, and image display. These settings can be adjusted based on individual patients.
- The image data can be postprocessed, adjusting the visibility of the anatomy being studied. The most powerful postprocessing technique is windowing, which allows adjustment of which CT numbers will be made visible.
- WW controls how many CT numbers will be assigned shades of gray (or black or white) and affects the image contrast.
- WL sets the midpoint of the window, determining which specific CT numbers will be included, and affects the image brightness.
- CT image quality is evaluated in terms of noise, spatial resolution, contrast resolution, and artifacts. Excellent image quality often has the tradeoff of increased patient dose.
- Quality-control testing must be done to ensure that the CT image has accurate information.
- Radiation dose caused by CT examinations is an important issue, especially as it relates to children. Technologists need to adjust technical factors, shield, and use pediatric protocols to protect the patient from unnecessary exposure. Radiation safety practices must also be in place to protect others who remain in the scan room.

## CRITICAL THINKING QUESTIONS

1. How does the process of creating a CT image differ from that of a radiographic image?
2. Why is the CT number a critical aspect of the CT imaging process?
3. How does the windowing process allow different tissues to be made visible in the CT image?
4. Why is it important to personalize the CT protocol to the patient size (e.g., pediatric versus adult)?
5. How would a change in the CT parameters affect the radiation exposure to the patient?

## REVIEW QUESTIONS

1. The circular structure that the patient and table travel through during the CT scanning process that encompasses the x-ray unit, data acquisition system, and the detector/detectors is the:
   a. donut.
   b. couch.
   c. magnet.
   d. gantry.

2. In a major improvement from single-slice CT acquisition, spiral (helical) CT allowed:
   a. continuous movement of the table and the patient through the gantry.
   b. the entire volume of tissue to be scanned in one acquisition.
   c. scan time to be reduced.
   d. all of the above.

3. The number of _____ in MSCT equals the number of slices per revolution.
   a. detector rows
   b. computers
   c. rows in the matrix
   d. protocol sequences

4. What is a key advantage of PCCT over conventional CT imaging?
   a. Reduced radiation dose to the patient.
   b. Faster scan times.
   c. Reduction of artifacts.
   d. Increased image noise.

5. The ____ controls how much of the detector is exposed during CT imaging, and severely limits the amount of scatter reaching the detectors.
   a. prepatient collimator
   b. postpatient collimator
   c. bowtie filter
   d. detector array

6. Logarithmic data from linear attenuation coefficients that is converted from analog to digital information by the analog-to-digital converter and sent to the computer for image reconstruction is the:
   a. raw data.
   b. filtered back projection.
   c. pixels.
   d. voxels.

7. What is the CT number of water?
   a. −2000
   b. 100
   c. 0
   d. 1500

8. Which of the following determines the actual anatomy that is imaged during the CT examination?
   a. SFOV
   b. DFOV
   c. FOV
   d. All of the above

9. Using a DFOV smaller than the SFOV results in a:
   a. magnified image.
   b. minified image.
   c. normal-sized image.
   d. computer system crash.

10. The amount of CT numbers that are visible in the image is known as the:
    a. window level (WL).
    b. window width (WW).
    c. raw data.
    d. histogram.

11. The ability of the image to differentiate between structures with very different attenuation characteristics (CT numbers) when they are very close together is known as the:
    a. patient dose.
    b. contrast resolution.
    c. edge enhancement filter.
    d. spatial resolution.

12. The ability to discriminate between structures with very similar attenuation characteristics (CT numbers) is known as the:
    a. patient dose.
    b. contrast resolution.
    c. edge enhancement filter.
    d. spatial resolution.

13. In CT imaging, ALARA encompasses which of the following?
    1. Patient dose is kept as low as reasonably achievable.
    2. Every exposure should have a benefit and justification.
    3. CT technologist must maintain required image quality needed for making a diagnosis (dose optimization).
    a. 1 only
    b. 1 and 2
    c. 1 and 3
    d. 1, 2, and 3

14. Ongoing adjustment of the mA based on patient size and tissue characteristics during the CT examination, used to maintain image quality while reducing dose, is known as:
    a. automatic exposure control (AEC).
    b. automatic tube current modulation (ATCM).
    c. filtered back projection (FBP).
    d. adaptive statistical iterative reconstruction (ASIR).

15. Inaccurate patient centering during a CT examination will degrade the image quality and increase the dose to the patient (especially with ATCM).
    a. True
    b. False

16. Which of the following statements is true regarding the use of lead shielding during CT?
    1. The AAPM recommends against using lead shielding in lieu of other methods of radiation protection.
    2. Lead shielding of radiosensitive tissues can be effective in limiting the radiation dose when the shields are placed appropriately outside the SFOV (out-of-plane).
    3. Lead shielding must completely surround the patient, because the tube(s) travel in a circular motion.
    4. Lead shielding must lie on the couch, because the radiation comes from the area around the table.
    a. 1 only
    b. 2 and 3 only
    c. 2 and 4 only
    d. All of the above

17. The dose notification and alert system occurs before patient scanning and can help protect patients from inadvertent use of excessively high $CTDI_{vol}$ and/or DLP.
    a. True
    b. False

# Answers to Review Questions

## CHAPTER 1

1. A
2. B
3. D
4. A
5. A
6. C
7. D
8. C
9. A
10. B

## CHAPTER 2

1. A
2. B
3. B
4. A
5. D
6. A
7. B
8. C
9. C
10. A

## CHAPTER 3

1. A
2. B
3. A
4. C
5. C
6. D
7. C
8. D
9. A
10. C

## CHAPTER 4

1. B
2. D
3. B
4. B
5. A
6. B
7. C

8. B
9. B
10. D
11. A
12. C
13. C
14. B

## CHAPTER 5

1. D
2. C
3. B
4. C
5. D
6. D
7. A
8. A
9. B
10. D
11. B

## CHAPTER 6

1. A
2. B
3. B
4. C
5. D
6. C
7. A
8. D
9. B
10. A

## CHAPTER 7

1. D
2. D
3. A
4. B
5. D
6. D
7. A
8. D
9. D
10. A

## CHAPTER 8

1. B
2. D
3. C
4. C
5. B
6. B
7. D
8. B
9. D
10. A

## CHAPTER 9

1. D
2. D
3. B
4. A
5. C
6. D
7. C
8. D
9. B
10. C
11. D
12. D
13. B
14. Q
15. A
16. D

## CHAPTER 10

1. A
2. C
3. C
4. D
5. A
6. A
7. B
8. D
9. D

## CHAPTER 11

1. C
2. D

3. D
4. D
5. D
6. B
7. B
8. A
9. B
10. B
11. C
12. 10 mAs × 2 = 20 mAs
13. 80 kVp @ 17.3 mAs, a 48-inch SID, and an 8:1 grid ratio
14. 30 mAs × 2 = 60 mAs

## CHAPTER 12

1. B
2. D
3. B
4. C
5. A
6. C
7. D
8. B
9. D
10. C

## CHAPTER 13

1. B
2. C
3. B
4. D
5. A
6. A
7. C
8. B
9. C
10. D
11. D
12. D

## CHAPTER 14

1. B
2. A

3. C
4. B
5. C
6. D

## CHAPTER 15

1. B
2. B
3. D
4. D
5. D
6. B
7. C
8. A

9. C
10. C
11. B
12. C
13. C
14. B
15. D

## CHAPTER 16

1. D
2. B
3. D
4. B
5. D

6. C
7. A
8. B
9. C
10. C
11. C
12. D

## CHAPTER 17

1. D
2. D
3. A
4. A
5. B

6. A
7. C
8. A
9. A
10. B
11. D
12. B
13. D
14. B
15. A
16. B
17. A

# Glossary

**15% rule:** Changing the kVP by 15% has the same effect as doubling the mAs or reducing the mAs by 50%.

**ABC:** See *automatic brightness control*.

**absorption:** The x-ray photons removed from the x-ray beam as a result of the uptake of their energy by body tissues.

**AC:** See *alternating current*.

**accelerating anode:** A positively charged electrode in the neck of the image intensifier that accelerates the electron stream to the output phosphor by maintaining a constant potential of approximately 25 kilovolts in the tube.

**actual focal spot:** Area of x-ray tube target actually bombarded with filament electrons.

**acute radiodermatitis:** A skin reddening and inflammation caused by prolonged exposure to ionizing radiation.

**adaptive statistical iterative reconstruction (ASIR):** A type of reconstruction technique in CT that begins to calculate data after a first-pass filtered back projection reconstruction, which shortens reconstruction time while maintaining much lower image noise. This technique reduces quantum noise substantially with no effect on spatial or contrast resolution.

**ADC:** See *analog-to-digital converter*.

**AEC:** See *automatic exposure control*.

**AERC:** See *automatic exposure rate control*.

**AI:** See *artificial intelligence*.

**air gap technique:** Method for limiting the scatter reaching the image receptor. Scatter will miss the image receptor if there is increased distance between the patient and the image receptor (increased object-to-image receptor distance).

**air kerma:** Specifies the intensity of x-rays at a given point in air at a known distance from the focal spot or source of x-rays.

**algorithm:** A sequence of computer operations for accomplishing a specific task.

**alpha particles:** A particle consisting of two protons bound to two neutrons with a net positive charge and the ability to ionize matter.

**alternating current (AC):** Electrical current that changes direction in cycles as the electric potential of the source changes.

**analog-to-digital converter (ADC):** A device that takes the analog signal and divides it into a series of bits (1s and 0s) that the computer "understands."

**anatomically programmed technique:** A radiographic system that allows the radiographer to select a particular button on the control panel that represents an anatomic area; a preprogrammed set of exposure factors is displayed and selected for use.

**annotation:** Additional information, such as a printed comment or label added to the digital image.

**anode:** The positive end of the tube that provides the target for electron interaction to produce x-rays; also an electrical and thermal conductor.

**anode heel effect:** Phenomenon resulting from the angling of the target face that causes the intensity of the x-ray beam to be less on the anode side because the "heel" of the target is in the path of the beam.

**aperture diaphragm:** The simplest type of beam-restricting device, constructed of a flat piece of lead that has a hole in it.

**array processor:** A component of the computed tomography computer that is dedicated to performing the calculations needed for image reconstruction.

**artifact:** Any unwanted image on a radiographic image.

**artificial intelligence (AI):** Machine intelligence as opposed to human intelligence: the ability of a machine to perform what is otherwise considered to be human functions such as conversation and decision-making.

**ASIR:** See *adaptive statistical iterative reconstruction*.

**ATCM:** See *automatic tube current modulation*.

**atom:** From the Greek word *atomos*, meaning "indivisible." The basic building block of matter composed of electrons, protons, and neutrons.

**atomic mass number:** The number of protons and neutrons an atom has in its nucleus.

**atomic number:** The number of protons an atom contains in its nucleus.

**attenuation:** Reduction in the energy or number of photons in the primary x-ray beam after it interacts with anatomic tissue.

**automatic brightness control (ABC):** A function of the fluoroscopic unit that maintains the overall appearance of the fluoroscopic image by automatically adjusting the kilovoltage peak, milliamperage, or both.

**automatic collimator:** Automatically limits the size and shape of the primary beam to the size and shape of the image receptor. Also called a *positive beam-limiting device*.

**automatic exposure control (AEC):** A device that uses an ionization chamber to detect the quantity of radiation exposing the patient and image receptor.

**automatic exposure rate control (AERC):** Automatically adjusts the tube current (mA), voltage (kVp), filtration, and pulse width to maintain radiation exposure to the flat panel detector.

**automatic tube current modulation (ATCM):** Technique used in CT that provides an ongoing adjustment of the mA based on patient size and tissue characteristics, maintaining image quality while reducing dose.

**backup time:** The maximum length of time the x-ray exposure will continue when using an automatic exposure control system.

**beam quality:** The penetrating power of the x-ray beam.

**beam quantity:** The total number of x-ray photons in a beam.

**beam-hardening artifact:** As the x-ray beam passes through the patient, especially through bone, the lower-energy photons are filtered out, resulting in beam hardening; results in inaccurate computed tomography numbers.

**beam-restricting device:** Changes the shape and size of the primary beam; located just below the x-ray tube housing.

**beam restriction:** Refers to a decrease in the size of the projected radiation field, also known as collimation.

**beta particles:** An electron that is emitted from an unstable nucleus with the ability to ionize matter.

**binding energy:** A force of attraction that holds the nucleus of an atom together and holds electrons in orbit around the nucleus. Also a measure of the amount of energy necessary to split an atom.

**bit depth:** Number of bits that determines the amount of precision in digitizing the analog signal, and therefore the number of shades of gray that can be displayed in the image.

**body habitus:** The general form or build of the body, including size. There are four types—sthenic, hyposthenic, hypersthenic, and asthenic.

**bone densitometry:** A specialized procedure using ionizing radiation to provide information on the condition of the skeletal bones.

**bowtie filter:** The filter frequently used in computed tomography with a shape and composition that serve to make the energy level of the photons reaching the detectors more consistent.

**bremsstrahlung (brems) interactions:** An interaction in which a filament electron is attracted to the nucleus, causing it to slow down and change direction. The energy loss is emitted as a bremsstrahlung photon.

**brightness:** The amount of luminance (light emission) of a display monitor.

**brightness gain:** An expression of the ability of an image intensifier tube to convert x-ray energy into light energy and increase the brightness of the image in the process.

**Bucky:** The Potter-Bucky diaphragm located directly below the radiographic tabletop, which contains the grid and holds the image receptor.

**Bucky factor:** Can be used to determine the adjustment in milliampere/second needed when changing from using a grid to nongrid (or vice versa) or for changing to grids with different grid ratios; also called the *grid-conversion factor*.

**calipers:** Devices that measure part thickness.

**camera tube:** One of two common devices used in a fluoroscopic system to convert the light image from the output phosphor to an electronic signal for display on a television monitor.

**C-arm:** Mobile unit that has fluoroscopic capabilities typically used in the operating room when imaging is necessary during surgical procedures. A video unit is also attached, offering both static and dynamic recording during the procedure.

**cassette:** A sturdy, light-proof container for film. Also a sturdy protective container for the photostimulable phosphor plate in computed radiography.

**cathode:** The negative end of the x-ray tube and source of electrons.

**cathode ray tube:** A partial vacuum tube that produced an electron stream and was used to study cathode rays and led to the discovery of x-rays.

**CCD:** See *charge-coupled device*.

**characteristic cascade:** This process of outer-shell electrons filling inner-shell vacancies, creating a cascading effect during a characteristic cascade.

**characteristic interactions:** An interaction in which a filament electron removes an orbital electron from an atom; to regain stability, an outer-shell electron fills the vacancy, giving up its excess energy as a characteristic x-ray photon.

**charge-coupled device (CCD):** A light-sensitive semiconducting device that generates an electrical charge when stimulated by light and stores this charge in a capacitor.

**classical interaction:** Also commonly known as *coherent scattering* or *Thomson scattering*. See *coherent scattering*.

**coherent scattering:** An interaction that occurs with low-energy x-rays, typically below the diagnostic range. The incoming photon interacts with the atom, causing it to become excited. The x-ray does not lose energy but changes direction.

**collimation:** Refers to a decrease in the size of the projected radiation field, also known as beam restriction.

**collimator:** Located immediately below the tube window where the entrance shutters limit the x-ray beam field size.

**comparative anatomy:** Similar anatomic parts can use similar exposure techniques to achieve diagnostic radiographs.

**complementary metal oxide semiconductor:** A scintillator device made up of a crystalline silicon matrix.

**compound:** The combination of elements in definite proportions.

**Compton effect:** Scattering that results from the loss of some energy of the incoming photon when it ejects an outer-shell electron from a tissue atom.

**Compton electron:** The electron ejected from an atom during a Compton scattering event.

**Compton scattering:** An interaction in which an incident x-ray photon enters a tissue atom, interacts with an orbital electron, and removes it from its shell. In doing so, the incident photon loses up to one-third of its energy and is usually deflected in a new direction.

**computed radiography (CR):** A digital imaging system that uses a cassette, a photostimulable phosphor plate, a plate reader, and a computer workstation to acquire and display a digital image.

**computed tomography (CT):** An imaging modality that uses an X-ray beam, computer, and equipment configuration to allow cross-sectional images of the body.

**CNR:** See *contrast-to-noise ratio*.

**conductor:** Material with an abundance of free electrons allowing free flow of electricity.

**cone:** Essentially an aperture diaphragm that has an extended flange attached.

**cone beam:** The shape of the beam in computed tomography imaging as the number of slices being imaged per revolution increases and the x-ray beam is opened.

**continuous emission spectrum:** A graphic representation of bremsstrahlung x-ray production.

**contrast medium:** A substance that can be instilled into the body by injection or ingestion.

**contrast resolution:** Used to describe the ability of the imaging system to distinguish between small objects that attenuate the x-ray beam similarly in digital imaging.

**contrast-to-noise ratio (CNR):** A method of describing the contrast resolution compared with the amount of noise apparent in a digital image.

**convergent line:** An imaginary line if points were connected along the length of a linear focused grid.

**convergent point:** An imaginary point, if imaginary lines were drawn from each of the lead lines in a linear focused grid.

**conversion factor:** An expression of the luminance at the output phosphor divided by the input exposure rate; its unit of measure is the candela per square meter per milliroentgen per second ($cd/m^2/mR/s$).

**covalent bond:** An atomic bond in which an outermost electron from one atom begins to orbit the nucleus of another adjacent atom in addition to its original nucleus.

**crossed grid:** Has lead lines that run at a right angle to one another.

**cross-hatched grid:** Has lead lines that run at a right angle to one another.

**CR:** See *computed radiography (CR) system.*

**CT:** See *computed tomography.*

**CT dose index in a volume (CTDIvol):** In multislice CT units, the CTDI measures mean absorbed dose in the scanned object volume and is adjusted for weighted index and pitch.

**CT number:** Value related to the attenuation characteristic of the tissue in the voxel but not an attenuation coefficient; also referred to as the *Hounsfield unit.*

**CT table:** Also known as the *couch*; a platform of which the top may be flat or curved and is used to move the recumbent patient through the gantry aperture. It can be raised or lowered to assist the patient in getting on and off.

**CTDI$_{vol}$:** See *computed tomography dose index in a volume.*

**current:** An expression of the flow of electrons in a conductor.

**cylinder:** Essentially an aperture diaphragm that has an extended flange attached to it.

**DAP:** See *dose-area product.*

**DAS:** See *data acquisition system.*

**data acquisition system (DAS):** Amplifies the weak signal produced by the detector-photodiode, converts it to logarithmic data, converts it from analog to digital data, and sends it to the computer.

**DBT:** See *digital breast tomosynthesis.*

**DC:** See *direct current.*

**dedicated units:** Radiographic units designed for specific imaging procedures.

**deep learning (DL):** The use of a series of neural networks to extract desired outcomes through a process similar to the way humans learn.

**deep learning reconstruction (DLR):** The use of a series of neural networks (see deep learning) to achieve mapping of image data and the image reconstruction process more efficiently.

**DL:** See *deep learning*

**DLP:** See *dose length product.*

**DLR:** See *deep learning reconstruction.*

**density controls:** Part of the automatic exposure control device that allows the radiographer to adjust the amount of preset radiation detection values, also known as exposure adjustment.

**derived quantities:** The combinations of fundamentals quantities to form velocity, acceleration, force, momentum, work, and power.

**detective quantum efficiency (DQE):** A measurement of the efficiency of an image receptor in converting the x-ray exposure it receives to a quality radiographic image.

**detector array:** The physical component consisting of multiple detectors that efficiently absorb the transmitted radiation and accurately convert it to an electrical signal for display on a computer workstation.

**detectors:** Radiation-measuring devices.

add electrons to exposed silver halide during film processing; also known as reducing agents.

**DFOV:** See *display field of view.*

**DICOM:** See *Digital Imaging and Communications in Medicine.*

**differential absorption:** The difference between the x-ray photons that are absorbed photoelectrically versus those that penetrate the body.

**digital breast tomosynthesis (DBT):** An advanced imaging technique available in many breast imaging centers. DBT is also known as three-dimensional (3D) mammography and is similar to CT. The x-ray tube moves over the compressed breast from one side to the other and creates multiple images of the breast from different angles. These multiple images are reconstructed (synthesized) in the computer to create a set of 3D images.

**Digital Imaging and Communications in Medicine (DICOM):** A common computer language that allows different systems of a picture archiving and communication system to communicate with each other.

**digital subtraction technique:** Increases the visibility of vasculature by creating images precontrast, postcontrast, and the subtracted image. The overlying structures such as bone and soft tissue are removed from the subtracted image, so the vasculature is better visualized.

**direct current (DC):** A type of electrical current that flows in only one direction.

**direct radiography (DR) systems:** A digital imaging system that uses a detector array in place of the Bucky assembly; the imaging-forming radiation is captured and transferred to a computer from the detector array for almost instant viewing at the control panel.

**direct square law:** Provides a mathematical calculation for adjusting the mAs when changing the SID, also known as exposure maintenance formula.

**discrete emission spectrum:** A graphic representation of characteristic x-ray production.

**display field of view (DFOV):** Setting that controls the area of anatomy seen on the monitor.

**distortion:** Results from the radiographic misrepresentation of either the size (magnification) or shape of the anatomic part.

**DLP:** See *dose length product.*

**dose alert value:** A value used in CT to trigger a message to the technologist when the cumulative dose at a location, plus the dose for the next planned and confirmed scan(s), is likely to exceed a preprogrammed value.

**dose descriptor:** A computed value of radiation dose received by the patient based on manufacturer and calibration phantoms.

**dose length product (DLP):** The measurement of energy absorbed per unit of mass over a scanned length (Z-axis).

**dose notification value:** A value used in CT to trigger a message to the technologist when a single planned and confirmed scan is likely to exceed a preprogrammed value.

**dose optimization:** The reduction of the radiation dose while maintaining the required image quality needed for making a diagnosis.

**dose rates:** A series of settings on a fluoroscopic unit, typically labeled as low, medium, and high, which allows dose changes by 50% between each.

**dose report:** In CT, the display of the CTDIvol and DLP indices before and after the CT study is performed.

**dose-area product (DAP):** A measurement of exposure in air, followed by a computation to estimate absorbed dose to the patient.

**DQE:** See *detective quantum efficiency*.

**DR:** See *direct radiography (DR) systems*.

**dynamic range:** The range of exposure intensities that an image receptor can respond to and acquire image data.

**EBCT:** See *electron-beam computed tomography*.

**Edge enhancement filter:** Makes all the information in the image appear sharper, including the noise.

**effective focal spot:** The x-ray beam area as seen from the perspective of the patient.

**electric potential:** The ability to do work because of a separation of charges.

**electrodynamics:** The study of electric charges in motion.

**electromagnetic induction:** The phenomenon of inducing an electric current in that conductor by moving a conductor through a magnetic field.

**electromagnetic radiation:** An electric and magnetic disturbance traveling through space at the speed of light.

**electromagnetic spectrum:** A way of ordering or grouping the different electromagnetic radiations. All of the members of the electromagnetic spectrum have the same velocity (the speed of light or $3 \times 10^8$ m/s) and vary only in their energy, wavelength, and frequency.

**electromagnetism:** The phenomenon of electricity and magnetism existing as two parts of the same basic force, electromotive force. A magnetic field is created by a flow of electricity, and a moving magnetic field can create an electric current.

**electron:** Subatomic particle with one unit of negative electrical charge and a mass of $9.109 \times 10^{-31}$ kg.

**electron shell:** A defined energy level at a distance from the nucleus within which electrons orbit.

**electron-beam computed tomography (EBCT):** A CT scanner developed for cardiac imaging, the EBCT reduces scan time to as little as 50 ms, fast enough to image the beating heart. EBCT is considered by many to be the fifth generation.

**electronic magnification:** Selection of a smaller field of view (FOV). When a smaller FOV is selected, an area smaller than the size of the detector is exposed by the x-ray beam, but the area is enlarged to fill the display monitor area magnifying the anatomic structures.

**electrostatic focusing lenses:** Negatively charged plates along the length of the image-intensifier tube that repel the electron stream, focusing it on the small output phosphor.

**electrostatics:** The study of stationary electric charges.

**element:** A substance that cannot be broken down into simpler parts by ordinary chemical means.

**elongation:** Refers to images of objects that appear longer than the true objects.

**exit radiation:** The attenuated x-ray beam leaves the patient and is composed of both transmitted and scattered radiation; also called *remnant radiation*.

**exposure adjustment:** Part of the automatic exposure control device that allows the radiographer to adjust the amount of preset radiation detection values, also known as density controls.

**exposure indicator:** Provides a numeric value indicating the level of radiation exposure to the digital image receptor.

**exposure latitude:** The range of exposure values to the image that will produce an acceptable range of densities for diagnostic purposes.

**exposure maintenance formula:** Provides a mathematical calculation for adjusting the mAs when changing the SID, also known as the direct square law.

**exposure technique chart:** Preestablished guidelines used by the radiographer to select standardized manual or automatic exposure control factors for each type of radiographic examination.

**fan-beam geometry:** In CT, the size, shape, and motion of the x-ray beam and its path, based on the divergent rays of the x-ray tube.

**FBP:** See *filtered back projection*.

**field of view:** The dimensions of an anatomic area displayed on the monitor.

**filament:** A coil of wire, usually 7- to 15-mm long, 1- to 2-mm wide, and usually made of tungsten with 1% to 2% thorium added.

**filament circuit:** Section of the x-ray circuit that consists of a rheostat, a step-down transformer, and the filaments.

**filtered back projection (FBP):** The most common reconstruction algorithm used in modern computed tomography that uses a computer or electronic filter to convert raw data from the DAS into image data.

**filtration:** The use of a material, usually aluminum (Al) or aluminum equivalent, to absorb the lower-energy photons from the x-ray beam.

**fixed kVp–variable mAs technique chart:** A type of technique exposure chart in which the optimal kilovoltage peak value for each part is indicated and the milliampere/second value is varied as a function of part thickness.

**fluoro loop save:** Saves single images or a fluoro sequence loop to memory and are maintained in the patient's permanent record.

**fluoroscopy:** The use of a continuous beam of x-rays to create dynamic images of internal structures that can be viewed on a display monitor.

**flux gain:** An expression of the ratio of the number of light photons at the output phosphor to the number of light photons emitted in the input phosphor; represents the tube's conversion efficiency.

**focal distance:** The distance between the grid and the convergent line or point. Also known as the *grid radius*.

**focal plane:** Same as the *object plane*; the plane where the area of interest lies, at the level of the fulcrum.

**focal range:** The recommended range of source-to-image receptor distance measurements that can be used with a focused grid.

**focused grid:** Has lead lines that are angled, or canted, to approximately match the angle of divergence of the primary beam.

**focusing cup:** A metal shroud that is made of nickel and surrounds the x-ray tube filaments on their back and sides, leaving the front open and facing the anode target.

**fog:** Unwanted exposure on the radiographic image that does not provide any diagnostic information.

**foreshortening:** Refers to images that appear shorter than the true objects.

**frame averaging:** Reduces overall patient dose and image noise by averaging multiple image frames together.

**frequency:** The number of waves passing a given point each second.

**fulcrum:** Also known as the *pivot point*; the fixed point during the movement of the x-ray tube, which lies within the plane of the anatomic area to be imaged.

**fundamental quantities:** The foundation units of measure of mass, length, and time.

**gamma rays:** A very high-energy electromagnetic radiation originating from a radioactive nucleus with the ability to ionize matter.

**gantry:** Part of the CT scanner that surrounds the patient and houses the x-ray tube and detectors.

**GCF:** See *grid conversion factor*.

**generations:** The major developments in x-ray beam and detector geometry in CT. CT generations represent advances in the operation of the x-ray tube and detectors, primarily to reduce scan time.

**generator:** Device that converts some form of mechanical energy into electrical energy.

**grayscale:** The number of different shades of gray that can be stored and displayed by a computer system in digital imaging.

**grid:** A device that has very thin lead strips with radiolucent interspaces; intended to absorb scatter radiation emitted from the patient before it strikes the image receptor.

**grid cap:** Contains a permanently mounted grid and allows the image receptor to slide in behind it.

**grid cassette:** An image receptor that has a grid permanently mounted to its front surface.

**grid conversion factor (GCF):** Can be used to determine the adjustment in milliampere/second needed when changing from using a grid to nongrid (or vice versa) or for changing to grids with different grid ratios; also called the *Bucky factor*.

**grid cutoff:** A decrease in the number of transmitted photons that reach the image receptor because of some misalignment of the grid.

**grid focus:** The orientation of a grid's lead lines to one another.

**grid frequency:** Expresses the number of lead lines per unit length in inches, centimeters, or both.

**grid pattern:** Refers to the linear pattern of the lead lines of a grid.

**grid ratio:** The ratio of the height of the lead strips to the distance between them.

**grounding:** A protective measure to neutralize an electric charge; also a process of connecting the electrical device to the earth via a conductor.

**half-value layer (HVL):** The thickness of absorbing material (aluminum or aluminum equivalent filtration) necessary to reduce the energy of the x-ray beam to one-half its original intensity.

**heat units (HUs):** A measure of the amount of heat stored in a particular device.

**hertz (Hz):** A unit of measure for frequency equal to one cycle per second.

**high subject contrast:** Tissues that attenuate the x-ray beam very differently.

**histogram analysis:** A process in which a computer analyzes the histogram using processing algorithms and compares it to a preestablished histogram specific to the anatomic part being imaged.

**Hounsfield unit:** Value related to the attenuation characteristic of the tissue in the voxel but not an attenuation coefficient. Also referred to as the *computed tomography number*.

**HUs:** See *heat units*.

**HVL:** See *half-value layer*.

**Hz:** See *hertz*.

**image artifact:** An unwanted patient or image object that detracts from the diagnostic quality of a radiographic image.

**image data:** The digital array of CT numbers based on the image matrix that results from raw data being reconstructed.

**image evaluation:** The process of systematically and critically evaluating an image to determine if it meets minimum diagnostic quality criteria.

**image intensification:** During fluoroscopy, the process of creating a brighter visible image.

**image intensifier:** An electronic vacuum tube used in fluoroscopy that converts the remnant beam to light, then electrons, then back to light, increasing the light intensity in the process.

**image receptor:** A device that receives the radiation leaving the patient.

**induction motor:** An electric motor in which the shaft is rotated through mutual induction.

**infrared light:** A low-energy, nonionizing electromagnetic radiation just above microwaves.

**input phosphor:** A layer of the image intensifier made of cesium iodide and bonded to the curved surface of the tube itself. It absorbs the remnant x-ray photon energy and emits light in response.

**insulator:** Material with very few free electrons prohibiting the flow of electricity.

**interspace material:** Radiolucent strips between the lead lines of a grid, generally made of aluminum.

**inverse square law:** The intensity of a source of radiation is inversely proportional to the square of the distance.

**ionic bond:** An atomic bond in which one atom gives up an electron and another atom takes the extra electron, and the difference in their electrical charge attracts and bonds the two together.

**ionization:** The removal of an electron from an atom.

**ionization/ion chamber:** A hollow cell that contains air and is connected to the timer circuit via an electrical wire.

**ionizing radiation:** Radiation with sufficient energy to ionize atoms.

**KAP:** See *kerma area product*.

**kerma area product (KAP):** The same as DAP; the product of the total air kerma and the area of the x-ray beam at the entrance of the patient.

**kilovoltage peak (kVp):** The potential difference applied to the x-ray tube that determines the energy (quality) of the x-ray photons produced.

**kVp:** See *kilovoltage peak*.

**last image hold (LIH):** Indicates the position of the collimator plates on the display monitor.

**latent image:** The invisible image that exists on the image receptor before it has been processed.

**lead mask:** Changes the shape and size of the projected x-ray field; similar to an aperture diaphragm.

**leakage radiation:** Photons produced in the x-ray tube that are traveling in directions other than toward the patient.

**LIH:** See *last image hold.*

**linear attenuation coefficient:** A measure of the probability that the x-ray beam will interact with the material while traveling in a straight path. The value is based on both the characteristics of the material and the energy of the x-ray photons. The linear attenuation coefficient is symbolized by the Greek letter μ.

**linear grid:** Has lead lines that run in one direction only.

**linear tomography:** An imaging procedure using movement of the x-ray tube and image receptor in opposing directions to create images of structures in a focal plane by blurring the anatomy located above and below the plane of interest.

**line-focus principle:** A principle that states by angling the face of the anode target a large actual focal spot size can be maintained and a small effective focal spot size can be created.

**low subject contrast:** Tissues that attenuate the x-ray beam similarly.

**luminescence:** The emission of light from the screen when stimulated by radiation.

**mA:** See *milliamperage.*

**machine learning (ML):** The configuration of computer systems to artificially create human learning processes using statistical modeling and algorithms rather than specific computer coding instructions.

**magnetism:** The ability of a material to attract iron, cobalt, or nickel.

**magnification:** An increase in the image size of an object compared with its true, or actual, size; also known as *size distortion.*

**magnification factor (MF):** Indicates how much size distortion or magnification is demonstrated on a radiograph. MF = source-to-image receptor distance divided by source-to-object distance.

**magnification mode:** A function of the fluoroscopic unit that increases the voltage to the electrostatic focusing lenses, resulting in only those electrons from the center area of the input phosphor interacting with the output phosphor and contributing to the image, giving the appearance of magnification.

**mammography:** *A specialized radiographic imaging procedure of the breast.*

**manifest image:** The visible radiographic image on the exposed detector after processing.

**mAs readout:** The actual amount of mAs used for an image is displayed immediately on an automatic exposure control panel immediately after exposure.

**matrix:** Combination of rows and columns (array) of pixels that make up a digital image.

**MF:** See *magnification factor.*

**microwaves:** A low-energy, nonionizing electromagnetic radiation just above radio waves.

**milliamperage (mA):** The current applied to the x-ray tube that ultimately controls the number (quantity) of photons produced.

**mini C-arm:** Provides a lower dose rate and greater equipment flexibility while providing quality images of extremities.

**minification gain:** An expression of the degree to which the image is minified (made smaller) from input phosphor to output phosphor.

**minimum response time:** The shortest exposure time that the automatic exposure control system can produce.

**ML:** See *machine learning.*

**mobile equipment:** Medical imaging equipment that is designed to be easily transportable and can be taken to the patient's bedside, to the emergency department, to surgery, or wherever it may be needed.

**modulation transfer function (MTF):** A measure of the ability of the system to preserve signal contrast (display the contrast of anatomic objects varying in size), and the value will be between 0 (no difference in brightness levels) and 1.0 (maximum difference in brightness levels).

**Moiré effect:** A zebra pattern artifact that can occur during CT imaging if the grid frequency is similar to the laser scanning frequency or if a grid cassette is placed in a Bucky.

**molecule:** Fixed ratios of each type of constituent atom resulting in a predictable mass.

**motors:** Device that converts electrical energy to mechanical energy through electromagnetic induction.

**MPR:** See *multiplanar reformation.*

**MSAD:** See *multiple scan average dose.*

**MSCT:** See *multislice computed tomography.*

**MTF:** See *modulation transfer function.*

**multiplanar reformation (MPR):** Operation by the computer to display the image data in coronal, sagittal, or oblique planes.

**multiple scan average dose (MSAD):** The average exposure dose estimated at a central point of multiple scans during table movement.

**multislice computed tomography (MSCT):** Instead of collecting the transmission data for one slice each time, the tube rotates around the patient and collects data for 4 to 320+ slices per revolution.

**neutron:** Subatomic particle with no electrical charge and a mass of $1.675 \times 10^{-27}$ kg.

**nonfocused grid:** Has lead lines that run parallel to one another; also called a *parallel grid.*

**nucleus:** The central core of an atom made up fundamentally of protons and neutrons.

**O-arm:** Provides both static and dynamic images along with 2D and 3D during surgical procedures. Equipment movement is motor controlled, gantry opens for easy patient access laterally, and specialized draping is used to maintain sterility when the gantry is closed.

**object plane:** Also known as the *focal plane*; the plane where the area of interest lies, at the level of the fulcrum.

**object-to-image receptor distance (OID):** Distance between the object radiographed and the image receptor.

**occupational exposure:** Radiation exposure received by radiation workers.

**OID:** See *object-to-image receptor distance.*

**optimal kVp:** The kVP value that is high enough to ensure penetration of the part but not too high to diminish subject contrast.

**osteoporosis:** A bone disease in which the bones become thinner and more porous and therefore are susceptible to fractures.

**output phosphor:** A layer in the image intensifier that absorbs the electron stream and emits light in response.

**PACS:** See *Picture Archiving and Communication System*.

**pair production:** An interaction occurs when the incident x-ray photon has enough energy to escape interaction with the orbital electrons and interact with the nucleus of the tissue atom, resulting in the creation of the positron and an electron.

**panoramic x-ray (panorex):** Unit is designed to image curved surfaces, typically the mandible and teeth.

**parallel grid:** Has lead lines that run parallel to one another; also called a *nonfocused grid*.

**partial-volume artifact:** During CT, inaccurate information that occurs when the voxel is so large it contains more than one type of tissue.

**particulate radiation:** High-energy particles with the ability to ionize matter.

**PBL device:** See *positive beam-limiting device*.

**PCCT:** See *photon-counting computed tomography*.

**penetration:** X-ray photons that are transmitted through the body and reach the image receptor.

**permanently installed equipment:** Medical imaging equipment that is fixed in place in a specially designed and shielded room.

**photocathode:** A layer of the image intensifier made of cesium and antimony compounds. These metals emit electrons in response to light stimulus.

**photoconductor:** A device that absorbs x-rays and creates electrical charges in proportion to the x-ray exposure received.

**photodetector:** A device used to sense the light released from the photostimulable phosphor plate during scanning.

**photodisintegration:** An interaction in which extremely high-energy photons interact with the nucleus of an atom, making it unstable; to regain stability the nucleus ejects a nuclear particle.

**photoelectric effect:** In the diagnostic range, the total absorption of the incident photon by ejecting an inner-shell electron of a tissue atom.

**photoelectric interaction:** An interaction in which the incident x-ray photon interacts with the inner-shell electron of a tissue atom and removes it from orbit. In the process, the incident x-ray photon expends all of its energy and is totally absorbed.

**photoelectron:** The electron ejected from an atom during a photoelectric interaction.

**photomultiplier (PM) tube:** An electronic device that converts visible light energy into electrical energy.

**photon:** A discrete bundle of electromagnetic energy.

**photon-counting computed tomography (PCCT):** A CT system that uses a detector technology that directly converts X-ray photons to an electronic signal.

**photostimulable luminescence:** The release of energy from trapped electrons by a laser during the scanning of a photostimulable phosphor plate.

**photostimulable phosphor (PSP) plate:** A plate made up of several layers that stores x-ray energy as a latent image for cassette-based digital systems.

**phototimer:** Automatic exposure control detectors that use a fluorescent (light-producing) screen and a device that converts the light to electricity.

**Picture Archiving and Communication System (PACS):** A secure network for transmitting and exchange of patient images and data, display (viewing and workstations), and storage (archive server) systems.

**pitch:** Identifies the relationship between slice thickness (single slice spiral) or beam collimation (MSCT) and the distance the table travels every time the tube rotates.

**pivot point:** Also known as the *fulcrum*; a fixed point during the movement of the x-ray tube and image receptor that lies within the plane of the anatomic area to be imaged.

**pixel:** Picture element; the smallest component of the matrix, which is represented as a single brightness level on a computer monitor.

**pixel bit depth:** Also called number of bits (e.g., 12, 14, or 16), it affects the number of shades of gray available for image display.

**pixel density:** Number of pixels per unit area.

**pixel pitch:** The pixel spacing or distance measured from the center of a pixel to an adjacent pixel.

**Planck's constant:** A mathematical value used to calculate photon energies based on frequency and equal to $4.135 \times 10^{-15}$ eV sec.

**plate reader:** A device equipped with a drive system and optical system that converts the stored image on a photostimulable phosphor plate to an electronic signal for display on a computer workstation.

**PM tube:** See *photomultiplier tube*.

**positive beam-limiting (PBL) device:** Automatically limits the size and shape of the primary beam to the size and shape of the image receptor. Also called an *automatic collimator*.

**postpatient collimator:** Located just before the detector array. This collimator controls how much of the detector is exposed.

**prepatient collimator:** Located between the tube and patient and limits the beam to a fan or cone shape.

**primary beam:** The x-ray beam upon exiting the collimator and exposing the patient.

**primary circuit:** Section of the x-ray circuit that consists of the main power switch (connected to the incoming power supply), circuit breakers, the autotransformer, the timer circuit, and the primary side of the step-up transformer.

**profile:** In computed tomography the transmission measurement for an individual detector and the composite electrical signal.

**protective housing:** A lead-lined metal structure that provides solid, stable mechanical support and serves as an electrical insulator and thermal cushion for the x-ray tube.

**proton:** Subatomic particle with one unit of positive electrical charge and mass of $1.673 \times 10^{-27}$ kg.

**PSP:** See *photostimulable phosphor*.

**pulse rate:** Number of pulses (exposures) that occur per second during fluoroscopic operation.

**pulse width:** Length of each pulse (length of exposure) during fluoroscopic operation.

**pulsed fluoroscopy:** A design of the unit that rapidly turns the x-ray beam on and off during operation.

**quality assurance (QA):** In medical imaging, a process of collecting and evaluating data to provide a high standard of health care.

**quality control (QC):** The evaluation of imaging equipment and other components used in the imaging process.

**quantum noise:** Visible as brightness fluctuations on the image. Caused by too few photons reaching the image receptor to form the image.

**radioactivity:** The process by which an atom with excess energy in its nucleus emits particles and energy to regain stability.

**radiographic contrast:** Differences in the brightness levels to differentiate among the anatomic tissues.

**radiologic quantities:** The special radiologic science category of measure for dose, dose equivalent, exposure, and radioactivity.

**radiolucent:** Descriptive of less dense structures that have a much lower probability of x-ray absorption.

**radiopaque:** Descriptive of dense structures that readily absorb x-rays.

**radiowaves:** The lowest-energy, nonionizing electromagnetic radiation.

**raw data:** The logarithmic data from the linear attenuation coefficient that is converted from analog to digital information by the analog-to-digital converter and sent to the computer for image reconstruction.

**rays:** Parts of the x-ray beam that fall on one detector.

**region of interest (ROI):** Selection of a region of the digital image data set for statistical analysis.

**remnant radiation:** The attenuated x-ray beam leaving the patient that is composed of both transmitted and scattered radiation; also called *exit radiation*.

**repeat analysis:** The process of analyzing a set of repeated images to determine repeat rate and categorize cause of errors.

**repeat exposure:** The necessity of a acquiring a subsequent image when the initial image does not meet the minimal diagnostic quality criteria.

**resistance:** That property of an element in a circuit that resists or impedes the flow of electricity.

**resolution:** The ability of the imaging system to resolve or distinguish between two adjacent structures and can be expressed in the unit of line pairs per millimeter (Lp/mm).

**ring artifact:** A circular-shaped artifact associated with a faulty detector in third-generation CT scanners. It was eliminated in fourth-generation scanners.

**road mapping:** Another digital subtraction technique that uses the maximum contrast filled image as a mask that can be subtracted from precontrast images. This technique provides a better method to navigate the catheter or wire through tortuous vessels.

**ROI:** See *region of interest*.

**rotor:** A part of an induction motor made of an iron core (iron bars embedded in the copper shaft) surrounded by coils and located in the center of the stators.

**saturation:** When the image receptor is extremely overexposed, cannot be properly processed, and the quality is severely degraded.

**scan field of view (SFOV):** SFOV in CT determines the actual anatomic area of interest as set by the technologist and imaged during the examination.

**scattering:** Incoming photons are not absorbed but instead lose energy during interactions with the atoms composing the tissue.

**scintillation-type detector:** Typically made of cadmium tungstate or a ceramic material; absorbs the transmitted radiation and produces a proportional flash of light.

**secondary circuit:** Section of the x-ray circuit that consists of the secondary side of the step-up transformer, the milliampere meter, a rectifier bank, and the x-ray tube (except for the filaments).

**secondary electron:** The ejected electron resulting from the Compton effect interaction; also called *Compton electron*.

**secondary photons:** Characteristic photons produced in ionized tissue atoms as outer-shell electrons fill inner-shell vacancies.

**SFOV:** See *scan field of view*.

**sharpness factors:** The accuracy of the structural lines is achieved by maximizing the amount of *spatial resolution* and minimizing the amount of *distortion*.

**SID:** See *source-to-image receptor distance*.

**signal-to-noise ratio (SNR):** A method of describing the strength of the radiation exposure compared with the amount of noise apparent in a digital image.

**slip-ring technology:** Located inside the CT gantry; allows the tube to continue to rotate without the need to rewind.

**smoothing filter:** A noise reduction filter that can change the appearance of the anatomy by smoothing out the image noise to make it less visible.

**SNR:** See *signal-to-noise ratio*.

**SOD:** See *source-to-object distance*.

**source-to-image receptor distance (SID):** The distance between the source of the radiation and the image receptor.

**source-to-object distance (SOD):** The distance from the source of radiation to the object being radiographed.

**space charge:** A cloud of electrons formed by the focusing cup as electrons are boiled off of the filament.

**space-charge effect:** The self-limiting factor caused by the space charge reaching a size commensurate with the current used and making it difficult for additional electrons to be emitted.

**spatial frequency:** Defined by the unit of line pairs per millimeter (Lp/mm). Small objects have higher spatial frequency and large objects have lower spatial frequency.

**spatial resolution:** A term used to evaluate accuracy of the anatomic structural lines.

**spiral (helical) CT:** Continuous rotation of the tube (and detectors) coupled with continuous movement of the table and patient through the gantry. Instead of collecting data one slice at a time, data are collected for an entire volume of tissue (such as the head or chest) at one time.

**stator:** A part of an induction motor made up of electromagnets arranged in pairs around the rotor.

**streak artifact:** A linear-shaped artifact that is caused by patient motion or the presence of metal in the anatomy being imaged during computed tomography.

**subject contrast:** Refers to the absorption characteristics of the anatomic tissue radiographed along with the quality of the x-ray beam.

**target window:** A thinned section of the x-ray tube enclosure that is the desired exit point for the x-rays produced.

**teleradiology:** An electronic system that allows patients' electronic records (medical information and imaging studies) to be accessed from various workstations within or outside of a facility.

**TFT:** See *thin-film transistor*.

**thermionic emission:** The literal boiling off of electrons from a filament by a flow of electrical current.

**thin-film transistor (TFT):** Electronic components layered onto a glass substrate that include the readout, charge collector, and light-sensitive elements.

**tissue density:** Matter per unit volume, or the compactness of the atomic particles composing the anatomic part.

**tomographic angle:** The arc created during total movement of the x-ray tube.

**transformer:** Device used to increase or decrease voltage (or current) through electromagnetic induction.

**transmission:** X-ray photons that pass through the body to expose the image receptor.

**ultraviolet light:** A low-energy, nonionizing electromagnetic radiation just above visible light.

**values of interest (VOI):** Established values within histogram models that determine what part of the data set should be incorporated into the displayed image.

**variable kVp–fixed mAs technique chart:** A type of exposure technique chart that changes the kilovoltage peak for change in part thickness.

**view:** During CT, a snapshot of all the transmission measurements from that anatomic location, composed of rays.

**virtual collimation:** Adjusting the collimator without exposing the patient to additional radiation.

**virtual grid:** The use of software and computer algorithms to minimize the effects of scatter radiation on the final radiographic image thereby achieving the same outcome as a physical grid.

**visibility factors:** Factors that make the anatomic structures visible and include the *brightness* and contrast of the image.

**visible light:** A low-energy, nonionizing electromagnetic radiation just above infrared light.

**VOI:** See *values of interest*.

**voxel:** Volume element; determined by the size of the pixel and the thickness of the slice, the actual small amount of tissue that will be represented by one pixel.

**voxel volume:** The dimensions of the small piece of tissue.

**wafer grid:** A stationary grid placed on top of the image receptor.

**wavelength:** The distance between the peak of one wave to the peak of the next wave.

**windowing:** Adjusting the window width (contrast) and window level (brightness) on the digital image. In CT, it adjusts how many CT numbers are visible in the image.

**window level (WL):** Sets the midpoint of the range of brightness visible in the digital image. In CT, the WL determines the midpoint of the range of CT numbers to be displayed.

**window width (WW):** A control that adjusts the radiographic contrast on the digital image. In CT, it adjusts how many CT numbers are visible in the image.

**WL:** See *window level*.

**WW:** See *window width*.

**x-ray emission spectrum:** A graphic representation of the x-ray beam as a whole, combining the relevant parts of the discrete and continuous emission spectra.

**x-ray scintillator:** A material that absorbs x-ray energy and emits visible light in response.

**x-rays:** A very high-energy electromagnetic radiation originating through interactions between electrons and atoms with the ability to ionize matter.

**Z-axis** Direction from head to foot in computed tomography imaging.

# Index

*Note:* Page numbers followed by *f* indicate figures, *t* indicate tables, and *b* indicate boxes.